Dysphagia and the Child with Developmental Disabilities

MEDICAL, CLINICAL, AND FAMILY INTERVENTIONS

Dysphagia and the Child with Developmental Disabilities

MEDICAL, CLINICAL, AND FAMILY INTERVENTIONS

Edited by
SUSAN R. ROSENTHAL, M.S., M.D.
University of Medicine and Dentistry of New Jersey
JUSTINE JOAN SHEPPARD, Ph.D.
Teachers College, Columbia University
and
Mary Lotze, M.S., R.N., C.S.
University of Medicine and Dentistry of New Jersey

SINGULAR PUBLISHING GROUP, INC
SAN DIEGO, CALIFORNIA

Singular Publishing Group, Inc.
4284 41st Street
San Diego, California 92105-1197

©1995 by Singular Publishing Group, Inc.

Typeset in 10/12 New Century Schoolbook by So Cal Graphics
Printed in the United States of America by McNaughton & Gunn

Library of Congress Cataloging-in-Publication Data

Dysphagia and the child with developmental disabilities : medical,
    clinical, and family interventions / edited by Susan R. Rosenthal,
    Justine Joan Sheppard, Mary Lotze.
        p.   cm.
    Includes bibliographical references and index.
    ISBN 1-56593-089-4
    1. Developmentally disabled children.   I. Rosenthal, Susan R.
II. Sheppard, Justine Joan,   III. Lotze, Mary
    [DNLM: 1. Deglutition Disorders—in infancy & childhood.
    2. Deglutition Disorders—therapy.   3. Deglutition—complications.
    4. Child Development Disorders—Complications. 5. Disabled—rehabilitation.
    WS 310 D998 1994]
    RJ135.D97   1994
    618.92'8—dc20
    DNLM/DLC
    for Library of Congress   94-28599
                                                      CIP

Contents

Foreword

Satisfying the hunger drive by eating not only brings relief but is an enjoyable experience. It is this reciprocal relationship between parent and child that allows survival.

Mothers nurture their infants by offering the feeding of nutrients. A satisfied infant looks upon the person responsible for the good feeling that comes with sucking, tasting, and swallowing as his or her protector who loves them.

Unfortunately, it often occurs that an infant with central nervous system dysfunction and his or her mother do not experience the rewards that come from a satisfying feeding relationship. Not only are nutritional needs at risk but the infant-parent dyad can suffer. The latter may lead to poor bonding, which in turn results in emotional maladjustments.

Some time ago I had the privilege of reviewing a videotape which showed a 24-hour-old infant who experienced mild hypoxia at birth but who appeared relatively normal when brought to his mother for the first feeding. The mother was experienced in breast-feeding having weaned three other normal children. She looked at her new son and a broad smile came over her face. He was a lovely baby. The mother picked up the baby from the supine position and placed him in a semisupine position in the crutch of her arm. This change from a supine to a semierect position elicited an exaggerated tonic labyrinth reflex (TLR), causing the baby to develop truncal hyperextension. It appeared as if the baby was "backing away" from the mother. The mother did not appear to be concerned about the baby's reaction and took the nipple of her breast and touched it to the baby's cheek to initiate a rooting reflex. This was successful but the turning of the head initiated an overactive asymmetrical tonic neck reflex (ATNR). The result was rigid extension of the arm ipsilateral to the side the chin was turned to. It appeared as if the infant was attempting to push the mother away. The hungry infant was experiencing a delay in his expected feeding and he cried lustily. This only exaggerated the primitive reflex reactions. The mother became agitated but finally succeeded in getting the nipple of her breast into the baby's mouth. What happened was unexpected. The baby literally spit the nipple out due to poorly coordinated sucking that resulted in a tongue thrust. The mother became distressed and exasperated and called for the nurse who took the baby from her without asking any questions as to what had transpired. If the nurse had observed the feeding, it could have been ascertained that this baby was showing signs of a mild and possibly reversible compromise of central nervous system functioning. If explained to the mother, it would have at least allayed her fears that her son was rejecting her or that she had failed him. As this book will point out, recognizing these types of feeding difficulties and offering simple remediation will enhance the normal emotional development of the infant and make the mother feel competent in nurturing her infant.

Sucking, chewing, and swallowing is the earliest evidence of organized motor activity. Dysphagia is often the first evidence that there may be difficulties with central nervous system organization and maturation. Attention to infants who have dysphagia or gastrointestinal dysfunction is essential. The editors of this book have emphasized how the problems in feeding that are seen in children with developmental disabilities may be recognized and remediated. Both mother and child can learn that there are ways to cope with a seemingly unsolvable and discouraging disorder.

I feel this book will enlighten health care professionals and alert them to the importance of listening to parents when they complain about how their infants are feeding. One cannot simply blame it on the size of the nipple opening, the shape of the nip-

ple, allergy to milk, or to an anxious mother. The editors have addressed in depth a subject that is given little attention in generic pediatric textbooks in spite of the frequency of dysphagia and other nutritional problems that occur in children with developmental disabilites. This book will provide professionals with a foundation as well as state of the art practice in caring for children with developmental disabilitites and dysphagia.

Lawrence T. Taft, M.D.
Professor of Pediatrics and
Chief, Division of Developmental Disabilities
University of Medicine and Dentisty of New Jersey
Robert Wood Johnson Medical School

Preface

Dysphagia and related feeding problems occur frequently in children with developmental disabilities. The disorder may be transient, resolving in infancy; episodic, related to exacerbation in the general disorder; or chronic and pervasive throughout the child's lifetime.

In this context the term *dysphagia* refers to problems with reception and oral preparation of a bolus, oral initiation of the reflexive components of swallow, pharyngeal phase coordination including airway protection, and the esophageal phase of swallowing.

The dysphagia may manifest as failure to thrive; distress during meals including coughing, choking, and refusal of feeding; chronic or episodic aspiration-related respiratory disorder; and failure to advance in development of feeding behaviors. In addition, control of oral secretions may be problematic with drooling or difficulty swallowing secretions. Swallowing behaviors may be further compromised by gastrointestinal disorders including gastroesophageal reflux.

Successful management of these issues is central to the child's well-being and ability to achieve his or her potential. Good nutrition predisposes a child to better health and consequently reduces the need for medical resources in the long run. Early attention to management and habilitation is most effective for achieving this end.

Management of these cases is frequently complicated· and involves considerable family resources, medical and nursing care, nutritional care, and education of the child and family. In this population, management is especially complex and may require consultation with a variety of professionals. Many of the references on this subject were written by specialists who did not address the full scope of needs for this population of children. In recognition of this need, the editors joined to assemble this comprehensive reference as a guide in their work with these children. An effort has been made to include the expertise of specialists with the necessary knowledge and skill for the total and comprehensive management of the child with developmental disabilities and dysphagia.

The material in this book is appropriate for medical, nursing, allied health, and education specialists who are interested in working with this challenging group of children. Parents may also find this reference helpful in answering the often difficult questions that arise in the management of their children.

In Chapter 1, Dr. Prontnicki introduces the reader to the range of etiologies of pediatric disability and the pathophysiology of dysphagia seen in each of the various categories. Bryan and Pressman discuss the dynamics of the diagnostic team in evaluating and developing the recommendations which emerge from the team process in Chapter 2.

In Chapter 3, Sheppard describes the clinical evaluation of dysphagia, mealtime management, and therapeutic strategies for habilitation and advancement of feeding skills. White, Mkandawire, and Rosenthal address the practical management of nutritional issues including tube feedings, concentration of formula, guidelines for determining nutrient needs, and catch-up growth in Chapter 4. Frequently reported nutritional problems and specific nutrient deficiencies with guidelines for supplementation are covered in depth.

In Chapter 5, Mkandawire addresses the unique nutritional problems in infants, toddlers, and older children with AIDS; and

Pressman shares her extensive experiences in diagnosis and treatment of dysphagia in children with AIDS in Chapter 6.

The psychologist's perspective on the causes of failure to thrive, assessment of psychological issues affecting the parent-child dyad, and family and child intervention is provided by Lachenmeyer in Chapter 7. In Chapter 8, Woods discusses the complex interactions between body postural control and feeding. She describes the considerations for assisting positioning, methods for achieving optimum function, and therapeutic interventions for improving underlying competencies.

The pivotal role of the radiologist in evaluating swallow is addressed by Marquis and Pressman in Chapter 9. They provide detailed procedures for managing the infant and child during the radiographic studies.

The otolaryngologist's perspective on clinical determination of head and neck causes of dysphagia and their management is provided by Haddad and Prestigiacomo in Chapter 10; and Cuasay and Mikkilineni describe respiratory conditions that may be caused by or may predispose children to dysphagia in Chapter 11. Procedures for medical management and prevention are discussed.

In Chapter 12 Mascarenhas and Dadhania review the clinical features and management of common gastrointestinal disorders that affect feeding behaviors. They focus on gastroesophageal reflux, motility disorders, peptic ulcer diseases, and constipation. The percutaneous endoscopic gastrostomy is discussed in detail. Ross and Hoffman follow in Chapter 13 with an in-depth overview of the surgical management of gastroesophageal reflux including the issues of fundoplication, pyloroplasty, and gastrostomy. Alternatives to antireflux surgery are presented as well.

In Chapter 14, Sonnenberg reviews some of the common problems encountered in providing dental care to children with physical handicaps, mental retardation, cleft lip and palate, and autism, and suggests behavioral techniques that can be used successfully in treatment of these children. He provides guidelines for a total dental treatment program with emphasis on prevention.

In Chapter 15, Alan Rosenthal discusses the importance of oral hygiene and the strategies for implementing programs. He gives special attention to children with Down syndrome, cerebral palsy, seizure disorders, and blindness.

In Chapter 16, Lotze examines parent-child interactions and feeding problems and reviews the role of family members and parental behaviors that facilitate feeding behaviors in the child from a nursing perspective. Breast-feeding, utensils for feeding, gastrostomy care, prevention of aspiration, CPR, and obstructed airway procedure and the Newborn Child Assessment Feeding Scale are topics covered in this chapter on nursing management.

The nature and needs of children with developmental disabilities are discussed by Handelman in Chapter 17. The impact of the child on the family system and steps to create effective family-professional relationships are presented. In Chapter 18, the ethical dilemmas involved in providing pediatric nutritional support to children with severe disabilities are laid out by Stolman for professionals and the family. The basis on which medical decisions are made, the role of the family, and allocation of scarce resources are discussed with sensitivity and clarity.

Contributors

Dorothy W. Bryan, M.D.
Medical Director
Tertiary Multidisciplinary Services
Childrens Hospital of New Jersey-
  United Hospitals Medical Center
Assistant Professor of Clinical Pediatrics
New Jersey Medical School-UMDNJ
Newark, New Jersey

Jay Dadhania, M.B.B.S.
Assistant Professor of Clinical Pediatrics
Division of Pediatric Gastroenterology
  and Nutrition
Robert Wood Johnson Medical School-UMDNJ
New Brunswick, New Jersey

Joseph Haddad, Jr., M.D.
Director of Pediatric ENT
Department of Pediatric Otolaryngology
Babies Hospital-Columbia Presbyterian
  Medical Center
New York, New York

Jan Handleman, Ed.D.
Director and Professor
Douglass Development Disabilities Center
Gibbons Campus, Douglass College
Rutgers University
New Brunswick, New Jersey

Mark A. Hoffman, M.D.
Chief of Liver Transplants
Department of Surgery
The Children's Hospital of Philadelphia
Philadelphia, Pennsylvania

Juliana Rasic Lachenmeyer, Ph.D.
Department of Psychology
Farleigh Dickinson University
Teaneck, New Jersey
North Shore University Hospital/Cornel
  University Medical College
Manhasset, New York

Lourdes Laraya-Cuasay, M.D.
Professor of Clinical Pediatrics
Division of Pediatric Pulmonology
Robert Wood Johnson Medical School-UMDNJ
New Brunswick, New Jersey

Mary Lotze, P.N.P., M.S.
Executive Director
Laurie Neurodevelopmental Institute
Assistant Professor of Pediatrics
Division of Developmental Disabilities
Robert Wood Johnson Medical School–UMDNJ
New Brunswick, New Jersey

James Marquis, M.D.
Director Department of Radiology
United Hospitals Medical Center
Clinical Professor of Radiology
New Jersey Medical School-UMDNJ
Newark, New Jersey

Maria R. Mascarenhas, M.B.B.S.
Assistant Professor of Pediatrics
Director of Nutrition Support Service
Assistant Director of Cystic Fibrosis Program
University of Pennsylvania Medical School
The Children's Hospital of Philadelphia
Philadelphia, Pennsylvania

Selina C. Mhango-Mkandawire, R.D., Ed.D.
Director
Pediatric Outpatient Nutrition Services
Children's Hospital of New Jersey-United
  Hospitals Medical Center
Newark, New Jersey

Sushmita Mikkilineni, M.D.
Assistant Professor of Clinical Pediatrics
Division of Pulmonology
Robert Wood Johnson Medical School–UMDNJ
New Brunswick, New Jersey

Cathy Y. Poon, Pharm.D
Philadelphia College of Pharmacology and
  Science and Pediatric Critical Care
The Children's Hospital of Philadelphia
Philadelphia, Pennsylvania

Hilda Pressman, M.A.
Director
Hearing and Speech Center
United Hospitals Medical Center
Newark, New Jersey

Cynthia Prestigiacomo, M.D.
Babies Hospital-Columbia Presbyterian
  Medical Center
New York, New York

Janice Prontnicki, M.D.
Assistant Professor
Division of Developmental Disabilities
Robert Wood Johnson Medical School-UMDNJ
New Brunswick, New Jersey

Alan Bennett Rosenthal, D.M.D.
Assistant Clinical Professor
New York University Dental School
New York, New York

Susan R. Rosenthal, M.S., M.D.
Associate Professor
Division of Pediatric Gastroenterology
  and Nutrition
Robert Wood Johnson Medical School-UMDNJ
New Brunswick, New Jersey

Arthur J. Ross III, M.D.
Professor
Department of Surgery and Pediatrics
University of Wisconsin Medical School
Director of Medical Education
Gunderson-Lutheran Medical Center
La Crosse, Wisconsin

Justine Joan Sheppard, Ph.D.
Department of Speech and Language
  Pathology and Audiology
Teachers College, Columbia University
New York, New York

Edward M. Sonnenberg, D.D.S.
Flanders Pediatric Dentistry
Flanders, New Jersey
Department of Dentistry
Morristown Memorial Hospital
Morristown, New Jersey

Cynthia J. Stolman, Ph.D.
Director of Medical Ethics
Department of Pediatrics
Children's Hospital of New Jersey-
  United Hospitals Medical Center
Assistant Professor
New Jersey, Medical School-UMDNJ
Newark, New Jersey

Lawrence T. Taft, M.D.
Director of Division of
  Developmental Disabilities
Director of Laurie Neurodevelopmental
  Institute
Professor of Pediatrics
Robert Wood Johnson Medical School-UMDNJ
New Brunswick, New Jersey

Kathleen R. White, M.S., R.D.
Pediatric Nutritionist
Division of Pediatric Gastroenterology
  and Nutrition
Robert Wood Johnson Medical School-UMDNJ
New Brunswick, New Jersey

Elaine K. Woods, M.A., P.T.
Cerebral Palsy Association of Middlesex County
Edison, New Jersey

Acknowledgment

This book was motivated by the problems of our patients and their families and the questions of our students. We are grateful to them for sharing with us their frustrations and successes as they met the challenge of coping with the child with dysphagia. Our sincere appreciation is extended to Patricia Murphy whose help at the outset was invaluable; to Patty Kress for her unstinting help with preparation of the manuscript; to Sandy Doyle, Marie Linvill, and Angie Singh for their assistance in bringing the book to publication, our thanks.

To my husband George and my children Rebecca, Aaron, and Johnathan Karp, without whose love and support, kindness and encouragement, this book would not have been realized; and to my parents, Mildred and Julius Rosenthal, thank you.

Susan Rosenthal

To Ron, Dan, and Mike Sheppard whose encouragement, patience, and support made this book possible.

Justine Joan Sheppard

To my husband Jim, my children Michael and Christine, and my mother Anne, thank you for always being there.

Mary Lotze

CHAPTER

1

Presentation: Symptomatology and Etiology of Dysphagia

JANICE PRONTNICKI, M.D.

CONTENTS

What Is a Developmental Disability?

Developmental disabilities can be defined many ways. In the Developmental Disabilities Assistance and Bill of Rights Act of 1991, it was defined as "any severe chronic disability of a person attributable to a mental or physical impairment or combination thereof that is manifested before the age of 22 years, is likely to continue indefinitely, and will result in substantial limitations of function in three or more of the following areas: (1) self-care, (2) receptive and expressive language, (3) learning, (4) mobility, (5) self-direction, (6) capacity for independent living, (7) economic self-sufficiency, and (8) need for combinations and sequences of special interdisciplinary or generic care, treatment or other services that are life-long or of extended duration and are individually planned or coordinated" (Public Law 98-527). In other words, it is a condition that interferes with a person's ability to function as expected for age. Areas so impaired may be physical, cognitive, communicative, or social.

What Is Dysphagia?

Dysphagia, a disorder of swallowing, can occur at any point during the passage of the bolus through the oral, pharyngeal, and esophageal structures. Any difficulty with swallowing that interferes with its safe and comfortable resolution or, overall, with nourishment of the individual or control of oral secretions is a symptom of dysphagia.

The act of swallowing consists of a complex series of events that, for the purposes of diagnosis and treatment, are divided into four phases: oral preparatory phase, oral initiation phase, pharyngeal phase, and esophageal phase. (Jones, 1988; Logemann, 1983). The oral preparatory phase includes the events associated with reception of the bolus into the mouth, its containment at the lips and at the juncture of the mouth and pharynx, its transport into place for initiation of the swallowing reflex, and its preparation for safe resolution of the remaining phases of swallow. During this phase, the bolus may be chewed, mixed with saliva, and partitioned into acceptable sizes for transit through the pharynx and esophagus. During the oral initiation phase of swallow, the tongue propels the bolus from the mouth into the pharynx, and the swallowing reflex is elicited. During the pharyngeal phase, a naso-pharyngeal seal is accomplished by the velum and superior pharyngeal constrictor. Airway closure is achieved by adduction of true vocal folds, approximation of the arytenoids to the base of the epiglottis, and downward movement of the epiglottis to seal the supraglottic vestibule. The upper esophageal sphincter (UES) relaxes; and the pharynx, UES, and larynx are elevated. The traction applied to the UES by the upward and anterior movement of the larynx opens it and holds it open until the tail of the bolus has passed (Cook et al., 1989; Shaker, 1992). As the bolus moves through the pharynx into the esophagus, it is followed by a wave of pharyngeal muscle contraction that strips the residuals of the bolus from the pharynx before the oral and pharyngeal structures return to their prior, resting alignments. The esophageal phase completes the swallow. Peristaltic action propels the bolus toward the stomach. The gastoresophageal sphincter relaxes to allow the bolus to pass into the stomach and then returns to its tonic state.

Neurological control for these events is coordinated in the medulla oblongata. Sensations related to swallow are mediated by Cranial Nerves V, VII, and X. Movement is mediated through Cranial Nerves V, VII, IX, X, XI, and XII. Sensory motor structures in mid-brain, cortex, and cerebellum contribute, as well.

Dysphagia may disrupt feeding and control of oral secretions to varying degrees and require varying levels of intervention for its management. In its mildest form, diet restrictions suffice to enable normal growth and airway protection. In its most severe form, alternatives to oral feeding and tracheostomy may be needed to maintain nutrition and respiratory health (See Chapter 13).

Why Is Dysphagia More Common in the Developmentally Disabled Population?

The process of feeding is complex, linking the physical process of eating with learned social interactions. The physical process requires a coordinated series of steps from the voluntary process of oral management to the swallowing reflex and involuntary esophageal peristalsis. This involves the autonomic nervous system, somatic nervous system, striated and smooth muscles, and sensory input. Any condition that hinders functioning of the relevant nerves or muscles can be problematic. Similarly, the social component requires a certain level of mental capabilities and communication skills. An impairment in any portion of the physical process or the social interaction can cause dysphagia.

This chapter will cover the developmental disabilities most commonly associated with dysphagia. For organizational purposes, the developmental disabilities have been divided into those causing problems primarily through neuromuscular control, cognitive impairment, interactive difficulties, or anatomic abnormalities. Some of these conditions can have a negative impact on more than one of these areas.

Dysphagia may be considered a "handicapping condition in and of itself" (Gustafsson & Tibbing, 1991). A reduction of functional capacity is described as a "disability." In turn, a disability is further characterized as a "handicap" if it limits the person's ability to achieve desired goals. Gustafsson and Tibbing found that dysphagia can interfere with a person's (physical, social, and mental) capabilities sufficiently to qualify for inclusion as a handicap.

Specific Developmental Disabilities

Neuromuscular Disease

Neurogenic developmental disabilities represent conditions in which abnormalities of brain or spinal cord cause dysphagia.

Cerebral Palsy

DEFINITIONS. Cerebral palsy (CP) is the most common cause of congenital neurogenic dysphagia. (Christensen, 1989). Cerebral palsy is a disorder of movement and/or posture, the result of a static encephalopathy with the insult to the brain occurring prenatally, perinatally, or during early childhood. (Taft, 1987). Cerebral palsy can be divided into types. The usual classification is based on clinical presentation as follows: spastic, dyskinetic, rigid, atonic/hypotonic, and mixed. These types are further qualified by degree (mild, moderate, severe) and areas of involvement. For example, the spastic type of CP may involve mainly the lower extremities (which is known as diplegia), the right or left side (hemisparesis), or all four limbs (quadriparesis). The dyskinesias can be subdivided into athetoid (slow writhing movements), choreiform (rapid, jerky movements), dystonia (relatively fixed posture), ballismus (flailing movements), or tremors (rhythmic alterations).

Because current diagnostic criteria are based on clinical presentation resulting from a static encephalopathy in a developing child, it is important to remember that the diagnosis can change over time. It is not unusual to see a hypotonic infant develop spasticity. Also, there are documented cases of infants diagnosed as having CP at 1 year of age who over time improved and "outgrew CP" (Nelson & Ellenberg, 1982).

Frequently, the clinical presentation is mixed and does not clearly fit into any one type. For example, a child could have a spastic-athetoid CP. Even children considered to have diplegia usually have some lesser involvement of the upper extremities. The lower extremity involvement, however, is much more pronounced. This picture is often seen in premature high-risk infants who develop CP.

CAUSES. Although all CP is assumed due to some type of brain insult, often a specific cause is uncertain. Any insult to the developing brain prenatally, perinatally, or in early childhood can be suspect.

In utero, maternal infections (i.e., toxoplasmosis, rubella, herpes, HIV), excessive radiation, toxic exposure, chromosomal abnormalities, or interruption of placental blood flow can all impair the developing brain. Timing of the insult determines whether there are gross brain malformations or more subtle problems.

Insufficient blood flow to the brain is the main cause of CP resulting during birth. Infants born prematurely are especially at risk for cerebral hemorrhage. Intraventricular hemorrhage (IVH) is common; but it is the hemorrhage extending into the brain parenchyma, and particularly any resulting brain tissue destruction causing cysts, that is most closely associated with CP (Graziani et al., 1986). The pyramidal tracts closest to the ventricles (and therefore most vulnerable) control the lower extremities. This explains the diplegia most characteristic of premature infants with CP.

Infections such as meningoencephalitis, anoxia (near-drowning), trauma, and toxins represent post-natal causes of CP.

PATHOPHYSIOLOGY. Diagnosis of CP in the first year of life is difficult. Later the characteristic findings of CP are more evident. In spasticity (the most common type of CP) findings include hypertonicity, hyperactive reflexes (including exaggerated gag), abnormal movements, unusual posture, and prolonged retention of primitive reflexes. Any and all of these features can interfere with normal feeding. In addition, children with CP are at increased risk for aspiration and gastroesophageal reflux. The incidence of dysphagia is high in the CP population. One study found 40% of patients with mild-to-severe CP had oromotor difficulties (Love, Hagerman, & Taimi, 1980).

PRIMITIVE REFLEXES. Primitive reflexes can be thought of as the earliest and simplest responses elicited by certain sensations. Many of these reflexes can be demonstrated even in anencephalic infants. Teleologically, it is believed that many of these reflexes initially had a self-survival purpose. For example, the palmar reflex is a grasping reflex which occurs when there is a sensation of pressure on the palm. The plantar reflex is similar. These reflexes are believed to have developed as a means to hold on to the mammalian mother during feeding. Several studies by Capute and colleagues, (1986) have shown that some of these reflexes begin as early as 28 weeks gestation. Hooker (1952) and Humphrey (1968) discuss the appearance of primitive oral reflexes in fetuses as early as 6.5 weeks gestation. With progressive maturation of the cerebral cortex, these reflexes become integrated (i.e., reflexes are progressively suppressed as the child's voluntary control of movements improve). In cases of cerebral dysfunction such as CP, however, there can be prolonged retention of these reflexes. They may remain obligate and become more prominent. That is, each time the sensory input is received, the reflex occurs outside of volitional control. This can further inhibit normal neuromotor development and, in turn, normal feeding patterns.

ASPIRATION. An additional problem for children with cerebral palsy is aspiration. Aspiration occurs when food matter incorrectly enters the larynx and lower respiratory tract rather than the esophagus. This problem occurs in children with cerebral palsy due to poor coordination of swallowing. In neurologically impaired children, the swallowing reflex may be completely absent (making oral feeding impossible) or more often delayed (Morris, 1989). In the latter case, the bolus enters the pharynx before the swallowing reflex is triggered and can enter the still-open airway which, prior to swallow, is the path of least resistance.

When the neuromotor coordination of swallowing is deficient, there may be gagging in some cases with associated vomiting or aspiration, choking, and pneumonia. These unpleasant sensations can cause further eating problems by triggering avoidance behaviors. Aspiration can also cause chronic lung disease which would result in changes in intrathoracic pressures. Such pressure changes may in turn cause gastroesophageal reflux. Food matter refluxing into the pharynx from the stomach can lead to further aspiration.

GASTROESOPHAGEAL REFLUX (GER). GER is the movement of food or acid from the stomach into the esophagus. The presence of gastric contents in the esophagus may be associated with an unpleasant, burning sensation. This can make the child associate feeding with pain; and he or she, in turn, will avoid feeding entirely. GER can also lead to aspiration. In severe cases of chronic GER, esophageal strictures may develop (Catto-Smith, Machida, Butzner, Gall, & Scott, 1991).

GER is common in children with neuromuscular coordination problems such as cerebral palsy and mental retardation. Studies have shown an incidence as high as 75% in children with severe CNS dysfunction (Byrne et al., 1982; Sondheimer & Morris, 1979). Proposed etiologic factors include supine positioning, scoliosis and kyphosis causing diaphragmatic distortion, spasticity, abnormalities of lower esophageal sphincter tone, motility disorders, and seizures. Medication used for seizure disorders can further exacerbate GI symptomatology (Whyllie, Whyllie, Cruse, Rothner, & Erenberg, 1986).

For more information regarding the pathophysiology of GER and its treatments, the reader is referred to Chapter 12.

CLINICAL CASE. A breastfeeding infant with spastic CP may present the following scenario. First the mother picks up the infant. An overactive tonic labyrinthine reflex may result in excess truncal extension. The baby appears rigid and tense to the mother. This limits the mother/child cuddling and interferes with the social component of feeding. When the mother pulls the child close, he may arch and hyperextend as if to pull away from her. (Increased extension tone is commonly seen in children with cerebral palsy.) Next, the baby's head is turned towards the breast. An obligatory asymmetric tonic neck reflex (one of the primitive reflexes) can be triggered. In this movement, the turning of the head to one side stimulates extension of the arm in the direction the child's head is facing with flexion of the opposite arm. The extension of the arm in the direction the child is looking may be misinterpreted as an attempt to push the mother away.

When a nipple is finally introduced into the mouth, the infant may show oral tactile defensiveness. This symptom may result from deprivation of pleasurable oral stimulation in the initial months of life while in the intensive care nursery. The infant may have been subjected to oral suctioning, intubation, and oral tube placement and feeding and have learned to associate oral sensation with these unpleasant experiences. The gag and primitive oral reflexes may be exaggerated. As a result, stimulus of the nipple or milk may elicit these reflexes. Gagging and tongue thrust may occur rather than rhythmic sucking movements necessary to empty the nipple. Because of the neuromotor involvement, the tongue may be thick and lack the rhythmic up-and-down movement, and the lips may not seal around the nipple. In the Intensive Care Nursery, the child may not have had the opportunity to suck and develop the ability to coordinate sucking and breathing. The child may breathe in when his mouth is full, or the child may hold his breath inappropriately long and become anxious. As a result of this poor coordination, children with CP are at risk for aspiration syndrome. With aspiration, pneumonitis may be caused by the food particles entering the lungs.

Once the child has swallowed the food, peristalsis moves it down the esophagus. If there is GER, the associated discomfort may cause the child to hyperextend. Sometimes turning the head stiffly to the side (Sandifer's syndrome) may occur. The child may become agitated and refuse to eat.

In older children with CP, the abnormalities of tone, position, and primitive postural and oral reflexes may persist and complicate feeding. Learned behavioral avoidance issues may also come to the forefront. Communication limitations will interfere with the social component of feeding. Although mental impairment is not necessarily part of the clinical picture of CP, co-existing mental retardation is not uncommon, existing in approximately 50% of children with CP.

Methods used to try to prevent feeding problems in the older child with CP include trying to make feeding as pleasant an experience as possible. In the earlier years, optimizing positioning, use of assistive devices, and dealing with the child on a communication and cognitive level he or she can understand are all important components of therapy.

SUMMARY. Children with CP usually grow poorly, often to the point of "failure to thrive." The causes are not fully understood, but certainly the difficulty in feeding these children plays some role in this process. It has been found that rapid improvement of nutritional intake by nasogastric or gastrostomy tube feedings can lead to improvement in circulation, healing, mood, and spasticity (Patrick, Boland, Stoski, & Murray, 1986). Preventing or treating dysphagia is therefore an important part of the child's care.

Post-Natal Brain Injury

DEFINITION. A different terminology is often used when brain injury occurs after early childhood. This injury is termed head trauma, cerebral hemorrhage, cerebral infarction, ischemia, or cerebral vascular accident, depending on the pathophysiology. When the insult results in a child's impaired functioning, the injury is referred to as a developmental disability.

Cerebral vascular disorders are much less common in children than adults in whom it is the most common neurologic disorder. A published survey showed an annual incidence of 2.52 cases of cerebral vascular disease per 100,000 children compared to 110 per 100,000 perinatal cases in the same population (Schoenberg & Schoenberg, 1980).

CAUSES. Hemorrhage into the brain can result from a variety of factors. Congenital disorders such as cerebral arteriovascular malformations or aneurysms, infections, blood dyscrasias, and trauma can all cause acute bleeding into the brain parenchyma.

Occlusive vascular disease causes direct disruption of blood flow to brain tissue with resulting infarction. Trauma to carotid arteries, cyanotic heart disease, hemoglobinopathy (such as sickle cell disease), infection, dehydration, and metabolic disease (such as homocystinuria) can lead to anoxia.

When there is acute bleeding, the introduction of blood into the confines of the skull causes increased intracranial pressure and reflex vasospasm. This, in turn, results in further damage through ischemia. (Seiler, Grolimund, Aaslid, Huber, & Nornes, 1986). In both hemorrhagic and occlusive insults, necrosis of tissue and neuron death result.

PATHOPHYSIOLOGY OF DYSPHAGIA WITH BRAIN INJURY. In children, cerebral vascular accidents usually affect the anterior circulation of the brain resulting in acute hemiplegia, that is, paralysis, weakness, and later spasticity of the right or left half of the body. Severity of involvement varies greatly. The spasticity can cause the spectrum of impairment in feeding discussed under cerebral palsy. Co-existing conditions include seizures and gastroesophageal reflux not unlike those seen in CP.

If the lower brain stem is the site of insult, pseudobulbar palsy can result due to interruption of the corticobulbar tracts supplying cranial nerves V, VIII, and IX–XII. As discussed previously, these are the cranial nerves receiving sensation from the oropharynx as well as controlling the musculature involved in swallowing. Symptoms of pseudobulbar palsy include dysphagia, drooling, problems with speech, nasopharyngeal regurgitation, and aspiration.

Spina Bifida/Meningomyelocele

OVERVIEW/DEFINITIONS. Spina bifida refers to a malformation of the vertebrae protecting the spinal cord. When associated with a meningomyelocele, nerve damage can be substantial. The most common site of this malformation is distally in the lumbosacral region. The incidence of spina bifida is 1 in 1,000 live births in the general population. There is increased risk in family members. The incidence is also increased in certain geographic areas such as Ireland. Recent research supports an association between folic acid deficiency and increased incidence, particularly in the at-risk population (Mills, et al., 1989; Milunsky, et al., 1989; Mulinare, Cordero, Erickson, & Berry, 1988).

Prenatal diagnosis is possible by sampling levels of alphafetoprotein in the maternal blood or amniotic fluid. When a case is diagnosed prenatally, planned Caesarean section lessens trauma to the nerve tissue.

Prognosis depends on many factors, especially the level of the lesion. Denervation with associated loss of sensation and motor control occurs. Flaccid paralysis is most common. Incontinence of urine and feces is frequent. Hydrocephalus often coexists. Mental retardation is not an expected component but can occur as a consequence of hdroephalus and its complications. Arnold Chiari malformations are not uncommon. This represents an elongation and herniation of the cerebellar tonsils into the foramen ovale at the base of the skull through which the spinal cord passes. Eighty-eight percent of children with lumbar or lumbosacral myelomeningocele have some type of abnormalities of the cervical spinal cord

(Gilbert, Jones, Rorke, Chernoff, & James, 1986).

TREATMENT. Treatment in the neonatal period consists of closure of the soft tissue defect. If hydrocephalus is present, a ventriculoperitoneal shunt is placed. Long-term management of the child with spina bifida is best served by a medical team approach. Management seeks to maximize potential and life satisfaction. Self-care skills, locomotion (independent or assisted ambulation or wheelchair access), minimization of joint contractures, and urine and bowel control are emphasized.

PATHOPHYSIOLOGY. Arnold Chiari malformations, as previously mentioned, are a relatively common occurrence in children with spina bifida. This malformation individually or in conjunction with hydrocephalus can lead to compression of the brain stem and lower cranial nerves (IX–XII) which are necessary for swallowing. Such compression results in neurogenic dysphagia, frequently the presenting sign of progressive compression. Pharyngeal and esophageal motility disorders, tracheoesophageal sensory impairment, and achalasia result (Pollack, Pang, Kochoshis, & Putnam, 1992).

In addition, dyspraxia is not uncommon in children with spina bifida. It represents an impairment of complex neuromuscular planning. As previously mentioned, the process of eating and swallowing can be hindered by such coordination difficulties.

Children with myelodysplasia are at higher risk than the general population for gastrointestinal malformations such as duodenal atresia, pyloric stenosis, and tracheoesophageal fistula as well as renal and cardiac abnormalities.

Hypotonia

OVERVIEW AND DEFINITION. Hypotonia is a symptom characterized by low muscle tone.

This means the child has limited resistance to passive movement of the joints and increased flexibility. Such children are often described as "floppy." Reflexes may be normal, exaggerated, or decreased, dependent on the underlying cause of the hypotonia.

Hypotonia is a feature of many developmentally disabling conditions including mental retardation, (especially Down syndrome) metabolic disorders, and early CP or may be an isolated condition.

ETIOLOGY/PATHOPHYSIOLOGY. Hypotonia is the clinical opposite of spasticity, yet the causes of these conditions are often the same. Brain insults, often more subtle than those causing CP, are the suspected cause. Early in the course of CP, infants may feel hypotonic but this usually evolves into a hypertonic state. Longstanding hypotonic CP is uncommon. Hypotonia is also noted in children with congenital myopathies or lower motor neuron disease, which will be discussed later in this chapter.

Fortunately, one of the most common causes of hypotonia in infancy is benign congenital hypotonia, a condition that improves in time. It is a difficult diagnosis to make, except in retrospect. With maturation, the hypotonia lessens and usually tone normalizes. Until this occurs, however, the low tone affects posture and neuromuscular coordination. There is frequently an open mouth posture with drooling, poor truncal stability, and difficulties with oromotor coordination resulting in dysphagia.

Hydrocephalus

DEFINITION. Hydrocephalus is a pathological increase in the volume of cerebral spinal fluid (CSF). This increase in volume, in turn, causes increased pressure on the brain.

ETIOLOGY. The most common cause of hydrocephalus is obstruction to CSF flow, preventing its reabsorption. Obstruction may occur at several sites in the ventricles. A common site of blockage is the fourth ventricle. Both Arnold Chiari malformation (as discussed in the section on spina bifida) and Dandy Walker syndrome cause such obstruction. In Dandy Walker syndrome, the fourth ventricle is grossly dilated, acting like a cyst or tumor to impede normal CSF flow. Tumors including choroid plexus tumors can also cause obstructive hydrocephalus. Meningeal inflammation can also inhibit CSF absorption. Oversecretion of CSF is a less common cause of hydrocephalus.

PATHOPHYSIOLOGY Hydrocephalus can cause dysphagia due to impaired lower brain stem functioning and damage to corticolbulbar tracts, causing signs of pseudobulbar palsy. These include poor suck in infancy and poorly coordinated eating skills in older children. There is often drooling, regurgitation, aspiration, and abnormalities of speech. The jaw jerk and gag reflexes are frequently exaggerated.

Spinal Muscular Atrophy

Spinal muscular atrophy (Werdnig-Hoffman disease) occurs with loss of anterior horn cells (motor neurons) in the spinal cord and brain stem. The results are marked muscle weakness, loss of deep tendon reflexes, and muscle atrophy with tongue fasciculations. The muscles needed for feeding are progressively involved because of denervation secondary to loss of cranial nerve nuclei.

Disease of Neuromuscular Junction/Myasthenia Gravis

Myasthenia gravis is a disease of the motor endplates (nerve-to-muscle junction) characterized by excess fatiguability of voluntary muscles. Dysphagia, choking, and aspiration are common. Frequently, the initial manifestation is progressive dysphagia. Swallowing is normal early in the meal, but becomes progressively more difficult. There is recovery of function with rest as well as after injection of intravenous edrophonium chloride (tensilon).

Disease of Muscle/Muscular Dystrophies

In addition to weakness of striated voluntary muscle, muscular dystrophies can also cause dysfunction of the smooth muscle. This can result in disorders of esophageal motility as well as problems with oral management of foods. Dysphagia is considered uncommon in muscular dystrophies except in relatively rare types, one of which can occur in children, myotonic dystrophy.

Miscellaneous Neurologic Conditions

RILEY-DAY SYNDROME OR FAMILIAL DYSAUTONOMIA. Familial dysautonomia is an inherited neurodegenerative disease mostly seen in Ashkenazi Jews. It affects not only the autonomic nervous system, but also peripheral sensory and motor neurons. Common features are excessive sweating, poor temperature control, indifference to pain, absent deep tendon reflexes, and motor incoordination (Riley, 1974). Poor or absent suck is present from birth as is excessive drooling and frequent regurgitation (Axelrod, Porges, & Sein, 1987). There is an abnormal swallowing reflex, impaired esophageal and gastric motility, and cyclic vomiting.

MOBIUS SYNDROME. Mobius syndrome is a congenital paralysis of the facial muscles. Causes include abnormal development of the brain (facial nuclei), facial nerve, or facial nerve musculature. Paralysis of the tongue, soft palate, and masseter muscles can occur and prohibit oral feeding.

Disorders of Cognition/ Mental Retardation

Definition

Mental retardation (MR) represents another major group of developmentally disabled children with dysphagia. Mental retardation is defined as significantly below average general intellectual functioning, accompanied by significant deficits or impairments in adaptive functioning with onset before 18 years of age. (American Psychiatric Association, 1987). IQ is 70 or below, and adaptive functioning including personal and social skills is deficient as defined by cultural and age expected norms.

The incidence of mental retardation in the U.S. is estimated at 2%. Male-to-female ratio is as high as 1.5 to 1.0

Cause

The causes of mental retardation are varied and in many individuals unknown. Generally, the less severe the MR, the less likely an identifiable cause will be found. Prenatal causes include chromosomal abnormalities (Down syndrome), disorders of brain development and intrauterine insults (alcohol, drugs, hypoxia). Perinatal causes include birth hypoxia, brain hemorrhage, and infection. Postnatally, CNS infections, trauma, and toxins (lead) are identified etiologic factors.

Pathophysiology

Mental retardation may occur in isolation or with a myriad of associated conditions which can interfere with feeding. Mental retardation may lead to impairment of communication skills. Thus the interactive component of feeding is hampered. Children with MR have more difficulty voicing food preferences and expressing feeding concerns.

There is delay in attainment of fine and gross motor coordination impeding the mechanisms of eating. Use of adaptive equipment and use of verbal instructions in therapy are more difficult than with the higher functioning child. Gastroesophageal reflux and rumination are more common than in the general population.

Interactive/Behavioral Problems

Pervasive Developmental Disorders/Autism

Pervasive developmental disorder (PDD) is a spectrum of disorders previously known as autism, childhood schizophrenia, and atypical ego development. Impaired social interaction, particularly in the area of verbal and nonverbal communication, is the principal feature. In severe cases (autistic subtype), social withdrawal, mutism, unusual preoccupation, and stereotypic behaviors such as hand flapping and rocking are seen. In less severe cases, relatedness to the environment is abnormal. There may be speech, but it is unusual in its speed, tone, or content and there is frequent echolalia.

Other commonly co-existing disorders include mental retardation, tone and postural abnormalities, mood disturbances, abnormal response to sensory input (e.g., high pain threshold, hypersensitivity to sound), and seizures in approximately 25% of affected children.

The prevalence is estimated at 10–15 children per 10,000. The most severe autistic subtype occurs with a prevalence of 5 cases per 10,000 children. Both PDD and the autistic subtype are more common in males with a ratio of 4:1.

CAUSE. The cause of PDD and autism is unknown. Etiology is believed to be multifactorial. There is an increased incidence of PDD and autism in individuals with Fragile X syndrome. PDD is more common in siblings of affected individuals than in the general population.

PATHOPHYSIOLOGY. A central feature of PDD is the impaired communication. As such, the child's ability to express hunger, fullness, dislike of food, or discomfort with eating is restricted. In turn, attempts at therapeutic intervention are thwarted by difficulties in explaining the therapies to the child.

These children often have very restrictive food preferences which are believed to be related to exaggerated sensitivity to food texture and may be part of the overall hypersensitivity of the senses. They frequently sniff, lick, or chew nonfood items as unusual interaction with their environment. Tone and postural abnormalities interfere with feeding as well.

Communication Handicap

Children with less severe communication handicaps such as language delays or those suffering from hearing loss may also have mild feeding impairments. This is believed due to limited expressive language resulting in inability to express their wants or needs. In turn, therapy is complicated by the difficulty with communication.

Lesch-Nyhan Syndrome

Lesch-Nyhan syndrome is a disorder of purine metabolism. It is sex linked. The gene involved is located on the long arm of the X chromosome. Degree of involvement is variable, depending on the activity level of the enzyme hypoxanthine guanine phosphoribosyltransferase (HGPRT). Affected individuals appear normal in infancy. There are progressive neuromuscular symptoms with resulting spasticity and/or athetosis. Their intelligence is not necessarily affected. Self-mutilation by biting of the fingers and lips is characteristic of the disease.

Prader-Willi Syndrome

Prader-Willi syndrome is characterized by obesity, hyperphagia, mental retardation, hypotonia, short stature, small hands and feet, and hypogonadism. Affected infants have low tone and feed poorly. In later years, hyperphagia can be extreme. There may be hoarding or stealing of food and binging.

High resolution banding techniques have found a partial deletion of chromosome 15 in a majority of patients with Prader-Willi syndrome.

Chronic Illness

AIDS

With improved medical treatment led by strong research efforts, children with AIDS are living longer lives. Children affected with the HIV virus leading to AIDS suffer a multitude of developmental disabilities, more so than the nonaffected population. Neurodevelopmental conditions can include spastic quadriparesis and associated severe mental retardation, mild mental retardation, developmental language disorders, attention deficit hyperactivity disorder, and conductive hearing loss. Fourteen percent of this population has significant feeding problems (Grosz, 1989).

The issue of dysphagia is discussed in a recent text *Management of HIV Infection in Infants and Children* (Yogev & Connor, 1992). The authors note that dysphagia and odynophagia (pain with swallowing) are frequently secondary to inflammation of the mouth or esophagus, resulting from opportunistic herpes or yeast infections. AIDS encephalitis can also result in pseudo-bulbar palsy (Pressman & Morrison, 1988).

Anatomic Abnormalities

Anatomic abnormalities involving the jaw, palate, and oral pharynx can cause dysphagia. Smith's textbook on recognizable human malformations (Jones, 1988) provides an excellent resource on the spectrum of such syndromes.

Cleft lip and palate are relatively common birth defects occurring in approximately 1:650 newborns (Morris, 1987). The degree of clefting is quite variable, and the abnormality may be isolated or part of a syndrome with associated defects. Affected newborns have feeding difficulties, particularly where there is a cleft palate. Cleft lip causes difficulty with good lip seal closure and decreases the effectiveness of sucking. Surgery to close the defect helps, but often does not obliterate later complications.

Pierre Robin sequence results in hypoplasia of the mandible. In severe cases, a small oral opening and retrognathia impedes normal oral intake. Treacher Collins syndrome includes mandibular hypoplasia and other facial malformations.

Esophageal atresia is a malformation which occurs in 1:4000 live births. It is associated with a tracheoesophageal fistula (TEF) in more than 75% of cases. Esophageal atresia occurs when the normal continuation of the esophagus to the stomach does not form prenatally; the esophagus ends in a blind pouch. If there is also a TEF, the food can enter the respiratory tract. Aspiration pneumonia may result.

The diagnosis of esophageal atresia should be made in the first day of life. These infants have excessive oral secretions and are unable to feed without choking or becoming cyanotic. The condition can be suspected prenatally in cases of maternal polyhydramnios. Diagnosis can be made by the inability to pass a catheter through the mouth or nose into the infant's stomach. The coiled catheter can be seen in the esophageal pouch on x-ray.

Esophageal atresia is a surgical emergency. The infant is maintained by intravenous feeding. A gastrostomy tube may be placed until surgical correction is possible.

Stenosis at the site of surgical anastomosis often occurs post-operatively, and esophageal motility is abnormal. This can mean a lifetime of gastroesophageal reflux, esophagitis, and aspiration.

Cornelia DeLange syndrome is a chromosomal condition characterized by growth retardation (pre- and postnatally), mental impairment, coarse cry, full eyebrows meeting in the midline (synophrys), hirsutism, small mouth, and abnormalities of the hands and feet. Abnormalities of the gastrointestinal tract can occur.

Summary

Children with developmental disabilities frequently suffer from dysphagia which may be caused by disorders of voluntary muscle control, pathological reflexes, autonomic dysfunction, and structural abnormalities. Nutrition and respiratory status may be compromised by the dysphagia. This chapter serves as an overview of some of these developmentally disabling conditions and their pathophysiology as it relates to dysphagia.

References

American Psychiatric Association. (1987). *Diagnostic and statistical manual of mental disorders* (3rd ed., rev.). Washington, DC: American Psychiatric Association.

Axelrod, F. B., Porges, R. F., & Sein, M. E. (1987). Neonatal recognition of familial dysautonomia. *Journal of Pediatrics, 110*, 946–948.

Byrne, W. J., Euler, A. R., Ashcroft, E., Nash, D. G., Siebert, J. J., & Golladay, E. S. (1982). Gastroesophageal reflux in the severely retarded who vomit: Criteria for and the results of surgical intervention in twenty-two patients. *Surgery, 91*, 95–98.

Capute, A. J. (1986). Early neuromotor reflexes in infancy. *Pediatric Annals, 15*, 217–226.

Catto-Smith, A. G., Machida, H., Butzner, J. D., Gall, D. G., & Scott, R. B. (1991). The role of gastroesophageal reflux in pediatric dysphagia. *Journal of Pediatric Gastroenterology and Nutrition, 12,* 159–165.

Christensen, J. R. (1989). Developmental approach to pediatric neurogenic dysphagia. *Dysphagia, 3,* 131–134.

Cook, I. J., Dodds, W. J., Dantas, R. O., Massey, B., Kerm, M. K., Lang, I. B., Brasseur, J. G., & Hogan, W. J. (1989). Opening mechanism of the human upper esophageal sphincter. *American Journal of Physiology, 20,* G748–G759.

Developmental Disabilities Assistance and Bill of Rights Act Amendments of 1991. U. S. Code 1988 Title 42, 6000, 6001, 6006, 6006 et seq., 6021 et seq., 6030 et seq., 6042., 6043, 6061 et seq., 6067, 6081 et seq. Nov. 6, 1978, P. L. 95-602, 92 Stat. 2955, Title 5 Oct. 19, 1984, P. L. 98-527, 98 Stat. 2662 Oct. 29, 1991, P. L. 100-146, 101 Stat.

Gilbert, J. N., Jones, K. L., Rorke, L. B., Chernoff, G. F., & James, H. E. (1986). Central nervous system anomalies associated with meningomyelocele, hydrocephalus, and Arnold-Chiari malformation: Reappraisal of theories regarding the pathogenesis of posterior neural tube closure defects. *Neurosurgery, 18,* 559–564.

Graziani, L. J., Posto, M., Stanley, C., Pidcock, F., Desai, H., Branca, P., & Goldberg, B. (1986). Neonatgal neurosonographic correlates of cerebral palsy in preterm infants. *Pediatrics, 78,* 88–95.

Grosz, J. (1989). The development and family services unit. In P. B. Kozlowski, D. A. Snider, P. M. Victze, & H. M. Wisniewski (Eds.), *Proceedings of the Conference on Brain and Behavior in Pediatric HIV Infection* (pp. 115–125). New York: Karger.

Gustafsson, B., & Tibbing, L. (1991). Dysphagia, an unrecognized handicap. *Dysphagia 6,* 193–199.

Hooker, D. (1952). *Prenatal origins of behavior.* Lawrence: University of Kansas Press.

Humphrey, T. (1968). The development of mouth opening and related reflexes involving the oral area of human fetuses. *Alabama Journal of Medical Science, 5,* 126–157.

Jones, K. L. (1988). *Smith's recognizable patterns of human malformations* (4th ed.). Philadelphia: W. B. Saunders.

Logemann, J. A. (1983). *Evaluation and treatment of swallowing disorders.* San Diego: College-Hill Press.

Love, R. J., Hagerman, E. L., & Taimi, E. G. (1980). Speech performance, dysphagia, and oral reflexes in cerebral palsy. *Journal of Speech and Hearing Disorders, 45,* 59–75.

Mills, J. L., Rhoads, G. G., Simpson, J. L., Cunninghan, G. C., Conely, M. R., Lassman, M. R, Walden, M. E., Depp, O. R., Hoffman, H. J., & the National Institute of Child Health and Human Development Neural Tube Defect Study Group. (1989). The absence of a relation between the periconceptional use of vitamins and neuraltube defects. *New England Journal of Medicine, 321,* 430–435.

Milunsky, A., Jick, H., Jick, S. S., Bruell, C. L., MacLaughlin, D. S., Rothman, K. J., & Willett, W. (1989). Multivitamin/folic acid supplementation in early pregnancy reduces the prevalence of neural tube defects. *Journal of the American Medical Association, 262,* 2847–2852.

Morris, H. (1987). Cleft lip and palate. In H. M. Wallace & R. F. Biehl (Eds.), *Handicapped children and youth* (pp. 273–280). New York: Human Services Press.

Morris, S. E. (1989). Development of oral motor skills in the neurologically impaired child receiving non-oral feedings. *Dysphagia, 3,* 135–154.

Mulinare, J., Cordero, J. F., Erickson, J. D., & Berry, R. J. (1988). Periconceptional use of multivitamins and the occurrence of neural tube defects. *Journal of the American Medical Association, 260,* 3141–3145.

Nelson, K. B., & Ellenberg, J. H. (1982). Children who "outgrew" cerebral palsy. *Pediatrics, 69,* 529–536.

Patrick, J., Boland, M., Stoski, D., & Murray, G. E. (1986). Rapid correction of wasting in children with cerebral palsy. *Developmental Medicine and Child Neurology, 28,* 734–739.

Pollack, I. F., Pang, D., Kocoshis, S., & Putnam, P. (1992). Neurogenic dysphagia resulting from Chiari malformations. *Neurosurgery, 30,* 709–719.

Pressman, H., & Morrison, S. H. (1988). Dysphagia in the pediatric AIDS population. *Dysphagia, 2*, 166–169.

Riley, C. M. (1974). Familial dysautonomia: Clinical and pathophysiological aspects. *Annals of New York Academy of Science, 228*, 283–287.

Schoenberg, B. S., & Schoenberg, D. G. (1980). Spectrum of pediatric cerebrovascular disease. In F. C. Rose (Ed.), *Clinical neuroepidemiology*. New York: State Mutual Books.

Seiler, R. W., Grolimund, P., Aaslid, R., Huber, P., & Nornes, H. (1986). Relation of cerebral vasospasm evaluated by transcranial Doppler ultrasound to clinical grade and CT visualized subarachnoid hemorrhage. *Journal of Neurosurgery, 64*, 594–600.

Shaker, R. (1992). *Functional relationship of the larynx and upper GI tract*. Paper presented to the Dysphagia Research Society. Milwaukee, WI.

Sondheimer, J. M., & Morris, B. A. (1979). Gastroesophageal reflux among severely retarded children. *Journal of Pediatrics, 94*, 710–714.

Taft, L. T. (1987). Cerebral palsy. In H. M. Wallace, R. F. Biehl, L. T. Taft, & A. C. Oglesby (Eds.), *Handicapped children and youth* (pp. 281–297). New York: Human Sciences Press.

Whyllie, E., Whyllie, R., Cruse, R. P., Rothner, A. D., & Erenberg, G. (1986). The mechanism of nitrazepam-induced drooling and aspiration. *New England Journal of Medicine, 314*, 35–38.

Yogev, R., & Connor, E. (1992). Gastrointestinal manifestation of pediatric HIV. In S. Manning (Ed.), *Management of HIV infection in infant and children* (pp. 376–388). New York: Mosby Year Book.

CHAPTER

2

Comprehensive Team Evaluation

DOROTHY W. BRYAN, M.D., AND HILDA PRESSMAN, M.A.

CONTENTS

Dysphagia symptoms frequently cross the traditional boundaries between professional disciplines (Bach et al., 1989; Ravich et al., 1985) which may make it difficult to decide which medical or therapeutic specialist a child needs to see. As a result, the multidisciplinary approach, which is becoming more common in medicine, is

15

especially useful in caring for children with dysphagia. In some facilities, following initial referral to a multidisciplinary diagnostic team, the members of the team see the child together and, after completing the diagnostic procedures, make joint recommendations on management. (Ravich et al., 1985). In others, team members may participate as consultants, as needed (Groher, 1984). Sometimes the issue of dysphagia is addressed by an existing team (Gritz, 1989); in other settings the team has been especially created to serve the child with dysphagia (Groher, 1984; Ravich et al., 1985). Whatever its form, the physical presence of the team has been noted to increase staff awareness of dysphagia issues (Jones & Altschuler, 1987).

In many facilities, the concept of a dysphagia team began with the collaboration between the feeding/swallowing specialist and the radiologist (Ott, Peele, Chen & Gelfand, 1990). Many teams add an occupational and physical therapist and a dietitian. Other teams have included, variably, the gastroenterologist, otolaryngologist, pulmonologist, neurologist, dentist/prosthodontist, attending physician, family member, nurse, medical social worker, respiratory therapist, thoracic surgeon, psychiatrist, and dental hygienist. (Bach et al., 1989; Gritz, 1989; Groher, 1984; Jones & Altschuler, 1987; Ravich et al., 1985).

The details of a dysphagia program in a particular institution will depend on the pediatric population served and the resources of the institution. The goals of the dysphagia team must be consonant with the goals of the institution in which it is located, and the team must be supported by the institution. Some thought must be given to whether the purpose of the evaluations will be primarily medical/diagnostic, focus on treatment strategies, or both. Children to be evaluated may be infants, children, or adolescents with varying levels of cognitive ability and physical size.

Children may be cared for as inpatients or outpatients. Educational and therapeutic facilities would require collaboration with a medical facility to obtain the radiologic capacity for videofluoroscopy. The makeup of the dysphagia team depends on the availability of individuals with sufficient interest and time to obtain the knowledge and skills required to understand and treat dysphagia. These individuals must be willing to work together to develop the interrelationships that are necessary for a successful team.

As an example, in a tertiary medical consultation model, children are seen for a single comprehensive consultation. The goals are primarily diagnostic, and the recommendations address medical diagnostic questions. There is also a therapeutic orientation as goals and suggestions for specific therapeutic techniques are generated from the evaluations. These include suggestions for equipment and positioning and types of foods to be used at mealtimes and at therapy time. Feeding options, (i.e., types of spoons and cups), techniques for presenting foods, and oral stimulation activities to improve function both for those who are being fed orally and those who are not are also addressed.

Development and Maintenance of a Multidisciplinary Diagnostic Team

Many different professionals have information and expertise pertinent to the function of swallowing and the study of dysphagia. The mouth, throat, upper airway, larynx, trachea, and esophagus are all involved. These contiguous anatomic areas are cared for by a number of medical subspecialists. Individuals from various therapeutic and psychosocial areas of rehabilitation are also involved with these children. These specialists must develop a new focus on the problems of feeding and swallowing. As busy professionals, they do not always have the desired time to exchange information. The individual professional may not be aware of all that other team members have to offer.

The team begins with a group of interested professionals who work in physical proximity and have some administrative connection with each other. Each discipline has its own procedures and standards of care as well as a unique cognitive structure for organizing information. Professionals interested in forming a team must feel compatible, demonstrate confidence in sharing what they know, and be open to expanding their knowledge. They may be seeing clinical problems which they are unable to solve completely within their own area of expertise and agree to share information and work in conjunction with each other.

The team comes to function almost as a family with members taking on certain roles according to their disciplines and personalities. The coordinator is the key to smooth team functioning and is the hub for information, particularly for informal communication between team members. All team members need to be comfortable with the coordinator. The member of the team who can bring a comprehensive view of the family and the child with developmental disability and dysphagia is the developmental pediatrician. This individual ensures the participation of all members of the team and ensures that all referral questions, both spoken and unspoken, are addressed.

Members of a well functioning multidisciplinary diagnostic team generate referrals from their own areas of expertise to the multidisciplinary team as well as to other individual team members. In a university setting, the team also serves as an educational model for students from many disciplines.

A well-defined and consistent program structure, maintained primarily by the program coordinator, is essential. Meetings must fit within all individual schedules and some flexibility may be needed. Changes in scheduling must be made well in advance to allow members to adjust their calendars. If essential team members cannot be present, other methods of gaining their input on specific topics may be necessary. Each team member needs to gain new insights and to feel that his or her input is respected. Time in team meetings needs to be set aside for individual members to update the team on what is happening in their particular areas of expertise. Socializing within or outside of the workplace may also help to keep the team cohesive. Team activities such as presentations and research projects also keep team members stimulated. There are multiple demands on the time of the team members, and administrative approval must sometimes be specifically sought to allow adequate time for their participation in this activity.

Members of the Team

Coordinator

The coordinator (Figure 2–1) integrates all team activities. For smooth functioning, the members of the team must be in agreement as to who will fill the role of coordinator. The individual must have time available. The coordinator must have experience in dysphagia and administration. It is essential that all communication to the team include the coordinator. It is the coordinator who receives and reviews all background information, decides, in consultation with the medical director, if the referral is appropriate for the team and defines the questions to be answered by the team. The coordinator must have good communication skills to interact with

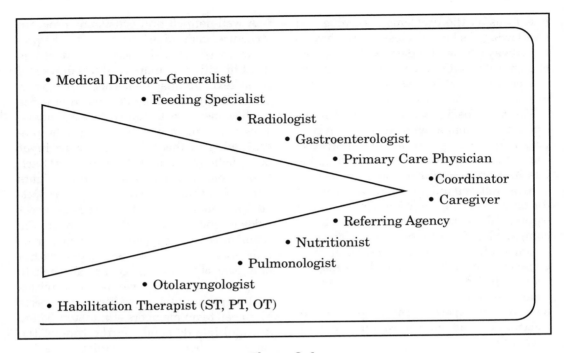

Figure 2–1.
The pediatric dysphagia team.

members of the team, the family, and outside professionals, including physicians and agency personnel.

It is the coordinator who facilitates the movement of the family and child through the diagnostic work-up which may involve multiple departments in the hospital. The coordinator schedules the various procedures needed and reassures parents and others who accompany the child. Family members have often anticipated this evaluation for quite some time and may be understandably anxious. Treating them with respect will reassure them that someone is listening to their concerns. For example, parents will tolerate delays in x-ray, if the coordinator keeps them informed as to the cause of the delay and the expected length of wait.

Medical Director/Generalist

The medical director brings a broad perspective to the team and should be involved in the general medical care of the type of individuals being evaluated. The individual may have specific expertise in gastroenterology, neurology, rehabilitation medicine, or developmental disabilities. A developmental pediatrician may be the person best qualified to serve as medical director for a team dealing primarily with developmentally disabled children. This individual will also be knowledgeable about the many emotional and psychosocial issues faced by families of such children (Christensen, 1989).

The medical director will be knowledgeable about different medical conditions which affect the well-being of the child.

Specific disorders characteristically are associated with varying types of developmental disabilities. The medical director may recognize and treat these disorders and facilitate further evaluations and treatment. Whomever is chosen to head the dysphagia team, however, should be experienced, interested in working on a multidisciplinary team, and able to function in a collaborative way with other professionals.

Prior to the consultation, the medical director reviews all medical and developmental background information to help clarify the questions to be answered by the consultation. Communication with the medical community both inside and outside the institution is necessary. A brief interview with the family can clarify the medical history, elicit information about previous evaluations, and determine parental expectations.

During the team discussions, the relationship between the child's feeding behavior and other medical conditions can be assessed. There are often differences between parental views of the child's needs and those of other professionals. The timing of the referral may have been precipitated by these differences of opinion. In addition, medical or family crises may have brought the child to the dysphagia evaluation. There are often unspoken agendas which need to be considered. These issues may be addressed by a social worker or psychologist on the dysphagia team. It is important, however, that they not be overlooked.

Feeding Specialist

The feeding specialist is most often a speech pathologist but may be an occupational therapist, a physical therapist, a nurse, or a dietitian. This specialist must review background information, conduct the clinical examination, refine the questions to be answered by the study, and define the plan for and assist in the radiological study.

Pediatric Radiologist

The pediatric radiologist must have experience in feeding disorders, as well as the relevant radiographic procedures, and should be a flexible individual. Radiologic studies of swallowing, as originally designed, maximized the possibility of aspiration. The modified study, although more difficult and time consuming, minimizes this risk (see Chapter 9). The radiologist has the primary responsibility for protection and support of the child during this procedure. In addition to assessing any anatomical abnormalities, the radiologist monitors the child for the extent of the aspiration. The radiologist then discusses the results with parents and team members and may recommend additional studies.

Pediatric Gastroenterologist

The pediatric gastroenterologist manages problems related to the GI tract. These include anatomic abnormalities and motility disorders in the esophagus, gastroesophageal reflux, abnormal gastric motility, diarrhea, peptic disorders, pancreatitis, hepatitis, and constipation. The pediatric gastroenterologist suggests further diagnostic procedures, recommends medical treatment, and/or alternative methods of feeding, including nasogastric tube, gastrostomy, or jejunostomy or the need for fundoplication and makes the referral for surgical consultation. In some hospitals, it is the gastroenterologist who performs percutaneous endoscopic gastrostomy. The pediatric gastroenterologist works closely with the nutritionist and communicates with gastroenterologists from other facilities. The gastroenterologist is a frequent source of referrals to the team.

Pediatric Pulmonologist

The pediatric pulmonologist manages airway hyperactivity, respiratory distress, and acute and chronic respiratory failure. This specialist evaluates children with congestion, pneumonia, and apnea. The pulmonologist monitors the adequacy of ventilation and oxygenation in children with respiratory problems who are on oral feedings. Deterioration of the child's respiratory status may indicate the need for an alternative method of feeding. Diagnostic studies which may be ordered to clarify pulmonary status include arterial blood gases, pulse oximetry, pulmonary function tests, chest radiographs, sleep pneumocardiograms, electrocardiograms, nuclear scans, gastroesophageal pH probe monitoring, and EEGs. The pulmonologist determines the need for tracheostomy or decannulation and often refers children for dysphagia evaluation to determine whether respiratory symptoms are feeding-related (see Chapter 11).

Pediatric Otolaryngologist

The pediatric otolaryngologist assesses structural abnormalities of the nose, mouth, and throat to determine their effect on swallowing and upper airway function. This specialist does a complete analysis of muscle structure and function (see Chapter 10). In addition, the specialist may utilize fiberoptic visualization of the pharynx and larynx to assess the child's swallow.

Pediatric Nutritionist

The pediatric nutritionist uses diet information obtained by other team members, including a 3-day recall diet, to assess intake. This specialist evaluates the information for calorie content and distribution and for adequacy of vitamins, trace elements, minerals, and fluids. The effect of medications must be taken into account. These children may have special needs secondary to spasticity, respiratory disorders and altered status, activity levels, and developmental status. Growth data and an-

thropometrics are used as well in formulating a diet recommendation. Such a recommendation includes total caloric needs, distribution of calories, total need for nutritional supplementation, and practical advice on achieving these goals. Parents are counseled in ways to modify their child's eating habits within the context of their culture (see Chapters 4 and 5).

Pediatric Habilitation Therapist

The pediatric habilitation therapist may be an occupational or physical therapist. This specialist assists in determining the best position for feeding equipment. Suggestions are made for therapeutic techniques that will increase or decrease tone to facilitate improved oral motor control for swallow. Adaptive equipment for self-feeding may also be recommended (see Chapter 8).

Other specialists who may participate on the team are the nurse (see Chapter 15) and the dentist (see Chapter 14).

Visiting nurse and home health agencies may be called on to assist in providing services in the home, carrying out the treatment plan, teaching families, and assisting in the daily care of the child with a chronic illness or handicapping condition.

Caregiver

The child's caregiver should be considered a primary member of the team so that family-centered care can be provided. Unless the family understands and accepts the recommendations of the team, the program will not be carried out. The caregiver provides background information regarding medical history, treatment history, positioning for feeding, and utensils used at home. Understanding of the caregiver's point of view is essential. Most importantly, caregivers provide emotional support for the patient throughout the diagnostic procedure. The caregiver is asked to feed the child during the clinical examination and, if possible, during the radiographic procedure. The x-ray study is reviewed with the caregiver to achieve a better level of understanding of the problem.

Referring Agency

The referring agency also is part of our team. Its staff can provide extensive and pertinent background information related to previous attempts at treatment and problematic foods. The referring agency may be a school, early intervention program, day training program, visiting nurse agency, a speech pathology department, or a physician. It is frequently the agency that identifies the problem and suggests the comprehensive dysphagia evaluation to the caregiver.

It is most helpful if someone from the referring agency accompanies the child to observe, contribute to the discussion, and help the child feel comfortable with the process. This individual may serve as the feeder during the study. Most frequently, the representative who comes is a speech pathologist, but may be an educator, occupational therapist, physical therapist, or nurse. In a consultative model, the referring agency, as well as the caregiver, will be responsible for carrying out the recommendations of the team and providing ongoing treatment.

Primary Care Physician

The primary care physician will implement the medical aspects of the team's recommendations. The family is encouraged to notify their physician of the evaluation. The guardian is asked to sign release forms to request information from the primary care physician and forward results. The family is referred back to their physician for management of related medical problems discussed during the evaluation. This physician integrates the diagnostic findings.

When to Refer to a Dysphagia Team

Three general concerns most commonly generate referral to a dysphagia team: aspiration, nutrition support, and therapeutic techniques for oral feedings (see Table 2–1). Questions specifically include: diet and position modifications, maintenance and introduction of oral feeds, and the safety of oral feeds in the child with a tracheostomy. Need for a cleft palate repair to improve swallowing, need for significant nutritional supplementation and/or tube feeding, and poor progress in dysphagia treatment are other reasons for referral. The team evaluation may be needed to rule out physiologic causes of food refusal and for resolution of disagreement between therapists and caregivers.

The following are pulmonary causes for referral for a dysphagia evaluation: coughing or choking during feedings and chronic respiratory congestion with wet breath and/or vocal sounds which may be exacerbated during feeding. A medical history

Table 2–1. Issues to be addressed in dysphagia evaluation.

Document safety of swallow

Demonstrate aspiration

Evaluate for tracheal decannulation

Assess need for diet modification

Identify need for nutritional rehabilitation

Determine need for change of PO status

Identify GI symptoms that may be contributing to problem

Resolve disagreements

that includes frequent respiratory infections, especially pneumonias, in dependent areas of the lung and/or reactive airway disorder or asthma, is suspicious of aspiration particularly when these symptoms are chronic and respond poorly to the usual pulmonary management.

Nutritional causes for evaluation include thinness and loss of subcutaneous fat in a child with dysphagia. Weight for length less than the 50th percentile is an objective measure of inadequate nutrition. Nutritional inadequacy may be manifested by frequent infections. Inadequate nutrition may be exacerbated by decreased intake during an illness. Prolonged feeding time may also place the child at risk for inadequate nutrition.

A broad range of therapeutic and intervention issues may precipitate a referral. Certain behaviors during feeding, such as: gagging, choking, skin color changes, or turning pale or blue, observed by the therapist and caregiver, may be physiologic indicators of an unsafe swallow. The child who refuses feedings entirely or accepts only specific textures may be protecting his airway. Concerns usually focus on the following: Is there a safe swallow? How is a safe swallow achieved? What positions are best for feeding? What food viscosities and textures can be given confidently?

The Referral Process

The initial referral to the team is made when the caregiver, physician, or agency contacts the coordinator to request evaluation. A referring physician's order is not necessary for the child to be seen by a team if the order for x-ray is written by the team medical director. The more active the involvement of the primary care physician, however, the more likely it is that the information obtained will be incorporated into the patient care plan.

The coordinator must generate the dysphagia history during the initial telephone contact (see Table 2–2). Detailed information is essential in determining if the referral is appropriate. The caller may, initially, give a long and possibly rambling story detailing medical history, therapeutic interventions, and dissatisfaction with others who have been involved in the child's care. This accumulated frustration needs to be turned into questions that can be answered. Symptoms given may be nonspecific or misleading, and careful questioning is needed to clarify these issues.

When the initial call is completed, permission is requested to contact other significant parties. If the first call is from an agency, it is important to determine what the parent has been told about the referral. The coordinator helps the referring agent and caregiver to define the questions that will need to be answered.

It important to determine why the child is being referred at this point in time. With the exception of inpatients who are referred because of acute conditions, most of the children seen by a dysphagia team have had symptoms of dysphagia for long periods of time. They frequently have been under treatment, and it is helpful to probe

Table 2–2. The referral process.

Inquiry by caregiver or agency personnel

Obtain demographic information

Dysphagia history taken by coordinator

Reports of previous medical and therapeutic evaluations obtained

Summary of intake information submitted to team includes:

    Relevant background information

    Clarification of key questions

    Plan for evaluation

for the issue that has brought them to evaluation. Reasons may be related to poor progress in treatment, a new individual service plan, or a change in medical status. Parental readiness to cope with the problem, frequent school absences, or frequent hospitalizations related to pneumonia or dehydration may also precipitate the referral. This background information is helpful in generating appropriate recommendations by the team.

At this point, the coordinator makes the preliminary decision as to whether a team referral is appropriate or, alternatively, if the child should be referred to individual medical specialists. For example, many children are seen for modified barium swallows but do not need the full team evaluation. If vomiting seems to be the primary issue, referral to the gastroenterologist alone may be indicated.

The team evaluation proceeds with collection of additional historical data from schools, agencies, physicians, and hospitals that have been involved with the child. The dysphagia history form (see Appendix A) is completed by the coordinator. The history form summarizes medical, feeding, and treatment information and leads to clarification of the questions to be addressed by the consultation. Attention is given to the family's concerns and their perception of the problem as well as the agency's concerns and the issues that they feel must be resolved. The reason for referral at the present time is addressed, and the need for nutrition evaluation is determined. The background information is reviewed by the medical director as well for an understanding of the etiology and course of the developmental disorder. This allows the medical director to comment on expected future course and prognosis. The medical director is interested in determining whether the neurologic condition is static or progressive; if a syndrome is present; and the child's developmental strengths and weaknesses.

Next, a tentative plan for the radiographic procedure is established. This is included in a brief summary of the medical and dysphagia history, which is prepared by the coordinator and distributed to all the members of the team. Instructions are given to the family, both verbally and in writing (see Appendix B), detailing the procedure on the day of the consultation. They are asked to bring the adaptive seat in which the child is fed, if possible, as well as the usual utensils (spoon and cup) that are used for feeding. The family is also instructed to bring a variety of foods, including those that are preferred and those that are known to cause difficulty. If nutrition appears to be an issue, a 3-day recall diet is requested, including foods eaten and quantity. The recall diet is best done for 3 consecutive days, one of which is a weekend when foods and schedules may vary. The family is also encouraged to bring other caregivers working with the child.

Evaluations

Children are scheduled for a clinical dysphagia evaluation, modified barium swallow, a developmental pediatric screening, and a concluding conference on the same day. This reduces the number of visits the family must make and allows them to have some immediate feedback. If a nutrition consultation is indicated, this may also be scheduled on that day. Throughout the consultation period, the focus is on the family as well as the child (see Table 2–3).

During the clinical dysphagia evaluation, the parent is observed while feeding the child to ascertain any position or technique which may be different than those previously described. The techniques to be used during the radiographic examination are determined during the clinical dysphagia examination (CDE); a determination is made as to which textures will be offered, which positions will be used, and the sequence of each, as well as compensatory strategies that may be tried. Gastroeso-

Table 2–3. Child's schedule for day of evaluation.

Clinical dysphagia evaluation

Nutrition consultation as needed

Modified barium swallow, and other radio–
graphic procedures, as needed

Developmental pediatric screening

Parent conference: Initial review of results and
preliminary recommendations

Total time = 3 hours

phageal reflux and gastric emptying stud-ies are planned if vomiting is present or a gastrostomy is anticipated. Following the study, portions of the videotape of the pro-cedure may be reviewed with the family to demonstrate any significant findings.

Next, the pediatric developmental screen-ing occurs. This gives the physician the op-portunity to clarify the medical history and complete a brief examination of the child. If aspiration has occurred during the radi-ographic procedure, the pediatrician pro-vides information to the caregiver as to pos-sible sequelae and treatment. Suggestions include maintaining hydration and maneu-vers to facilitate clearing of aspirated mate-rial, such as postural drainage and chest physical therapy. The caregiver is advised to call the primary pediatrician should symptoms of aspiration pneumonia occur. The family is given the opportunity to ask questions and express their views of the child's feeding problem and their own fam-ily priorities. Interaction among family members and accompanying professionals can be observed during this time.

An underlying concern of the developmen-tal pediatrician is clarification of the type of developmental disability and the medical etiology for it. The focus, however, remains on the problems of dysphagia. Growth para-meters are plotted, and weight for length is determined during this brief screening.

After the examinations are completed, a concluding conference with the speech pathologist and coordinator provides im-mediate feedback to the family regarding findings. It is stressed that the recommen-dations given are preliminary as the video-tape of the x-ray procedure will be re-viewed further and the team will meet to formulate final recommendations. The family is encouraged to raise any questions that they may have. Questions that cannot be answered immediately are discussed with the team, and the answers are pro-vided to the family at a later time. Once again, if there are any signs of aspiration, a diagram is used to explain the findings more concretely to the family.

Specific therapeutic recommendations are made, including seating, positioning, diet, and utensils. Feeding techniques are demonstrated, and the parent is given a chance to feed the child in the recommend-ed way. Food with the recommended vis-cosities and textures is presented so that there is no confusion over terminology and everyone agrees, for example, what thick puree looks like. If thickening of liquids is recommended, specific proportions of thick-ener to liquid are given. Notations of these instructions are given to the family before they leave. When it appears that a gastros-tomy tube may be one of the recommenda-tions, this is discussed with the family. In this instance, a treatment plan for main-taining acceptance of oral stimulation and oral motor competency for controlling se-cretions is described.

Team Meeting

The team meets following the evaluation (see Table 2–4). The core members of the team are present, including the coordinator,

Table 2–4. Team meeting agenda.

Medical and therapeutic history
  Coordinator

Summary of evaluations
  Each specialist who saw child

Review of videotape

Discussion
  Medical issues
  Nutritional issues
  Therapeutic issues
  Psychosocial issues

Generation of recommendations

Sequence of appointments to be scheduled

Summary

speech pathologist, medical director, dietitian, and gastroenterologist. Other team members attend as their schedules permit. The referring agency representative is also welcome to attend. After presentation of the referral questions, summaries of findings from individual evaluations, and review of the videotape, the team then enters into a discussion, which culminates in setting priorities and negotiating a set of final recommendations. It is important for team members to agree on what is practical in a particular situation and also how to present recommendations to the family and the agency. Each member of the team brings not only information in his or her area of expertise, but also a unique style of problem solving and patient counseling. This process leads to comprehensive and practical final recommendations.

The issues dealt with by the team may be organized on three levels, from the most concrete to the most abstract. The first level of discussion and interaction centers around the specific issues related to swallowing adequacy. These issues are concern about aspiration, concern about adequate nutrition, and concern about the oral motor and feeding programs.

The second level of issues is psychosocial. Because the feeding and nurturing of a child by any caregiver is a basic social activity, a disruption in this process generates intense feelings in caregivers. The ability to adequately feed a child is one of the basic elements in the caregiver's self-concept as a nurturer of the child. Feeding time is a critical time for parent-child interaction and may set the tone for other areas in the relationship. Compromise regarding conflicts between professional and family are addressed here. Oral feeding may be very difficult for both parent and child to give up, and this is an important psychological issue.

Lastly, there are what might be called political or community issues. Discussions about these issues include the resources in the child's community for carrying out team recommendations, financing the treatments, and other issues of access for the family such as transportation and care for other children. Observation, during the assessment day, of the relationship between family and other caregivers, including home nurses and professionals, provides important clues to guide the formulation of recommendations that are practical and can be carried out.

Team Report

Written reports are prepared and, with parental permission, are sent to the family, the referring agency, the primary care physician, and any other professionals designated by the family as well as other subspecialists to whom the child is being referred (see Table 2–5). Separate reports are prepared by the feeding specialist, developmental pediatrician, and radiologist. These are summarized in, and supplemented by, the team meeting report which is co-signed by the coordinator and the medical director.

This report concludes with a plan that addresses medical, surgical, nutritional, therapeutic, and equipment issues and prioritizes needed follow-up services, based on the level of urgency. In the report, we point out that the videofluoroscopic examination is a limited sample of the child's swallowing abilities and may not reflect the child's performance with larger amounts of foods or when fatigue influences swallowing. In considering the findings, it is important to keep the history in mind, because what is seen in an examination may not be what is happening all the time. The history allows the team to judge how demonstrated aspiration is tolerated by the child and whether it is safe to use a conservative "wait and see" approach. This would determine whether we recommend that oral feedings be discontinued immediately or if trial modifications will be employed (see Table 2–5).

A recommendation for re-evaluation is made based on achievement of specific goals. A formal re-evaluation may be scheduled, or a request for feedback from the referring agency or the child's physician may be solicited, before deciding whether re-evaluation is indicated.

Follow-Up

Further evaluations which have been recommended are scheduled by the coordinator

Table 2–5. Outline of team report.

Names of participants

Background information

Summary of evaluations

Summary of team discussion

Impressions

Recommendations

Distribution list for copies of reports

---

if the family agrees and may include medical appointments such as pediatric gastroenterology or pediatric otolaryngology or therapy appointments for treatment or selection of appropriate seating. Families are sent a Patient Satisfaction Questionnaire 3 to 6 months following their appointment (see Appendix C). The family is asked to rate, on a scale from 1 to 5, how helpful each of the individual evaluations were. Each subspecialist is listed including follow-up appointments such as gastroenterology, ENT, or surgery. The caregiver is also asked to comment on any difficulties that they or the therapists may be having in carrying out the recommendations and whether any additional tests or procedures were necessary. Comments are solicited regarding the child's general health and his or her current weight. The family may elect to put the child's name on the form or to respond anonymously. A follow-up letter and questionnaire are sent 2 weeks later if the first has not been returned. If the child's name appears on the form, a letter acknowledging receipt of the form is sent to the family. Generally, families have indicated that they found the consultation useful but had some difficulty in finding therapists who could implement the recommendations.

However this complex consultation is evaluated, it is important to realize that achieving full oral feeding is a narrow goal by which to measure success. A consultation is considered successful if the information generated by the evaluation and/or the discussion sheds an objective light on the questions asked. If the information proves useful to the therapist and caregiver, as documented by the patient satisfaction questionnaire, or if it helps ease the intense conflict between professionals and caregivers, the consultation has been worthwhile.

Case Summary

The following brief case summary will serve to clarify the process of a tertiary consultation dysphagia model as well as to illuminate the collaboration possible between several pediatric subspecialists and demonstrate the important role played by the caregiver.

The child was a 2-year, 7-month-old male referred for dysphagia consultation by the speech-language pathologist seeing him for individual therapy at home. The therapist's concerns were the refusal of liquid, increased congestion following feeding, chronic respiratory problems, and recurrent pneumonias.

The child had been diagnosed as having cerebral palsy, a seizure disorder, and developmental delay. His functioning was at less than a 6-month level. He was not yet sitting independently. He was on both anticonvulsant medication and nebulized medication for wheezing. He had been seen by the Immunology Clinic at this hospital for work-up of a possible immune disorder. He had been enrolled in an early intervention program for developmental facilitations, however, he had not been attending because of his chronic respiratory problem. The child was fed orally by the mother although he had been fed with an NG tube while hospitalized. Feedings lasted for one half to one hour. He was given soft and blenderized table food; coughing was noted during feeding, and the child often refused liquids.

Past records were requested from the child's local hospital, neurologist, and pediatrician. Our hospital chart was reviewed, and information was requested from the early intervention program. Additional information stated that the etiology of this child's neurologic disorder was related to meconium aspiration at birth associated with asphyxia, seizures, and respiratory distress in the neonatal period. There had been several admissions to a local hospital for seizure control and respiratory problems. One admission resulted from a respiratory arrest and required mechanical ventilation.

The clinical dysphagia evaluation revealed severe deficits in oral preparatory, oral initiation, and pharyngeal stages of swallow. These deficits were associated with oral facial paralysis and severely impaired body postural control for eating. Coughing and wet breath sounds occurred following swallowing of both solids and liquids, and liquids were generally refused. Control of secretions was problematic with intermittent wet breath sounds and coughing associated with pharyngeal accumulation of secretions. The sequence for the modified barium swallow was to evaluate for thick purees, thick liquid, and thin liquid, in the upright position. If aspiration was seen, the plan was to proceed to evaluate for reflux and stomach emptying.

The modified barium swallow revealed very poor oral transport with virtually no posterior displacement of the tongue. The barium passed over the tongue into the pharynx by gravity, and pharyngeal swallow was then initiated. With thick barium, of a cereal consistency, no tracheal aspiration was noted. However, there was poor clearing of the pharynx after swallow. When the fluoroscopic equipment was turned on again, prior to the ingestion of the thinner preparation, barium was noted in the trachea indicating tracheal aspiration presumably of the thick or semi-solid material had occurred following swallowing. In light of this, the plan was modified; and thick liquids were not given. With ingestion of thin barium, tracheal aspiration was noted. No cough reflex was noted at the time of aspiration.

The developmental pediatric evaluation reviewed the child's birth history as well as the complex multidisciplinary medical care required by this severely handicapped youngster. The mother felt that he had regressed somewhat in his social skills, possibly related to his frequent illnesses. Physical examination found a child whose weight for length was in the 50th percentile;

lungs were clear. The developmental pediatrician's recommendations included attending a combined Pulmonary Immunology Clinic if respiratory symptoms persisted or worsened. The mother requested additional information regarding the immune disorder. She was also urged to re-enroll the child in the early intervention program (EIP).

During the concluding conference, the mother was advised to feed the child only thick semi-solids while maintaining him in an upright position. Feedings were to be short, and he was to be kept upright or prone following the feedings. It was recommended that all foods be swabbed from his mouth after the meal. All liquids were to be of pudding consistency. Some suggestions were made to improve his sitting position. It was recommended that the physical therapist at his EIP assess the suggestions and arrange for implementation. In the team discussion it was felt that a gastrostomy should be considered due to the severity of the child's respiratory problems and the documented aspiration. The child was referred to the GI Clinic for GI series and milk scan to assess whether or not fundoplication should also be done. Consultation reports accompanied these referrals and were sent also to the mother, primary care physician, referring therapist, and the school program.

The child attended the GI Clinic on one occasion. Milk scan showed some gastroesophageal reflux but no aspiration. The child attended the Pulmonary Clinic, and in the following 4 months the child's respiratory status improved markedly. When the pulmonologist felt that the lungs were clear and surgery could be considered, the mother then requested reconsideration of the recommendation for gastrostomy. She pointed out that his meal times had decreased to one-half hour. He was congested only after being given his anti-convulsant medications, and he had had an adequate weight gain. The mother was also very pleased with the improvement of his respiratory status. The team concurred with the mother's

assessment that the child's overall situation had greatly improved with the mother's careful following of the feeding suggestions. The mother requested a repeat clinical examination and modified barium swallow to clarify whether there was a safe swallow for liquid. Although the study was scheduled on two occasions, the appointment was not kept, and the dysphagia team had no further contact with this family.

Follow-up information provided by the school indicated that subsequent study at another facility revealed aspiration of both thick and thin liquid when given by cup. Therefore, continued thickening of all liquids to pudding consistency for spoon feeding was recommended. The youngster continued to be in good health and to attend school on a regular basis.

In conclusion, this child was appropriately referred for dysphagia consultation based on his symptomatology and severe respiratory problems. The dysphagia consultation documented the aspiration and provided some suggestions to the mother for minimizing it. It was the feeling of the professional team, however, that placement of a gastrostomy was indicated. With continued multidisciplinary management of this child as well as careful following of the therapeutic suggestions by the mother, the child's general condition improved to the point that he could be maintained on oral feedings. His nutrition was adequate at the time of the consultation and good weight gain had been seen in the interim. The involvement of this thoughtful and very motivated mother significantly shaped this child's good progress.

References

Bach, D. B., Pouoget, S., Belle, K., Kilfoil, M., Alfieri, M., McEvoy, J., & Jackson, G. (1989, Fall). An integrated team approach to the management of patients with oropharyngeal dysphagia. *Journal of Allied Health*, pp. 459–468.

Christensen, J. R. (1989). Developmental approach to pediatric neurogenic dysphagia. *Dysphagia*, *3*, 131–134.

Gritz, J. M. (1989). Assessment and intervention techniques for the dysphagia patient in the home setting. *Journal of Home Health Care Practice*, *1*(4), 51–65.

Groher, M. E. (Ed.). (1984). *Dysphagia: Diagnosis and management*. Stoneham, MA: Butterworth.

Jones, P. L., & Altschuler, S. L. (1987) Dysphagia teams: A specific approach to a nonspecific problem. *Dysphagia*, *2*, 200–205.

Ott, D. J., Peele, V. N., Chen, Y. M., & Gelfand, D. W. (1990). Oropharyngeal function study: Radiologic means of evaluating swallowing difficulty. *Southern Medical Journal*, *83*, 191–193.

Ravich, W. J., Donner, M. W., Kashima, H., Buckholz, D. W., Marsh, B. R., Hendrix, T. R., Kramer, S. S., Jones, B., Bosma, J. F., Siebens, A. A., & Linden, P. (1985). The swallowing center: Concepts and procedures. *Gastrointestinal Radiology*, *10*, 255–261.

APPENDIX 2A

History Form

Name:_____ Date of Birth:_____

UH#:_____ Age: _____

Date:_____

Presenting Problem:

Patient's Medical Diagnosis:

Current feeding history

Is patient fed orally ☐ NG ☐ GT ☐

Position for feeding: _____

Special Positioning equipment:_____

Utensils: _____

Adaptive Utensils: _____

Independent or dependent feeder?_____

Persons who feed child _____

Number of meals/day_____Number of snacks/day_____

Duration of meals: _____

Foods taken: (obtain 3 day diet recall)

Are liquids thickened? _____

Are purees jarred or prepared from table food at home? _____

Problems during feeding:

Coughing/choking during ☐ after ☐ meals

Nasal regurgitation _____

Refusal of certain foods or textures

Vomiting or excessive spitting up during ☐ or after ☐ meals

Increased mucous production during ☐ or after ☐ meals

Limited intake_____

History Form
Page 2

Slow feeding_____

Crying _____

Has patient ever been fed   orally ☐   NG ☐   GT ☐   TPN ☐

Growth Parameters	Present	1 Year Ago	Birth
Height	_____	_____	_____
Weight	_____	_____	_____

Current motor control

Independent sitting? _____

Adaptive Seat? _____

Mental/Cognitive status _____

_____

Medical History

Pneumonia/bronchitis _____

Noisy breathing_____

Wheezing/asthma _____

Middle ear infections _____

Seizure Disorder _____

Medications _____

Allergies _____

Surgeries_____

Other _____

Family History

Family members in household _____

APPENDIX 2B

Parent Appointment Letter

UNITED HOSPITALS MEDICAL CENTER
HEARING AND SPEECH CENTER
TERTIARY MULTIDISCIPLINARY SERVICE (TMDS)
PEDIATRIC DYSPHAGIA PROGRAM
15 SOUTH 9TH STREET
NEWARK, N.J. 07107
HILDA PRESSMAN, M.A., CCC S-LP
COORDINATOR
(201) 268-8140

Dear Parents,

Your child has been scheduled for a dysphagia or swallowing consultation by our pediatric dysphagia team. We have scheduled the assessment for Monday, October 19, 1992 and ask that you be here at 12:00 Noon. Please come to the Hearing and Speech Center in the basement of the Annex Building. Directions to UHMC are enclosed. It is important that you arrive on time so that we can accomplish all that we have to do. Please bring your insurance information and forms to assist in the registration process. Your child may have a light breakfast at 7:00 AM, but nothing to eat after 7:30. It is alright to give scheduled medicine, however.

After registering, you will be seen by Dr. Sheppard, who is a speech pathologist specializing in the care of children with swallowing difficulties. This initial evaluation will help us to plan how to proceed in the x-ray portion of the consultation. In order to accommodate the two children scheduled to see the dysphagia team on the same day, a delay between evaluations does occur.

Following Dr. Sheppard's evaluations we will go to the x-ray department where we will make final preparations for the study. You are welcome to be in the room during the x-ray procedure and to help us if you wish, unless you are pregnant. This procedure is under the direction of Dr. Marquis, a pediatric radiologist.

During the x-ray procedure, your child will be offered barium which is a white substance that comes in liquid and paste forms and allows us to see what happens when the child swallows. It has a mild flavor and may be mixed with cereal, fruit or chocolate flavoring. If your child has a particular taste preference please discuss this with the Coordinator before the date of the evaluation. The barium may be given by spoon, cup, bottle or tube. We will discuss this with you further when you see Dr. Sheppard.

Appendix 2B *(continued)*

Following the x-ray procedure, you will be seen by Dr. Bryan who is a developmental pediatrician and the Medical Director of our program. Dr. Bryan will have reviewed all of the records that were submitted. She will discuss any significant medical and educational, issues with you and examine your child briefly.

You will then see Dr. Sheppard again to discuss preliminary results of the morning's assessment and recommendations for intervention. As your child will have had little to eat, we suggest that you bring food. The food can be given at this time, and may be part of the demonstration of intervention techniques.

You can expect to be finished by 3:00 pm. It is often helpful to parents to bring a friend or family member and we certainly encourage you to invite the speech pathologist or other specialist who works on feeding with your child. As space is limited we can only accommodate 4 adults in the actual examination rooms. Because it is a long day, it is best to leave other children at home, if possible. Throughout the day, and at any time before or after the evaluation, we urge you to ask any questions or discuss any concerns that you may have.

Many parents ask if their child will have any reaction to the barium. In our experience, barium does not cause either constipation or diarrhea. We usually give a small amount of barium, but you might want to decrease the quantity of the next meal slightly. As always, if you have any concerns about your child's health you should contact your pediatrician.

To complete the consultation, the dysphagia team will meet to further discuss the evaluations and to formulate final recommendations. Reports will then be written; you should receive them approximately two weeks after the visit. Copies will be mailed to you and with your written permission, to the medical and educational professionals whom you designate.

If you have any questions regarding the above or any other aspect of the assessment, please feel free to call the Coordinator. We look forward to meeting you and your child and hope that this assessment will provide information useful in your child's care.

Hilda Pressman, M.A.,CCC
Coordinator

Dorothy W. Bryan, M.D.
Medical Director

APPENDIX 2C

Consumer Satisfaction Questionnaire

Child's name (optional) _____

Name of person filling out this form (optional) _____

Read each item carefully and **circle** the one answer that is best for you.

SA – Strongly Agree	**N** – Neutral	**SD** – Strongly Disagree
A – Agree	**D** – Disagree	**NA** – Not Applicable

1. The Dysphagia (Feeding-Swallowing) assessments were helpful to me.

    A. Clinical Dysphagia Evaluation   SA   A   N   D   SD   NA
        (Ms. Pressman, Dr. Sheppard)

    B. Videofluoroscopy (x-ray)   SA   A   N   D   SD   NA
        (Dr. Marquis)

    C. Developmental Pediatric Screening   SA   A   N   D   SD   NA
        (Dr. Bryan)

    D. Nutritional Assessment   SA   A   N   D   SD   NA
        (Dr. Mkandawire, Ms. Meicke-Taylor)

    E. Gastroenterology Evaluation   SA   A   N   D   SD   NA
        (Dr. Nord, Dr. McLoughlin)

    F. Surgical Consultation   SA   A   N   D   SD   NA
        (Dr. Falla)

2. The post assessment conference at   SA   A   N   D   SD   NA
    the end was helpful to me.

3. The written reports were helpful.   SA   A   N   D   SD   NA

4. The evaluations were helpful to the   SA   A   N   D   SD   NA
    child's physician.

5. The evaluations were helpful to the   SA   A   N   D   SD   NA
    therapists who work with the child.

Appendix 2C *(continued)*

Customer Satisfaction Questionnaire   **Page 2**

Child's name (optional) _____

Please comment on your above responses. In what way were the evaluations helpful or not helpful? How can the evaluations, post assessment conference and reports be improved? (Feel free to attach additional pages.)

Are you having any difficulty following through with the recommendations?

Have the child's therapists been able to carry out the recommendations?

What additional tests or procedures were carried out, relative to the dysphagia (feeding-swallowing) problem?

Has the child's general health improved, stayed the same, become worse?

Present weight_____

Additional comments:

CHAPTER

3

Clinical Evaluation and Treatment

JUSTINE JOAN SHEPPARD, Ph.D.

───────────── **CONTENTS** ─────────────

Clinical management of pediatric dysphagia includes the pediatric equivalent of the "bedside" evaluation and the management program. The examination determines the contributing causes of the swallowing disorder and which treatments will best improve the functional adequacy of feeding and swallowing behaviors (Logemann 1983). In infants and children with developmental disability, the primary dysphagia is caused by anatomical abnormalities and sensorymotor deficiencies. However, it is frequently complicated by secondary consequences of dysphagia and by co-occurring disorders. The assessment considers these secondary and co-occurring causes, as well. The management program includes therapeutic exercise to improve swallowing and advance the child to more mature eating behaviors as well as a plan for current management of oral secretions and nutritional intake.

The Clinical Presentation of Dysphagia

The functional behaviors addressed in the swallowing program are (a) control of oral secretions; (b) oral management of liquid, nonchewable solid foods, and chewable solid foods in suckling, cup drinking, and spoon feeding; (c) the ability to chew and otherwise soften and moisten the food in preparation for oral-pharyngeal and esophageal transit; and (d) the ability to swallow safely and effectively during dependent and self-feeding. The functional adequacy of swallow is stated in terms of related medical outcomes in respiratory health, nutrition and hydration, psychological satisfactions that arise from ease of eating and satiation of hunger, developmental level of feeding skills, and normality of the oral motor and respiratory coordinations themselves.

Secondary and Co-occurring Deficiencies

Deficiencies that co-occur or are secondary to dysphagia complicate its management. Frequently occurring problems examined in the clinical dysphagia evaluation include impaired praxic competency, sensory defensiveness, deprivation of timely and ap-

propriate experiences, and traumatically conditioned effects. Co-occurring medical problems that affect swallow and the management of dysphagia are dealt with elsewhere in this book.

Praxic Deficiencies

Studies of swallowing competencies in adults following left cerebrovascular accident (CVA) have revealed a symptom complex with severity correlated with the presence of oral and/or verbal apraxia. These deficits interfered with oral and pharyngeal events in swallow and were discussed as a primary cause of dysphagia (Robbins & Levine 1988). In children, praxic deficiencies, likewise, have been observed to affect swallowing and interfere with acquisition and performance of developmental feeding skills. In some cases oral praxic deficiency is seen as a secondary disorder resulting from deprivation of the normal amount and variety of oral, sensory-motor experiences. In other cases it appears as a primary oral apraxia causing or co-occurring with dysphagia. In children who exhibit praxic deficiencies, the neuromuscular degradation of swallow is exacerbated. In children without primary neuromuscular disorder or diminished sensory acuity, there may be difficulty with suckling, slow acquisition of developmental skills, and persistent drooling. The differential diagnosis of praxic disorder in the developmentally disabled child is difficult and the symptoms are easily overlooked.

Oral Sensory Defensiveness

The problem of intolerance of the sensory experiences associated with eating was discussed first by Mueller (1972). She noted an "exaggerated response to oral stimulation" in children with cerebral palsy that was "destructive for feeding" (p. 297). She recommended exercise prior to feeding to diminish these responses. Oral sensory defensiveness appears as a catastrophic response to the sensory array associated with eating and with touch to mouth and face. Responses may include crying, facial grimacing, and associated, increased, overall muscle tone and movement. Symptoms of oral sensory defensiveness occur in children who exhibit (a) hyperactive primitive oral reflexes (Sheppard, 1964), (b) apraxia, (c) irritability, (d) poorly controlled physiological homeostasis, (e) deprivation of timely experience with the variety of food types and utensils, and (f) distress during eating caused by primary disorders in the oral initiation, pharyngeal, or esophageal phases of swallow or related gastrointestinal conditions. It is important to determine the cause of the defensiveness in order to select appropriate intervention strategies.

Deprivation of Experience

Deprivation of timely and appropriate developmental eating experiences has been observed to complicate later attempts to advance eating skills. Illingworth and Lister (1964) hypothesized a critical or sensitive period for acquisition of eating skills. They observed that children who were not given chewable foods in the first year had difficulty accommodating to them and learning to chew. In the child with developmental disabilities, medical and developmental problems in the first year may disrupt the orderly sequence of feeding experiences including those with varieties of food types, modification of body postures for eating, and use of variety of utensils. The effects of deprivation may appear as refusal to advance eating skills or as praxic difficulties with planning and organizing new feeding behaviors.

Traumatically Conditioned Effects

The child who has experienced prior difficulty with swallowing may acquire a conditioned fear of eating, a feeding phobia. The difficulty may have resulted from dysphagia that has since resolved, severe gastroesophageal reflux, a choking incident, odynophagia, or repeated, uncomfortable oral procedures. These traumatically conditioned dysphagias (Di Scipio & Kaslon 1982; Di Scipio, Kaslon, & Ruben 1978) appear as refusal of specific textures or types of foods, rigid eating behaviors, restricted amount of food intake, and, in the child who is tube fed (NPO), as refusal of oral feeding. Treatments may be needed for both traumatically conditioned effects and co-occurring physiologic dysphagia.

The Clinical Dysphagia Evaluation

In the clinical dysphagia evaluation, oral, pharyngeal, and thoracic anatomy, oral reflex reactivity, voluntary movement patterns, bolus motility, and developmental eating skills are examined. This examination of swallow is limited, however, to oral, cervical, and thoracic events that can be observed directly. Overall adequacy of swallow for nutrition and airway protection is deduced from the patient's history and from observed behavioral and sensory-motor events which, when associated with swallow, suggest pharyngeal, respiratory, or gastro-esophageal competency. Symptoms that indicate the possibility of oral initiation, pharyngeal, and esophageal dysphagia are coughing, gagging, regurgitation, increased respiratory rate, skin color change, gurgling breath or vocal sounds, and self-restricted bolus size, viscosity, or amount of intake, among others.

The clinical assessment rules out, or confirms, the dysphagia and motivates referrals for assessments to rule out or manage related behavioral, medical, maxillo-facial, or nutritional problems. In addition, the results are useful in determining the need for, and planning appropriate procedures for, x-ray and other instrumental studies of the dysphagia. The clinical dysphagia examination, therefore, is frequently the first procedure scheduled in a team evaluation.

Published Clinical Assessments

There are few published clinical assessments for pediatric dysphagia, although the topic has drawn considerable attention in the literature (Arvedson & Brodsky, 1992; Cooper & Stein, 1992; Gisel, 1991; Sheppard, 1987; Tuchman, 1989; Wolf & Glass, 1992). The *Neonatal Oral-motor Assessment Scale* (NOMAS) is an evaluation of adequacy of nutritive and non-nutritive suckling that discriminates normal from abnormal suckling and quantifies degree of abnormality (Braun & Palmer, 1985–1986; Palmer, Crawley, & Blanco, 1993). Items describe normal and abnormal movement components of suckling in jaw and tongue as "disorganization," lack of overall rhythm of total sucking activity, and "dysfunction," interruption of suckling by abnormal movements of tongue and jaw (p. 19). The *Oral-Motor / Feeding Rating Scale* (Jelm, 1990) is a checklist and rating scale for adequacy of lip/ cheek, tongue, and jaw movement in breast, bottle, spoon, cup, and straw conditions and during biting and chewing on soft and hard cookies. Implicit in both of these assessments is the assumption that dysfunction in the oral initiation, pharyngeal, and esophageal phases of swallow will be reflected in the functional movements of the oral preparatory phase. Neither assessment localizes the dysfunction by phase of swallow or is diagnostic of contributing causes. The *Assessment Scale of Oral Functions in Feeding* (Ottenbacher, Dauck, Gevelinger, Grahn, & Hassett 1985; Stratton, 1981) rates movement adequacy, in jaw, lips, and tongue, with additional items for containment of liquid and solid food, ability to sip from cup, and coughing, gagging, or "hypersensitivity" associated with swallow. A checklist is provided for abnormality in selected oral structures, oral reflexes, positioning, diet, utensils and feeding time. *The Prespeech Assessment Scale* (Morris, 1982) is a rating scale which includes examination of both vocal and swallowing behaviors from birth through 2 years old. In the section that addresses swallowing, duration of meal, amount of intake, food consistencies, positioning, sucking from nipple and sipping from cup, coordination of suck, swallow, and breathing, spoon feeding, biting and chewing, and control of breathing are rated. Oral movements in lips, tongue, and jaw and "swallow" are rated separately for each food type. Summaries include analyses of the quality of movement patterns (i.e., extent of abnormality) and developmental level of behaviors.

Examination Procedures

The examination procedures for NPO children and those who are nourished by oral feeding (PO) differ, but both are constrained by a child's limited capabilities for cooperation. The children are generally unable to perform tasks on command, have limited stamina, and have not experienced the behaviors that are to be tested. The examination items are, therefore, structured to gain information about sensory-motor competency and level of skill by inference and by observation of response to probes of spontaneous performance rather than requested demonstrations (Sheppard, 1987) (see Figure 3–1).

The History

As in the clinical dysphagia evaluation for adults, the foundation of the pediatric dysphagia evaluation is the patient's history (Groher, 1992; Logemann, 1983). Information is gathered regarding onset and symptoms of swallowing disorder; nutritional,

STEP A
HISTORY

Onset and description of disorder
Nutritional and other medical disorders/problems
Prolonged hospitalization & surgery
Ages of acquisition of developmental feeding skills
Adequacy of feeding and mealtime behavior

STEP B
BASIC OBSERVATIONS

ANATOMY
Malformations
Deformations

REFLEXES
Swallow
Gag
Primitive oral reflexes

RELATED BEHAVIORS
Body postural control
Oral postural control
Voice
Oral imitation & blowing skills

SECRETIONS
Drooling
Oral pooling
Pharyngeal pooling
Pooling at tracheostoma

STEP C
EXAMINATION OF BOLUS SWALLOW

THE NPO CHILD
1 to 3 ml clear liquid
1 to 3 ml semisolid

THE PO CHILD
Nipple: usual liquid bolus
Spoon: smooth semisolid
                 textured semisolid
                 viscous, smooth solid
Fingers: chewable food
Spoon: soft chewable food
                 complex soft chewable food
                 hard chewable food
Cup: thick liquid
                 thin liquid

STEP D
EXAMINATION OF STATE DURING FEEDING

Alertness
Level of activity (quiet, active, crying)
Receptiveness to feeding

Figure 3–1. Observations for pediatric clinical evaluation of dysphagia.

gastrointestinal, and respiratory compromise; medical diagnoses and conditions that might be precipitating, contributing, or maintaining causes; related surgical procedures; medications that may be affecting swallow; previous evaluations for dysphagia; current management strategies for nutrition and hydration; current medical management; and dysphagia therapy. In the child with chronic disorder, the history of ongoing respiratory and nutritional health supplement the direct observations in the clinical evaluation as indicators of the functional adequacy of swallow.

Anatomy

Oral and thoracic structures are examined for malformations or deformations that may contribute to the disorder and for abnormalities of muscle tone and muscle mass. Palatal and labial clefts, palatal webs, micrognathia, deviant dental occlusions, ankyloglossia, trismus, scoliosis, and pectus excavatum are some of the more frequently seen anomalies. Although these may be readily compensated for swallow by the normal child, they can be significant contributing causes of dysphagia in the child with developmental disabilities who may have co-occurring neuromotor, cognitive, and behavioral involvements. Neuromuscular features of joint laxity or stiffness, muscle tightness or weakness, and involuntary movements, such as athetosis or tremor, that may affect adequacy of swallow are examined by palpation and observation of spontaneous activity (see Table 3–1).

Oral Reflexes

Examination of oral reflexes includes swallow, the protective reflexes, (i.e., cough and gag), and a selection of primitive oral reflexes. Spontaneously occurring swallow is palpated for timeliness of initiation, symmetry, and excursion of laryngeal movement. Its occurrence and coordination with the respiratory cycle may be examined by auscultation. Spontaneously occurring cough is observed for effectiveness or, in the child with pharyngeal hyporeflexia, may be stimulated with a soft probe to test its reactivity. Gag and primitive oral reflexes are elicited in a standardized manner (Sheppard, 1964; Sheppard & Mysak, 1984). The reflex examination is, in part, the pediatric equivalent of the touch localization and oral movement tasks used in the bedside examination of adults. In young infants, the examination provides evidence of the presence or absence of the sensory-motor pathways associated with suckling and swallow. In older, developmentally disabled infants and children with persistent primitive oral reflexes, the reflex responses reveal patterns of abnormal movement that may interfere with swallowing (Sheppard, 1964). In addition, they reveal the oral, sensory-motor repertoire that is available to the child (Sheppard, 1987). The reflexes included in the test are selected to examine the sensory fields and structures involved in eating (see Table 3–2).

Respiratory Function

Examination of respiration includes observation of the thoracic and abdominal movement patterns associated with breathing, and upper airway sounds. Symptoms of deficiency include sternal retraction, asynchronous thoracic and abdominal movements, and sounds of congestion or breath obstruction that are associated with blockage by oral and pharyngeal structures, accumulating oral secretions, or foods. The acoustics of swallow may be examined without instrumentation. However, there is a growing interest in the use of auscultation of swallow (Vice, Heinz, Giuriati, Hood, & Bosma, 1990) for examining the timing of

Table 3–1. Procedures for examining oral and thoracic anatomy.

Anatomical Feature	Examination Technique
Oral-facial features	Examine at rest and during spontaneous movement. Observe muscle tone in superficial facial and labial muscles.
Buccal muscles and gingival mucosa	Spread cheek with tongue blade and slide blade slowly along inner surface of cheek toward lips. Avoid touching vertical gingiva. Observe rebound of buccal and labial muscles and palpate range of movements and muscle tone.
Mandible Laxity	Palpate anterior-posterior range at ramus. Observe for habitual open-mouth posture and lateral instability during activity.
Reduced mandibular range of motion	Observe range during gag reflex and during spontaneous movements.
Retrognathia	Displace mandible forward at ramus and upward. Observe alignment of mandible with maxilla.
Velo-pharyngeal deformity gag reflex/velar reflex	To open mouth: stabilize head, stroke or press vertical gingiva, slide tongue blade posteriorly along raphe to uvula. Press tongue dorsum or stroke pharyngeal wall to elicit gag. Observe symmetry and range of velar, pharyngeal, lingual, and mandibular movements as reflexes are elicited.
Thoracic deformity and respiratory movements	Examine in upright and reclining, at rest, and during vocal behavior. Observe for bony deformities of spine, sternum, and ribs. Observe coordination between thoracic and abdominal respiratory movements. Observe for sternal retraction and flared lower ribs.

swallow, respiratory sounds as they are co-ordinated with swallow, and sounds associated with pharyngeal stasis of the bolus. Another promising technology is pulse oximetry, which has been used during clinical evaluation of developmentally disabled children and adults to detect hypoxemia associated with eating (Rogers, Arvedson, Msall, & Demerath, 1993; Rogers, Msall, & Shucard, 1993).

Oral Postural Control and Voice

Additional information about underlying oral and pharyngeal neuromuscular control can be gained from observing oral postural

Table 3–2. Stimulus areas and movement responses for oral reflexes.

Reflex	Stimulus Area	Movement Response
Gag	Tongue dorsum Posterior pharyngeal wall	Mouth opening; tongue protrusion and grooving; velar elevation; pharyngeal wall displacement; and head ventroflexion.
Cough	Laryngopharyx, glottis, trachea	Mouth opening; tongue protrusion and grooving; velar elevation; and vocal fold adduction.
Rooting	Perioral area	Head rotation to side of stimulation, plus other movements of head, eyelids, mandible, lips, and tongue.
Lip	Labial	Lip shaping movement, plus other movements of head, eyelids, mandible, and tongue.
Mouth opening	Anterior vertical gingiva	Mandible depression, lip separation, plus other movements of head, eyelids, and tongue.
Biting	Mandibular molar table	Mandible elevation, plus other movements of head, eyelids, tongue, and lips.
Lateral tongue	Lateral lingual margins	Lateral tongue movement toward side of stimulation, plus other movements of head, eyelids, mandible, and lips.
Babkin	Bilateral pressure to palms	Mandible depression, head ventroflexion, and eye closure, plus other movements of tonue and lips.

control and voice. When the mouth is not engaged in a specific action oral postural alignments are such that lips, mandible, tongue, palatal velum, pharynx, and vocal folds are stabilized to maintain a closed mouth and a patent naso-tracheal airway. This is a dynamic stability that is maintained against the forces of head-neck movement and gravity. Vocal quality and duration of phonation are features that reflect control of vocal fold adduction and adequacy of respiratory support. Although the neurological organization for oral postural control and voice differ from that for swallow, control of the motor subsystems observed in posture and voice is evidence of the underlying sensory-motor competency that is available for swallow and may be recruited

through treatment. If these behaviors are competent, it is an indication that paralytic involvement, if present, is probably not severe enough to interfere with basic control of oral and pharyngeal behaviors (Sheppard, 1987).

Praxis

Oral praxic capabilities also can be probed in nonfeeding tasks. Praxic competencies are apparent in infants when they begin to engage in reciprocal social vocal exchanges, imitate oral sounds, such as cough and sneeze, and mouth objects held in their hands. The older infant and child will purposefully eject an unwanted pacifier or an object, such as a Toothette, that is placed in its mouth or blow on a simple horn or whistle. If neuromuscular capabilities appear to be adequate in oral postural control and vocal behaviors and no other primary limiting deficits are apparent, early oral imitation and oral manipulation behaviors are expected to be present. If by history or examination they have not developed, then praxic competency is suspect and should be probed in the examination of eating behaviors (Sheppard, 1987).

Oral Secretions

Direct observations of swallow begin with examination of control of oral secretions. If the child is placed in a reclining position, secretions will be carried by gravity into position for oral initiation of swallow. This eliminates from consideration questions of the competency of labial containment and oral transport. Pooling in the posterior oral cavity, therefore, indicates a problem with swallow initiation. If, when the tongue dorsum is depressed, secretions are seen to have pooled in the laryngo-pharynx, adequacy of

lingual bolus propulsion and pharyngeal phase coordinations are suspect. Nasal discharge of foamy secretions, secretions exuding from a tracheostoma, and need for frequent suction are symptoms of incompetent or absent swallow for secretions. The oral reflex examination itself, because it stimulates increased salivary flow, tends to stress the child's ability to swallow, thereby probing a higher level of competency.

Once oral initiation and pharyngeal stage problems for controlling saliva are ruled out, the oral preparatory phase competencies are examined in upright postures. Drooling may reflect difficulty with neuromuscular or sensory competencies in lips, cheeks, tongue, and mandible (see Table 3–3). In addition, oral praxis may be inadequate to sustain control of secretions during stresses of co-occurring movement behaviors, discomfort, or attending behaviors.

Swallowing for Nutrition

Adequacy of swallow for nutrition can be probed in the child who is not receiving oral

Table 3–3. Task components for control of oral secretions and associated sensory and motor deficiencies.

Task Component	Deficiencies
Sensory appreciation of accumulation of secretions at the lips and on the tongue body	Impaired sensory acuity or perception.
Anterior and posterior containment	Impaired motor competency for labial and lingua-velar closure.
Collection of secretions and bolus formation	Impaired mandibular stability and lingual dexterity. Impaired praxis.
Initiation of swallow	Reduced reflex reactivity because of sensory and/or motor deficits.
Pharyngeal transit	Impaired lingual propulsion, pharyngeal stripping action, laryngeal elevation and/or cricopharyngeal relaxation. Impaired sensation.

feeding (NPO) and in the orally-fed (PO) child . The clinical examination for swallow of food boluses involves observing typical eating patterns and probing the child's potential capabilities. During the examination, the child's responses to typical eating conditions are compared to the responses elicited when optimum conditions are provided. In the NPO child who demonstrates adequate oral initiation and pharyngeal phases of swallow for secretions, swallowing adequacy for food can be probed with small test boluses.

SPECIAL CONSIDERATIONS FOR THE NPO CHILD. In the NPO child, the history of ongoing respiratory and nutritional health is not related to eating. In the absence of this history, adequacy of airway protection during swallow of a food bolus can be determined only by instrumental examination. The Modified Barium Swallow and the Salivagram are the tests used most frequently to make this determination. In this instance the clinical examination provides inferential information regarding relative swallowing competencies for oral secretions and liquid and semisolid boluses which may be used to select the appropriate instrumental tests and test procedures (Bryan, McLoughlin, Pressman, & Sheppard, 1989; Heyman & Respondek, 1989).

Before beginning the clinical evaluation of swallow for nutrition an order from the child's physician, indicating prescribed limits of the examination with reference to bolus size and type (e.g. clear liquid, 1 ml, or puree, 1 to 3 ml), should have been obtained. Implicit in this order is the physician's judgment that the medical risk from such an examination is acceptable. However, during the examination, decisions of whether, and how, to continue must be made by the examining clinician. If oral initiation and pharyngeal phases of swallow appear to be incompetent for secretions, introduction of food boluses should be deferred. If the child has

demonstrated competent oral initiation and pharyngeal phases of swallow for secretions but incompetent oral preparatory phase skills, a 1 ml bolus is introduced by pipette into the posterior oral cavity. If bolus formation is functional, then the bolus can be offered at the lips or spooned onto the tongue. In clinical assessment of the NPO child, food boluses should be restricted in size to no more than 3 cc, in viscosity to liquid and semisolid, in texture to puree, and in amount to 30 ml. It is advisable to have suctioning equipment available to relieve the child of the residual bolus or accumulated secretions if there is distress.

If the child has been NPO because of prior difficulty in oral feeding, boluses are limited to 1 to 3 ml of clear liquid and thin semisolid. If an infant is NPO because of preterm birth, but has responded well to introduction of the 1 to 3 ml bolus, trial nippling of breast milk or formula may be examined, preferably with a nipple that limits flow, such as a Haberman feeder (Haberman, 1988; Mathew, 1990). The amount of the feeding given the NPO infant or child in the assessment trial should be limited to allow time to rule out adverse respiratory effects from the feeding before advancing further. This can be accomplished by dispensing liquid into the nipple by syringe as the infant suckles (Pressman, personal communication, 1992). The infant should be referred for modified barium swallow or oral feeding deferred if a problem with airway protection is suspected. Use of auscultation to augment palpation and visual observations of swallow are useful during this procedure.

SPECIAL CONSIDERATIONS FOR THE CHILD WITH TRACHEOSTOMA. The child with tracheostoma may experience transient, recurrent, or persistent dysphagia. The swallowing disorder has been associated with diminished vocal fold function for airway protection, diminished effectiveness of cough, and mechanical limitations of laryngeal excursion and head movement caused by the tracheostoma, the cannula, and the cannula tapes, and deviant coordination of respiration and swallow (Bonanno, 1971; Myers & Stool, 1985; Shaker, Milbrath, Pen, Hogan, & Campbell, 1992; Simon, Fowler, & Handler, 1983). In the child with co-occurring anatomical or neuro-motor abnormalities, dysphagia is more likely to be recurrent or long-term. Many children with tracheostoma have also been tube fed and have suffered the effects of deprivation of timely eating experiences and traumatic oral experiences that can complicate attempts to advance oral feeding (Simon, Fowler, & Handler, 1983).

The tracheostoma is a subglottic window for detecting aspiration. If the child is NPO, a preliminary test for aspiration of secretions and small food boluses can be conducted using Evans (methyline) blue dye (Cameron, Reynolds, & Zuidema, 1973). The dye is placed on the tongue or is fed, mixed with a food bolus. Appearance of the dye at the stoma or in material suctioned from the trachea after succeeding swallows confirms deglutive aspiration.

Tracheostomy speaking valves, which direct exhaled air through the vocal folds, have been reported to aid in reducing nasal and oral accumulations of secretions and to direct tracheal accumulations orally for expectoration (Passy, 1986). Informal observations in children indicate that use of the valve may improve the effectiveness of swallow. If a tracheostomy valve is determined by the physician to be appropriate for the child, it can be tried during evaluation as a compensatory strategy.

FEEDING THE CHILD. Examination of the typical eating patterns in the PO child is best done by observing the caregiver offering several tokens of each food type and using each utensil as in daily feeding. This part of the evaluation may be deferred if, because of

patient or caregiver, it appears that it will interfere with the probe of optimum function.

The child should be positioned optimally for eliciting normal swallowing coordinations (Bergen, Presperin, & Tallman, 1990; Morris & Klein, 1987; Trefler, 1984). The infant from birth through 3 to 4 months old—corrected age if the child was born prematurely—and the infant or child who is unable to transport a bolus into position for oral initiation may be positioned semi-reclining to allow bolus transport to be assisted by gravity. The infant may be swaddled tightly with flexed extremities for feeding in lap or placed in an infant seat with the lateral trunk and head-neck supports needed for stable body alignment. Clinical observations of 4- to 5-month-old infants reveal increasing difficulty controlling oral bolus transit and oral initiation of swallow for spooned foods in a semi-reclining position. The changes are associated with changes in oral and oral-pharyngeal anatomy. These difficulties appear to be exacerbated by neuromuscular and praxic deficiencies seen in infants of the same age who are at risk or developmentally disabled. The position of choice, therefore, is upright sitting in an appropriately sized chair with upper body weight supported on elbows and lateral trunk and head-neck supports provided as needed for stable body alignment. If assistance is needed to stabilize the head for reception and oral transport of the bolus, the face should be vertical or tipped forward slightly to facilitate oral movements that contain and transport the bolus posteriorly. This position prevents the bolus from being carried into the oral pharynx by gravity. Utensils, bolus size, food texture and viscosity for liquids and solids, and feeding techniques are selected to elicit optimum coordinations for swallow (Sheppard, 1987). Bolus types and utensils that may be used to examine the patient include liquid, smooth semisolid, textured semisolid, nonchewable solid, chewable solids, and thickened or thin liquids from nipple, spoon, cup, and straw. The food types are introduced in order from best tolerated and easiest to swallow to most difficult, as indicated by history and presenting symptoms. Only food types that are considered to be within the child's current capabilities for management or for advancing are offered. Trials with other food types are deferred. Swallow is examined in dependent and self-feeding behaviors for each food type as permitted by the child's motor capabilities (Sheppard, 1987).

Praxic competency can be probed during examination of eating behaviors by observing the child's ability to accommodate to new feeding strategies, to use novel utensils, such as a Doidy cup or molded handle spoon, and to learn a new eating skill, such as straw drinking, chewing, cup drinking, or self-feeding. Cuing and assistance to motivate the child and facilitate a successful trial should be provided (Sheppard, 1987).

Interactive behaviors and "state" (Als, Lester, Tronick, & Brazelton, 1982; Brazelton, 1973) during eating are observed. Typically an infant or child is alert, quiet, and receptive when feeding is initiated. Somnolence, decompensation, physical avoidance, refusal of food, and rigid or restrictive eating routines or diet preferences are all symptoms that suggest there may be a behavioral component of the feeding disorder, and should be noted.

The effects of compensatory strategies on eating competency should be observed. Compensatory strategies that have been found to improve swallow include modifications of head-neck and body position; specially designed nipples and other utensils; special bolus presentation techniques, including pacing and bolus placement; bolus characteristics, especially size, texture, and viscosity; and environmental facilitators, such as music (Logemann, 1983; Morris, 1989; Sheppard, 1991) The prescription for mealtime procedures or in the case of the

NPO child for prefeeding therapy, is derived from the results of these probes (see Table 3–4). If modified barium swallow is anticipated, selection of feeding and compensatory strategies to be used in that test will be based on these results, as well. The clinical diagnosis of dysphagia is made if there are deficiencies in oral preparation of the bolus and/or symptoms of, or previously confirmed deficiencies in, oral initiation, pharyngeal, or esophageal phases of swallow that have potential or ongoing consequences for nutrition, respiration, ease of eating, or acquisition of the developmental skills needed for safe ingestion of an unrestricted diet. The severity of the dysphagia in terms of the functional consequences of the disorder and of the complexity of the management strategies that are needed may be designated through staging. A model for staging pediatric dysphagia can be seen in Table 3–5.

Figure 3–2 illustrates a test form which can be used in conjunction with this examination model. Observations can be recorded on this form with descriptive comments or with binary scoring for normal and abnormal findings.

Dysphagia Therapy

In the normal child, the apparently seamless acquisition of developmental eating skills is an expression of emerging oral-pharyngeal and postural neuromotor competency, psychosocial and self-regulatory behaviors, and cognition (Christensen, 1989). When dysphagia occurs, a therapy program may minimize disruption of development in these domains, improve nutrition and respiratory health, improve swallow and feeding coordination, and improve the behaviors associated with feeding.

Goals of the Management Program

In the long term, the aims of the treatment program are to improve underlying sensory-

Table 3–4. Selected compensatory strategies for trial use during pediatric clinical evaluation of dysphagia.

Variable Affecting Swallow	Compensatory Strategy
Body posture	
High postural tone	Hip flexion >90°. Shoulder girdle stabilization by elbows and forearms on tray/table. Face mid-line and vertical or tipped forward.
Low postural tone	Hip flexion at 90°. Reclining <10° with vertical face alignment.
Impaired cervical stability/ hemiparesis	Head turn toward side. Face vertical. Assist stabilization at crown of head.
Impaired oral initiation and pharyngeal swallow	Chin tuck (capitol flexion). Chin down.
Retrognathia	Bottle feeding in prone position.
Utensils	
Uncontrolled mouth closure/biting on utensil	Hard plastic or coated spoons. Plastic tumbler. Firm plastic straw. Firm-walled nipple.
Tonic bite reflex	Smaller spoon.
Impaired lip pucker and dribbling during drinking	Cut out cup/tumbler, appropriately sized for mouth.
Disorganized or dysfunctional suckling	Controlled flow nipple.
Weak suckling	Soft-walled nipple. Nipple expressed by biting (Ross cleft palate nipple). Cup drinking with thick liquids. Spoon feeding.
Bolus characteristics	
Impaired airway protection or containment and nasopharyngeal reflux	Thicker bolus (syrup, honey or pudding consistency), and smaller bolus.
Oral, pharyngeal, or esophageal stasis	Thinner bolus (nectar, syrup or honey consistency), smaller bolus, and smoother bolus.
Disorganized oral preparatory swallow	Smoother bolus.
Reduced oral sensory acuity	Increased viscosity, texture, and size of bolus.
Bolus presentation	
Respiratory changes; disorganized oral preparatory swallow	Pacing rate of intake; rhythmic bolus presentation.
Reduced stability in lips, mandible, and tongue	Firmer contacts between oral structures and spoon, cup or nipple. Slower entry and exit of utensil. External stabilization of jaw.
Tonic bite reflex or reduced mobility in lips, mandible, and tongue	Light contacts between oral structures and spoon, cup, or nipple. Rapid entry and exit of utensil.
Impaired chewing	Place chewable pieces toward side of mouth. Use crisp, soft-chewable food.
Impaired biting	Rest piece on mandibular table for biting. Use thicker piece of food
Impaired cup drinking	Slide cup onto mandibular dental arch. Pause for sip. Withdraw cup for swallowing.
Environmental facilitators	
Distractibility, disorganization, or irritability	Use familiar background music. Reduce distractions. Use repetitive verbal cuing and praise.

Table 3–5. Model for staging functional adequacy of pediatric dysphagia.

Stage of Swallowing Competency		Functional Adequacy
I	Not dysphagic	Competent oral, pharyngeal, and esophageal management of all food categories and oral secretions.
II	Mild dysphagia	Dysphagia is compensated by diet restrictions or medications. Nutritional and respiratory status, as related to swallow, are good.
III	Moderate dysphagia	Dysphagia is compensated by diet restrictions and special feeding strategies. Nutritional and respiratory status, as related to swallow, are good.
IV	Severe dysphagia	Diet restrictions and special feeding strategies are needed to facilitate oral feeding. Nutritional and/or respiratory, status, as related to feeding, are marginal or unsatisfactory.
V	Profound dysphagia	Nonoral feeding is needed for supplemental or total nourishment.

Source: Adapted from Managing dysphagia in mentally retarded adults by J. J. Sheppard, 1991. *Dysphagia, 6,* 83–87.

motor competency for swallowing saliva and food, train more mature and appropriate swallowing and eating skills, facilitate appropriate functional compensations for deficits, and establish mealtime routines that satisfy the needs of both caregivers and their charges. In the short term, the program goals are to establish routines that will promote optimum swallowing and feeding behaviors for control of secretions, nourishments, and ingestion of oral medications and prevent the development of maladaptive motor patterns and secondary behavioral, respiratory, nutritional and dental problems. An effective and efficient program is symptom specific, that is, appropriate strategies are selected to treat the specific causes of the disorder.

The Caregiver's Role in Treatment

The role of the caregiver in shaping the feeding behaviors of infants and young children has been discussed most often with reference to children who present with nonorganic failure to thrive (Mathisen, Skuse, Wolk, & Reilly 1989; Satter 1990). Feeding skills and self-regulatory behaviors emerge from caregiver-child interactions. Positive mealtime interactions are recognized as important to the developmentally disabled infant as well (Pridham, 1990; Satter, 1990). Oral motor dysfunction, lack of feeding skills, and the often co-occurring communication difficulties may affect nutrition by distorting requests for food, interfering with expressions of hunger and food preference, and preventing foraging (Reilly & Skuse, 1992), as well as by interfering with food intake. Stresses experienced by the caregivers of children who are difficult to nourish may interfere with successful management of the problems, especially if the child's problems persist past the first year (Barnard, 1981; Jones, 1989; Mathisen et al., 1989; Reilly & Skuse, 1992). Caregiver knowledge and compliance with management programs may also be a problem. Reilly and Skuse (1992) compared caregivers of children with cerebral palsy to caregivers of normal, age- and sex-matched children. The caregivers of children with cerebral palsy

CLINICAL DYSPHAGIA EVALUATION

Justine Joan Sheppard, Ph.D.
Teachers College, Columbia University

NAME ______________________________ DOB ____________ DATE ____________

DIAGNOSIS ______________________________

	COMMENT	SCORE 0 = normal 1 = abnormal
CURRENT STATUS		
FEEDING MODE		
❑ ngt ❑ gt ❑ oral		
DIET		
Texture		
Supplements		
FEEDING		
Duration		
Frequency		
FEEDING REFUSAL		
❑ solids ❑ liquids		
DISTRESS/SOLIDS		
❑ gag ❑ cough ❑ choke		
DISTRESS/LIQUIDS		
❑ gag ❑ cough ❑ choke		
SPECIAL FEEDING TECHNIQUES		
SPECIAL UTENSILS/NIPPLES		
SPECIAL SEATING		
INDEPENDENCE		
CONTROL OF ORAL SECRETIONS		
❑ drooling ❑ congestion		
❑ coughing on secretions		
RESPIRATORY DISORDER		
REGURGITATION		
❑ vomiting ❑ nasal regurgitation		
PERIPHERAL SPEECH MECHANISM		
LIPS		
MANDIBLE		
TONGUE		
MAXILLA & PALATE		
OROPHARYNX		
THORAX		

Figure 3–2. Recording form for caregiver comments on current status, examination observations and evaluation conclusions.

	COMMENT	SCORE
RELATED BEHAVIORS		
ORAL POSTURAL CONTROL		
VOICE		
PRAXIS		
❏ ejects Toothette ❏ voluntary imitated cough		
❏ voluntary swallow ❏ other tasks		
CONTROL OF ORAL SECRETIONS		
DROOLING		
POOLING IN MOUTH		
POOLING IN PHARYNX		
ORAL PREPARATORY PHASE SYMPTOMS		
SUCKLING		
SPOONED NONCHEWABLE SEMISOLID		
SPOONED NONCHEWABLE SOLID		
Smooth		
Textured		
MASTICATION & BITING		
CUP DRINKING		
STRAW DRINKING		
BEHAVIOR		
ORAL INITIATION PHASE SYMPTOMS		
MOUTH CLOSURE		
POSTERIOR CONTAINMENT		
BOLUS TRANSPORT		
❏ gagging ❏ piecemeal swallow		
PHARYNGEAL PHASE SYMPTOMS		
CONGESTION		
❏ wet vocal sounds ❏ wet breath sounds		
COUGHING		
❏ solids ❏ liquids		
MULTIPLE SWALLOWS		
RESPIRATION CHANGES		
	TOTAL SCORE	

Figure 3–2. *Continued*

Page 3 CLINICAL DYSPHAGIA EVALUATION – J.J. SHEPPARD

CONCLUSIONS

SUMMARY OF SWALLOW

ORAL PREPARATORY PHASE __________

ORAL INITIATION PHASE __________

PHARYNGEAL PHASE __________

RELATED DISORDER __________

SUBSYSTEM DYSFUNCTION

BODY POSTURAL CONTROL __________

❑ head/neck ❑ thorax __________

BREATH CONTROL & AIRWAY PATENCY __________

LIPS & CHEEKS __________

MANDIBLE __________

TONGUE __________

OTHER __________

ASSOCIATED FACTORS

NEUROMUSCULAR __________

PRAXIC __________

ANATOMICAL __________

PSYCHOSOCIAL __________

EXPERIENTIAL __________

STAGE OF DISORDER

I. NORMAL

Functioning WNL

II. MILD DYSPHAGIA

nourished with special dietary/medical management

III. MODERATE DYSPHAGIA

nourished with dietary management & adaptive strategies

IV. SEVERE DYSPHAGIA

inadequate nourishment and/or airway protection in spite of management

V. PROFOUND DYSPHAGIA

non-oral feeding is required

Figure 3–2. *Continued*

positioned them poorly, even when appropriate equipment was available. Growth problems in the children studied were associated with inadequate diets. Observation of the communicative interactions during mealtimes of poor feeders revealed differences from those experienced by normal controls (Mathisen et al., 1989). These results indicate that the caregiver has a significant effect on the outcome of the dysphagia program. In response to their needs, special programs for caregivers have been provided as an adjunct to their children's therapy program. These special programs include feeding support groups (Harris 1989) and supervised practice of the physical handling and social interactive aspects of feeding (Geertsma, Hyams, Pelletier, & Reiter, 1985; Morris, 1981). Consideration of the caregiver when developing a program maximizes the likelihood that the caregiver will be motivated and able to comply.

Treatment Approaches

The treatment program may include a combination of therapy approaches. "Oral motor" exercise approaches use sensory modalities, including massage, resistance to movement, muscle stretch, touch cues, assisted maintenance of body positions, and assisted movements to improve sensory tolerances and neuromotor competency (Alexander, 1987; Morris & Klein, 1987; Palmer & Horn, 1978). Behavioral approaches provide practice opportunities for task components of eating with selected reinforcements to increase the occurrence of desirable responses and decrease the occurrence of undesirable ones. In this approach, positive reinforcements and punishments may be used. In the compensatory approaches, strategies are sought which may improve function quickly by circumventing the physiological deficits or, when used in conjunction with oral motor or

behavioral approaches, by expediting functional improvements.

In the child with developmental disabilities, multiple stresses often affect swallowing and feeding behaviors. These may include medical, neuromotor, behavioral, developmental, and environmental issues that complicate management and slow resolution of feeding problems. An eclectic approach is often needed, one that incorporates oral motor, behavioral, and compensatory approaches (Morris, 1987; Sheppard, 1987).

Oral Motor Exercise

The aims of oral motor exercise in dysphagia therapy are to improve strength, stability, range of movements, and coordination in the structures used during eating. The motor subsystems of interest for swallow are those that control body posture for sitting, respiration, and pharyngeal-laryngeal, labio-buccal, mandibular, and lingual structures. The oral motor approach is used for infants and children who exhibit neuromuscular and praxic deficiencies that interfere with swallowing and with advancing feeding behaviors. There are two elements to the approach. First, routines that incorporate assisted and active oral and body movements and sensory stimulation are used prior to direct work on swallowing as "priming" (i.e., preparatory activities and exercises that facilitate more competent motor coordinations in the swallowing activities that follow). Second, hands-on assistance and touch cues are used during swallowing and feeding practice to facilitate the desired modifications in the movement patterns. When oral motor exercises are used with the NPO child, swallowing practice may be restricted to spontaneous swallows of the enhanced flow of saliva that has been stimulated by the exercise procedures or to swallows of small boluses (1 to 3 ml) of sterile liquid or clear juice as prescribed by the physician (see Table 3–6).

Table 3–6. Selected oral motor exercise strategies used for preparatory activities and swallowing practice.

Symptom	Preparatory ("priming") Strategies	Swallowing Practice Strategies
Impaired body postural control	Handling and gross motor exercise	Maintain desired postures with positioning equipment and assistance. Facilitate orienting movements for the approaching bolus.
Impaired breath control	Handling. Exercise for upper extremity support, and abdominal and thoracic mobility and/or stability.	Shoulder girdle stabilization with elbows on tray, controlled bolus size, and pacing bolus presentation.
Oral motor dysfunction	Resistance exercise for stability and mobility of oral and cervical structures. Oral manipulation of sham bolus.	Prescribed head and body postures. Assisted stabilization and movement of oral structures. Touch cues and resistance with spoon, cup, and nipple. Chewing and cup drinking practice.
Velopharyngeal and hyo-laryngeal dysfunction	Thermal stimulation. Exercise for cervical and mandibular stability and mobility.	Prescribed head and body postures. Cold formula and tart ices. Pacing. Tracheostomy speaking valve.

BODY POSTURAL CONTROL FOR EATING. It is easier to control food in the mouth, swallow, and self-feed when positioned with moderate flexion in upper and lower limbs, stable thorax, stable shoulder girdle, and head-neck posture that incorporates sufficient cervical extension to align cervical and thoracic vertebrae and sufficient flexion of the head on the neck to achieve a moderate chin tuck (i.e., capitol flexion). These postural elements enhance the ease of coordinating breathing and swallow, closing the mouth, maintaining tongue in the mouth, and executing the pharyngeal-laryngeal coordinations needed for swallowing (see Chapter 8).

Assisted body movement, assisted maintenance of postures, and gentle rocking, bouncing, and joint compression are used as the readiness exercises. Specific aims are "neck elongation" and chin tuck (Alexander, 1987; Morris & Klein, 1987); balanced muscle tone in trunk and limbs for sitting, or in young infants semireclining (Morris, 1987; Morris & Klein, 1987); and balanced muscle tone and stability in the shoulder girdle (Nelson & De Benabib, 1991).

These priming exercises are followed by eating practice. During this practice specially selected seating equipment and assistance facilitate the desired adjustments of body posture. Practice routines develop the needed stamina for maintaining the appropriate postural controls during eating. Stabilization in a well-fitted chair with hip belt, lateral trunk supports, cut-out tray, and foot rests, for example, may allow the child to practice swallowing more effectively and develop the tolerances needed to use these postures for mealtimes. The more involved child may need swaddling or hands-on assistance for head-neck stabilization or for steadying elbows on the tray (Bergen et al., 1990; Finnie, 1975; Morris & Klein, 1987).

BREATH CONTROL FOR SWALLOWING. The ability to coordinate breathing and swallowing is essential for airway protection during swallow (Groher, 1992; Logemann, 1983). In the normal adult swallow, the period of apnea between cessation of respiration and its resumption occurs primarily during the expiration cycle. In young, normal infants, these coordinations are not well developed (Bramford, Taciak, & Gewolb, 1992). In children with cerebral palsy, this coordination differs from that of normal children in duration and timing of cycles (Casas, Kenny, & McPherson, 1994; Kenny, Casas, & McPherson, 1989). Breath control issues arise most frequently during the transitions for advancing feeding behaviors. In infants, coordination of suckling, swallowing, and breathing may be a problem in advancing infants from tube to bottle feedings (Morris, 1989; Vandenberg, 1990). Clinical experience indicates that it may also be a problem when advancing from bottle to spoon feeding in children who have been maintained for prolonged developmental periods solely on bottle feeding.

Body movement, handling, and gross motor exercises are used in priming routines to improve the underlying competencies needed for breath control during swallow. These exercises promote balanced, appropriate, muscle tone in thorax, abdomen and pelvis; stability in the shoulder girdle; and ability to elevate and stabilize the rib cage. Following the exercises, the child is encouraged to practice the problematic eating task. Task difficulty is regulated to facilitate competent swallows. The child may be positioned, with swaddling or in appropriate sitting, to carry over the effects of priming and preliminary exercise for use in

swallowing food. Small boluses are offered using controlled flow nipples, such as the Haberman feeder, a pipette, spoon, or cup. Presentation is paced to encourage breath holding prior to swallow, resumption of breathing following swallowing, and return to basal breathing rate. The nipple may be withdrawn periodically to control suckling burst length and to prevent decompensation. An upright position with tongue ramped toward the lips is preferred to avoid inadvertent entry of the bolus into the pharynx before breath holding and to promote active propulsion of the bolus into the pharynx by the tongue.

ORAL COORDINATIONS FOR SWALLOWING. In the oral preparatory and oral initiation phases of swallow, lips, cheeks, mandible, and tongue receive the bolus into the mouth, contain, process, transport it, and, finally, propel it through the pharynx. The movements of these structures are guided by sensory information from the bolus. The strategies selected by the child to accomplish these tasks are learned (adaptive) behaviors that have resulted from the influences of the child's neuromotor, self-regulatory, and cognitive capabilities in combination with the caregiver's regulation of the child's eating experiences. Abnormal movement patterns, therefore, can express an amalgam of primary oral, sensory-motor, and structural deficiencies; learned, maladaptive patterns; and compensations for oral, pharyngeal, esophageal, gastrointestinal, pulmonary, or infectious conditions. Oral motor strategies are appropriate treatments for the sensory-motor and structural deficiencies and, in combination with behavioral strategies, may be used to modify learned, maladaptive movement patterns and sensory defensiveness.

The priming routines and preliminary exercises that have been recommended to improve desired oral movements and movement coordinations include massage; vibration; stroking; muscle stretch; pressures to muscle, tendons, and joints; resisted and assisted movement; and touch cues. The types and sites of stimulation are selected to improved the specific movement abnormalities that have been observed during reception, bolus formation, and initiating swallow for food or saliva. Stimulation may be varied with respect to duration, rhythm, speed, and intensity for specific effects on muscle and behaviors (Farber, 1982; Morris & Klein, 1987; Nelson & De Benabib, 1991; Palmer & Horn, 1978). Handling and positioning have been recommended to improve alignments of head, neck, and oral structures in preparation for eating (Alexander, 1987; Case-Smith, 1988; Morris & Klein, 1987) and thereby facilitate improved oral motor coordinations. Oral manipulation of a nonfood bolus, such as a Toothette or small toothbrush, can improve underlying competencies for bolus manipulation with only the additional stress on swallowing of the increased salivary flow.

During therapeutic practice of oral preparation for, and initiation of, swallow, the structures will respond to the movements of the bolus. Typical movement patterns in lips, tongue, and mandible are generated when a bolus is drawn by gravity toward the lips and has to be actively contained in the mouth and transported toward the pharynx. Positioning the child with tucked chin and face vertical or tipped forward has been observed to facilitate these more normal oral coordinations. (Morris & Klein, 1987; Sheppard, 1987).

The jaw mobilizes to open and close and stabilizes in open, intermediate, and closed positions variably during reception and oral transport of the bolus and during initiation of swallow for both solids and liquids (Stolovitz & Giesel, 1991). Strategies that have been recommended to improve these coordinations are applying pressure to chin (i.e., "jaw control") (Morris & Klein, 1987); touch cues with spoon, cup, or nipple (Shep-

(pard, 1987; Vandenberg, 1990); firm contacts of cup or spoon to dental arch with slow withdrawal of utensil to enhance stabilization ; and rapid, light contacts and rapid withdrawal to enhance mobilization of jaw (Sheppard, 1982, 1987). Chewing practice can be used in combination with resisted movement to enhance biting, masticatory force, and jaw protraction and retraction during opening and closing, respectively, and the lateral jaw movements that assist in transporting the bolus to the molar table as the jaw elevates (Sheppard, 1982; Sheppard & Mysak, 1984).

The muscles that control lip and cheek movement work together to mobilize these structures, to assist in opening and closing the mouth, and to control bolus movement into and out of the buccal cavities (Stolovitz & Gisel, 1991). The structures stabilize for reception of the bolus (sealing on nipple and cup or stripping food from spoon), for containment, and for directing the bolus onto the tongue. Strategies that have been observed to improve these functions are touch cues and firm contacts with nipple, cup, or spoon to gain lip opening, lip shaping to the contours of the utensil and lip closure; pressing the cheeks lightly against the dental arches during suckling; and stretching the cheeks with small chewable pieces as they are placed onto the molars for chewing (Sheppard, 1982).

The tongue changes its shape and its position relative to surrounding structures to receive, form, and transport the bolus into place for swallowing (Stolovitz & Gisel, 1991). It manipulates the bolus to mix it with saliva and, during chewing, coordinates with mandible and cheek to collect and reposition the bolus on the molar table for each masticatory cycle (Gisel, 1991). On initiation of swallow it propels the bolus through the pharynx and into the esophagus (Cerenko, McConnel, & Jackson, 1989). In the suckling infant, this is accomplished by an anterior-inferior displacement of the tongue base (Ardran, Kemp, & Lind, 1958). In mature swallow it is accomplished by posterior displacement of the tongue base to the pharyngeal wall (Groher, 1992; Logemann, 1983). Tongue movements, therefore, restrain the bolus from falling toward the lips, control the size of the bolus to be swallowed, and regulate the timing and force of its delivery into the pharynx. Head position, specifically position of the tongue surface with respect to gravity, influences the lingual movement patterns that will be used for oral transport and for propelling the bolus through the pharynx.

Priming strategies that have been observed, informally, to improve lingual coordinations for swallow are pressures to superior, inferior, lateral, and anterior tongue surfaces and tapping, stretch, vibration, and pressure to muscle surfaces in sublingual and submental areas. These strategies are used to elicit stabilization and movement against resistance, improve range of movement, and develop more precise coordinations (Farber, 1982; Morris & Klein, 1987; Nelson & De Benabib, 1991; Palmer & Horn, 1978).

During eating, head position is modified to increase anterior or posterior displacement of the tongue body as needed for controlling the bolus. The site of placement for spoon and cup, and the firmness of the contact between the utensil and the lips, mandible, and tongue as it enters and is withdrawn from the mouth are varied to facilitate tongue stabilization for reception of the bolus and appropriate movements for containing and transporting it into place for initiation of swallow (Morris & Klein, 1987; Sheppard, 1982). Chewing practice, in which the food is placed on the molar table or the side of the tongue, is used to increase the range of lateral tongue movements, its dexterity, and the ability to coordinate tongue and jaw movement (Morris & Klein, 1987; Sheppard, 1982). Strategies that have

been observed to improve tongue action for control of the bolus and its propulsion during oral initiation of swallow are increasing chin tuck, encouraging head turn to the side, and assistance in stabilizing the jaw in a closed position.

VELOPHARYNGEAL AND HYO-LARYNGEAL COORDINATIONS FOR SWALLOWING. Velopharyngeal closure, elevation of the hyoid and larynx, adduction of the vocal folds, and pharyngeal muscle contractions that shorten the pharynx during bolus transit and strip the residual bolus into the esophagus at the end of swallow are components of the pharyngeal phase of swallow. Adequate seal between the velum and the posterior pharynx prevents reflux of the bolus into the nasopharynx, an occurrence that disrupts feeding in infants (Plaxico & Loughlin, 1981) and makes eating more difficult in older children. Timely hyo-laryngeal elevation is a pivotal component of swallow that pulls open the cricopharyneal segment and holds it open for passage of the bolus into the esophagus. The upward and forward movements of these structures into position under the tongue base and inverted epiglottis, in combination with vocal fold adduction, guard the airway from bolus penetration and aspiration. Pharyngeal muscle contraction strips the residuals of the bolus into the esophagus. Priming exercises that promote head-neck and shoulder girdle stability, stabilize closure of the jaw, and facilitate capitol flexion provide appropriate stability and alignment in the structures that support velar elevation, displacement of the pharyngeal wall, and hyo-laryngeal elevation (Groher, 1992).

Priming exercises include stimulation of anterior faucial pillars with cold probe (i.e., "thermal stimulation") (Helfrich-Miller, Rector, & Straka, 1986; Lazzara, Lazarus, & Logemann, 1986; Logemann, 1993); use of muscle stretch, vibration, and massage in cervical and submental areas (Farber, 1982; Palmer and Horn, 1978); and assisted body movements and positioning (Alexander, 1987; Morris & Klein, 1987). Helfrich-Miller, Rector, & Straka (1986) found that a priming program that incorporated both thermal stimulation and oral motor exercise prior to eating improved airway protection for swallow in older developmentally disabled children and young adults.

During feeding the use of refrigerator-chilled formula has been observed to decrease aspiration in infants with bronchopulmonary disorders (Davis, Glass, Hayden, & Wolf, 1988). In adults with hemiparesis, maximum head rotation to the paretic side has been observed to increase both the percentage of bolus that is swallowed and the diameter of the upper esophageal sphincter during swallow (Ekberg, 1986). In children, the head rotation strategy has been informally observed to reduce pharyngeal phase symptoms. In addition, it may enhance stabilization of the head and neck in children with instability in neck and thorax .

Other strategies that have been informally observed to improve the pharyngeal swallow in children are: (1) positioning in more upright postures with face aligned vertically or tipped forward in order to enhance control of bolus for initiation of swallow; (2) increasing head-neck (capitol) flexion and assisting head-neck stabilization by resting a hand on the crown of the head in order to enhance stabilization of structures in the head and neck; (3) stroking the velum prior to offering a bolus in order to increase velar muscle tone and facilitate its elevation during swallowing (Farber, 1982); (4) stroking the laryngeal area and lightly resisting laryngeal elevation to enhance its upward movement during swallowing; and (5) regulating bolus size and viscosity to accommo-

date the specific symptoms (Ekberg, 1986; Kahrilas, Dodds, Dent, Logemann, & Shaker, 1988).

Compensations

Specially designed equipment and contrived feeding strategies are frequently used when immediate short-term assistance is needed to achieve functional oral feeding or when underlying competencies have been found, in the long-term, to be inadequate.

POSITIONING AND UTENSILS. Strategies related to positioning for feeding and special utensils are used most commonly to facilitate compensation. Infants with micrognathia and retrognathia have been observed to benefit from feeding in prone position (Lewis & Pashayan, 1980; Takagi & Bosma, 1960). Nasopharyngeal reflux has been observed to improve in infants with cleft palate or other palatal dysfunction when they are nippled in upright sitting position (Clarren, Anderson, & Wolf, 1987). Custom-designed adaptive seating devices have been found to reduce dribbling of liquid and solid foods and to facilitate advancing from bottle to cup and from puree to table food textures (Hulme, Shaver, Acher, Mullette, & Eggert, 1987). Specially designed nipples, bottles, and devices to assist the breast-feeding infant have been found to aid compensation for cleft palate in neonates (Clarren et al., 1987) and to improve feeding in neonates who are poor feeders, fretful, or experiencing strangling during feeding (Thornton, 1985). Specially designed spoons and cups and assistance, such as jaw control, have been observed to reduce dribbling and improve oral management of solid and liquid foods (Finnie, 1975; Morris & Klein, 1987).

PROSTHESES AND ORTHODONTIC APPLIANCES. Devices to compensate for palatal abnormalities have been used to improve feeding in neonates and young infants. Obduration of cleft palates in neonates achieved immediate normal feeding using standard nipples in 11 subjects and no delay, as compared to normal infants, in discharge from hospital (Markowitz, Gerry, & Fleishner, 1979). Selley and Boxall (1986) described the short-term use of a "palatal training appliance," a palatal plate with wire loop that, when adjusted, supports and stimulates the velum, in 12 babies who were experiencing sucking and swallowing difficulties and did not respond to other treatments. Improvement in function was seen in 1 to 3 weeks. Children with persistent drooling, swallowing, and chewing problems were seen to improve with orthodontic treatment that included use of palatal plates and orthodontic appliances in combination with oral motor approaches (Limbrock, Hoyer, & Scheying, 1990).

Behavioral Training and Motor Learning

Developmental eating behaviors are learned in a gradual process of modification and accommodation of existing patterns to environmental demands. For example, to master suckling the neonate learns to modify innate sensory-motor responses to accommodate the nipple size, shape, and firmness and the flow characteristics of the delivery system (Ingram, 1962; Mysak, 1980). As new feeding positions, new utensils, and new foods are introduced, new ingestion strategies are acquired. Illingworth and Lister (1964) found that unfamiliar eating tasks were tolerated and the skills were acquired without special difficulty when introduced during a sensitive period for acquisition of these skills.

Typically, the child with a developmental disability will experience some difficulty in acquisition of eating behaviors because of problems in the related domains of sensory-motor competency, psychosocial and regulatory behavior, and cognition. More practice time, carefully graded experiences, assis-

tance, and special motivators may be needed. Special medical problems and atypical experiences may exacerbate these difficulties, however, and complicate management. For example, the typical flow of experiences may have been disrupted, thereby delaying a child's experience with all or some eating skills beyond the sensitive period. The child's learning experience may have been atypical, or compensations may have been needed. The resulting skills may, therefore, contain maladaptive patterns, that is, habitual movement strategies that interfere with refinement of the existing skill or with advancing to more mature behaviors. Furthermore, the child may have experienced uncomfortable or frightening events which have been associated with swallowing or eating and resulted in traumatically conditioned dysphagia. The primary problem may have improved or resolved, but the conditioned expectation, and associated fear, remain to interfere with eating (Di Scipio, et al., 1978; Di Scipio & Kaslon, 1982). Children who are deprived of appropriate and timely experience or who experience traumatically conditioned dysphagia will need special training to acquire mature eating behaviors. These problems may present as sensory defensiveness, that is, intolerance of the sensory experiences associated with learning more advanced eating skills or, in the NPO child, with difficulty advancing to oral feeding. Or they may present as a phobia-like condition in which fear of eating is the primary manifestation. In these children, introduction of the eating task may be associated with decompensation, gagging, food refusal, and consequent failure to master the needed skills. Behavioral therapy (Kaplan & Sadock, 1988) and motor learning theory (Singer, 1972) provide the theoretical framework for programs that promote acquisition of mature behaviors in these children. Because developmental and behavioral problems frequently co-occur with anatomic, neuromotor, and medical problems in developmentally disabled children, behavioral approaches are most often used in combination with oral motor, compensatory, and medical treatments.

ORAL-FACIAL DESENSITIZATION. As with oral motor approaches, priming or readiness activities may be used to prepare the child for practicing target eating behaviors. To improve the child's tolerance of novel sensory arrays (Morris, 1987) and to modify the child's state for improved learning (Nelson & De Benabib, 1991), facial and oral areas may be stroked, massaged, and otherwise stimulated with toys (Alexander, 1987; Jones, 1989; Morris, 1985, 1987; Simon & Handler, 1981). The stimuli are graded to avoid decompensation. The child may be encouraged to use his or her mouth to explore objects and to explore their mouth with fingers (Morris & Klein, 1987).

TOLERANCE FOR THE EATING EXPERIENCE. Tolerance for the sensory arrays that are associated with specific eating behaviors can be encouraged during eating practice. Typically, as infants develop they acquire tolerances for the interactive social and communicative routines associated with eating (Stroh, Robinson, & Stroh, 1986); for modification of body position from reclining to sitting; for advancing from nipple to spoon to cup; for advancing from baby foods and formula to table food tastes, textures, and viscosities; and for advancing from dependent feeding to the synchronous hand-mouth activity required for self-feeding. When behavioral problems are associated with eating, it may be necessary to grade practice tasks by gradually modifying only one of these variables at a time (Palmer & Horn, 1978).

AUDITORY AND COMMUNICATION ENVIRONMENTS. The auditory environment associated with eating has been discussed by Morris (1981), Morris and Klein (1987), and Geertsma et al. (1985) as a modality for modifying behavior. They recommend musical

selections that facilitate the desired modification in the child's state prior to and during feeding practice and a communicative environment that enhances social experience and permits the child to express immediate needs and wants without decompensating.

ADVANCING EATING BEHAVIORS. Behavioral management programs for advancing eating behaviors in children with developmental disabilities have been used to facilitate acquisition of more mature eating skills, to increase food intake, and to facilitate the transition from tube to oral feeding. Programs have been reported that rely on positive reinforcements for incremental mastery of components of the target tasks (De Scipio et al., 1978; Palmer & Horn, 1978; Palmer, Thompson, & Linscheid, 1975; Simon & Handler, 1981); include both positive reinforcements and "time out" for failing to comply (Handon, Mandell, & Russo, 1986; Larson, Ayllon, & Barrett, 1987); and take a more forceful approach that may include elements of forced feeding (Blackman & Nelson, 1987; Imhoff & Wiggington, 1991; Pipes & Holm, 1980).

Advancing eating behaviors in children who are older than 1 year involves training the components of the behaviors. For example, to master cup drinking a child first must learn to stabilize lip and jaw on the undersurface of the cup and close his or her mouth as the cup is withdrawn. Sipping, and sequential sipping and swallowing on a single breath, must be mastered. The final step is learning to pause to take a breath and, with cup and liquid still in the mouth, resume the sequential sip-swallow. The child with a developmental disability learns these skills through a slow process of trial, error correction, and habituation instead of the apparently effortless acquisition experienced by normal children who have enjoyed a timely and typical introduction to eating behaviors. The general principles for training motor skills have been observed to apply to acquisition of eating skills by children with developmental disabilities. Mastery depends on experiencing a sufficient number of practice trials, receiving feedback on trial adequacy, having opportunities for error correction , motivation , and task modifications that facilitate learning (Singer, 1972).

Table 3–7 describes the developmental sequence experienced by the normal child as eating skills are advanced during the first year of life. Although the child engages in all of these activities within the first year, the quality of performance continues to im-

prove in the second and third years. Further refinements of eating skills are apparent as the child ages and masters more complex eating tasks.

Table 3–8 describes the progression of food textures and viscosities experienced by the normal child. With the exception of the final level, regular diet, all food types are introduced gradually during the first year. Firm, fibrous foods which are harder to chew and form higher viscosity boluses typically are introduced gradually, at older ages.

Table 3–7. Sequences for advancing developmental eating behaviors.

Optimal Posture[1]	Eating Skill and Food Examples
Semi-reclining in arms	Suckling. Liquids as prescribed by physician. Dependent feeding.
Semi-reclining in infant seat/ in arms	Spoon feeding smooth, semisolids (infant cereals, fruit purees, etc.) as prescribed by physician. Dependent feeding.
Infant seat at highest setting or supported upright in high chair	Tolerating texture. Textured nonchewable food (solids)—cottage cheese, pastina, mashed ripe banana. Dependent feeding. Self-feeding during suckling and biting. Bottle fed liquids with or without bottle straw and teething biscuits.
Upright sitting in high chair	Biting and chewing single pieces. Soft chewable food—soft moist cookies, followed by soft fresh or canned fruits (e.g., banana, peach, pear) and soft cooked vegetables without skins (e.g., carrots, potatoes). Dependent feeding. Cup drinking. Thick liquids fed from cup—fruit nectars, milk shakes, liquid yogurts, followed by introduction of thin juices, milk, and water Dependent feeding. Spoon feeding chewable foods. Soft foods that form cohesive, chewed bolus—macaroni, poultry, fish, meatloaf, soft cooked vegetables, soft canned or fresh fruit. Self finger feeding. Soft chewable foods—soft cookies and pieces of cold cereal followed by bite-sized pieces of soft vegetables, fruit, or meat, followed by sandwiches with soft fillings that form cohesive bolus when chewed.
Upright sitting in high chair, booster seat, or toddler chair	Self cup feeding. Thicker liquids as preferred, followed by thin liquids. Self spoon/fork feeding. Nonchewable foods followed by soft chewable foods, followed by chewable mixtures. Straw drinking. Liquids as preferred.

[1]These are necessary conditions for learning the skill with normal movement patterns.

Table 3–8. Progression of food texture and viscosity for advancing eating behaviors in children.

Food Type	Examples
Thick liquids: Suspended sediment, slower, more cohesive flow.	Fruit nectars, liquid yogurt.
Thin liquids: Clear, faster, less cohesive flow.	Water, clear juices.
Puree food: Smooth texture. Progress from semisolid to solid viscosity.	Jarred baby food, strained food, yogurt, pudding.
Fine chopped/ground food: Grainy textured solids in a creamy sauce. Lower viscosity than mashed food.	Foods processed in blender, stage 2 jarred food.
Mashed food: Mechanically soft foods, fork mashed to a rice-textured, cohesive, moist mass.	Cottage cheese, mashed banana, tuna fish and egg salads.
Mechanically soft chewable food: Easily chewed food, forms a cohesive, higher viscosity bolus during chewing.	Cooked vegetables, fish, poultry, pancakes, soft and cooked fruit.
Unrestricted diet: Soft and firm chewable foods that may be crumbly and/or high viscosity when chewed.	Fibrous meats, raw vegetables, crisp fruits and nuts.

Table 3–9 describes procedures for advancing the child with developmental disability and dysphagia who has demonstrated adequate swallow for maintenance of nutritional needs and airway protection. The developmental sequence begins with bottle feeding and ends with self-feeding using utensils. Before attempting to advance to a higher level, the child should demonstrate consistent, compliant performance at the current level of achievement and generalization at that level to a variety of foods and feeding environments. Before advancing to self-feeding, the child should have demonstrated an acceptable level of competency during dependent feeding for oral management of the food type that is to be self-fed.

Advancing feeding skills of a child with a disability requires both strategies that facilitate more adequate body postural control and oral management for feeding and behavioral strategies for facilitating learning. The treatment options in Table 3–9 include both. Table 3–10 presents some general rules for facilitating learning.

Table 3–9. Procedures for advancing feeding in the developmentally disabled child with dysphagia.

Symptom	Treatment Strategies and Sequences
Failure to advance to bottle feeding	Adaptive positioning. Non-nutritive sucking with pacifier that is same shape as bottle nipple. Pacifier dipped in formula offered prior to bottle. Use nipple with regulated low flow. Withdraw nipple to regulate duration of suckling burst and swallowing sequence.
Failure to advance from bottle to spoon feeding	Position in upright posture with vertical face alignment. Support as needed for thoracic, shoulder, and cervical stabilization. Use infant or toddler size spoon. Offer small boluses (one half spoonful) and small amounts. Spoon feed when child is not very hungry (i.e., snack time or middle to end of meal). Give same food daily for at least 1 week before introducing next new food. Increase bolus size and amount offered gradually, as accepted. Offer habituated foods as part of mealtime diet to maintain acceptance.
Failure to advance from puree to nonchewable solid	Position in upright sitting with elbows on tray to support upper body and face vertical or tipped forward. Increase viscosity of preferred purees with baby cereal or graham cracker crumbs. Introduce pureed semi-solid table foods. Introduce mashed moist transition foods. Follow procedures outlined above under "spoon feeding" for introducing new foods.
Failure to advance from bottle to cup	Position in upright sitting with face vertical or tipped forward. Use open cup with cut out rim to improve control for placement in mouth and dispensing. Introduce thickened liquids before introducing thin liquids. Introduce preferred liquid tastes first.
Failure to advance from mashed to chewable food	Adjust sitting position as above for advancing from puree to nonchewable solid. Introduce crisp soft chewable by finger feeding small pieces to side of mouth. Introduce crisp soft chewable by spoon placed toward side of mouth. Begin with single piece. Introduce soft chewable by finger followed by spoon as above. Introduce complex spooned soft chewable bolus. Introduce firm chewable finger food. Introduce firm chewable food by finger, followed by spoon as above.

(continued)

Table 3–9. *(continued)*

Symptom	Treatment Strategies and Sequences
Failure to advance from dependent to self-feeding	Adjust sitting position as above for advancing from puree to nonchewable solid. Encourage finger feeding of teething biscuit and holding own bottle (use bottle straw if needed). Encourage finger feeding of bite sized pieces and cookies if child can chew. Encourage holding cup to assist during drinking. Select toddler-sized utensil with built-up handle. Encourage holding spoon during dependent feeding. Select smoother textured, nonchewable, preferred foods for self-feeding. Encourage self-feeding at snack or end of meal. Guide hand movements to assist as needed to get food onto spoon and into mouth. Provide daily practice with same or similar foods.

Table 3–10. General rules for advancing feeding skills in infants and young children.

1. Maintain child in an alert, quiet state. Avoid attempting the practice task when child is in a somnolent or agitated state.

2. Practice with new foods and procedures when child is not very hungry. Snack time or midway through a meal is best.

3. Provide daily experience with the practice task. Practice for 10 minutes or less if child is resistant.

4. Introduce only one new item each week. If there is resistance, gradually change the characteristics of the foods within the week.

5. Begin with small amounts of food to avoid decompensation. Offer small boluses and be ready with the next bolus as soon as the child has swallowed the previous one.

6. Praise each acceptance, even if it does not end in swallowing the food. Gradually shape the total behavior to include swallowing.

7. Provide feeding assistance when introducing new food.

8. End practice on a successful trial. Do not push the child to the limit of his or her tolerance.

9. Finish each practice session with preferred food as reward.

10. The child should demonstrate tolerance for the task and moderate competency during practice before incorporating the step into mealtimes and beginning the next level of practice.

A child who becomes ill or experiences distress in a newly acquired behavior can be expected to regress to a lower level of performance. When the illness or distress is severe or prolonged and the behaviors are poorly established, the child may be resistant to returning to the prior performance level. As a general rule, it is easier to regain a behavior than to learn it for the first time. In the child with developmental disability and dysphagia, however, it will usually require retraining.

Transitions from Tube to Oral Feeding

Children with developmental disabilities and dysphagia experience special difficulties in transition from tube to oral feedings. Bazyk (1990) found that the duration of the transition from tube to oral feeding in a randomly selected group of children who were fed by nasogastric tube prior to 1 year old was related to the number of medical complications experienced by the child. There were positive correlations between the number of days until oral feeding was achieved and the number of digestive, respiratory, and cardiac complications. "Good feeders" transitioned in 2 to 58 days (Mean, 11.59). Children with special difficulties, six "poor feeders" in the Bazyk study, a child on hyperalimentation because of ilea atresia and complications (Geertsma et al., 1985), and three children with fetal alcohol syndrome (Van Dyke, Mackay, & Ziaylek, 1982) were reported to take from 6 to 36 months to achieve the transition, and, in four cases, failed to achieve oral feeding (Bazyk, 1990).

Preparing the Child for Transition

The child's readiness for implementing the transition is determined initially by examination of adequacy of swallow. Adequate pharyngeal competency for airway protection and esophageal and gastroesophageal competency for ingestion of a mealtime bolus are needed (Bryan et al., 1989). To facilitate a prompt transition, treatment to prevent and mitigate iatrogenic problems may be initiated at the onset of tube feeding (Geertsma et al., 1985; Morris, 1989; Van Dyke et al., 1982). Early experiences with oral tactile stimulation, tastes, smells (Geertsma et al., 1985; Morris, 1989), and non-nutritive suckling during tube feedings (Schwartz, Moody, Yarandi, & Anderson, 1987) have been observed to have a positive effect on later transition to oral feedings. A program that focuses on developing oral, sensory tolerances, oral exploration of non-food objects, and stimulation of variety of oral movements may precede the introduction of feeding by several months (Geertsma et al., 1985; Morris, 1989; Vandenberg, 1990; Van Dyke et al., 1982). If the swallowing reflex is considered to be inadequate for secretions or for oral feeding, exercises that increase the frequency of swallow have been observed to improve competency. These exercises include oral stimulation routines, thermal stimulation, and introduction of 1 ml boluses of clear liquid into the mouth to elicit swallows (see Table 3–11).

Implementing the Transition

Transition to oral feeding may be facilitated by assigning one primary caregiver to implement the program, avoiding invasive oral procedures (Geertsma et al., 1985), and modifying tube feeding schedules to promote mealtime hunger-satisfaction cycles (Dowling, 1972; Morris, 1989; Vandenberg, 1990). During the transition food tastes are associated with satiation of hunger by offering small amounts for swallowing during tube feedings (Van Dyke et al., 1982). Readiness activities prior to feeding include assisted movement and positioning to improve muscle tone for body postural control (Case-Smith, 1988; Morris, 1989), gentle

Table 3–11. Selected strategies for improving oral prefeeding skills in the NPO child.

Diagnosis	Skill	Practice Activity
Esophageal atresia	Oral management of liquid and puree semisolid	Sham feeding.
Oral-pharyngeal, neurogenic dysphagia	Tolerance of smells and tastes	Kitchen and mealtime exposure to smells and 1 ml bolus tastes.
	Oral bolus manipulation	Ejecting, holding and moving a Toothette, or other absorbent, tethered bolus.
	Increased frequency of swallow	Thermal stimulation. Oral manipulation of nonabsorbent bolus. Tasting bolus from pacifier, toothbrush, or play object.
	Tolerance for sitting, utensils and meal routines	Kitchen and mealtime experiences without eating.
	Improving oral and pharyngeal reactivity	Oral and pharyngeal stimulation and resistance exercise.
Traumatically conditioned dysphagia	Establish mealtime hunger-satiation cycles Increase intake of preferred foods	Adjust tube feeding schedule. Establish routine feeding sessions of preferred foods, using preferred utensils and feeding mode on a meal time schedule prior to tube feeding. Increase intake with preferred foods. Introduce new foods with similar viscosity, consistency and taste (see Table 3–10). As intake increases decrease tube feeding by 25% of total calorie needs in four stages. Expand the variety of foods tolerated and advance skills once tube feeding is discontinued.

stroking in the oral-facial area, and encouragement of mouthing of soft rubber objects to improve adaptive responses to oral sensory experiences (Geertsma et al., 1985; Morris, 1989; Van Dyke et al., 1982; Vandenberg, 1990). If the infant is fed by nasogastric tube, frequent removal of the tube for oral feedings has been suggested (Van Dyke et al., 1982; Vandenberg, 1990). Drops of food may be offered from finger, pacifier, or Nuk-type stimulators prior to nippling or spooning (Morris, 1989; Vandenberg, 1990). Geertsma and colleagues (1985), Morris (1989), and Vandenberg (1990) emphasize the importance of maintaining social verbal stimulation as a positive reinforcement during the therapeutic feedings and of responding to the child's communicative signals. Care should be taken to provide a comfortable environment for the feedings. Morris (1989) suggests the use of music as an aid to maintaining appropriate state. The child's preferred foods and utensils are used during the transition. For example, Geertsma et al., (1985) and

Van Dyke et al., (1982) describe cases in which the transition was accomplished with cup and spoon, rather than nipple, and chopped, rather than pureed solids. The duration of the feeding and the amount of food should be increased gradually as tolerated by the child. Reductions in tube feeding should be regulated to maintain nutrition while advancing oral feeding (see Table 3–11). Vandenberg (1990) emphasizes that feeding sessions should end before the child decompensates.

In contrast to the strategies reviewed above, a program in which a force feeding approach was the primary therapy component was reported by Blackman and Nelson (1987). Eleven children, eight of whom were developmentally disabled, were hospitalized for 2 to 3 weeks for the purpose of inducing oral feeding. During the hospitalization, the children were fed frequently by staff and parents. At discharge 20 of the 11 patients had advanced to oral feeding. Following discharge, however, two patients suffered serious consequences of aspiration, and oral feeding was discontinued. This program for rapid induction of oral feeding through forced feedings is controversial because of the short- and long-term risks of aspiration and the potential long-term psychological effects on the child and parents. From a motor learning perspective the approach does not allow sufficient time for acquisition, habituation, and generalization of the skills needed for long-term successful oral feeding.

It is generally agreed that the most efficient approaches to this problem are to prevent aversion to oral feeding through earlier attention to the emerging psychological effects of deprivation of oral feeding and to introduce prefeeding activities that will permit acquisition of subskills needed for oral feeding. Failing that, approaches that shape appropriate behaviors during feeding through positive reinforcements, state management, and environments that facilitate motor learning are more generally accepted.

Chronic Illness and Dysphagia

A dysphagia program for the child who is chronically ill and disabled differs from one for the child who is healthy and disabled. The chronically ill child experiences exacerbations and remissions of the systemic illness and associated variations in swallowing competency. The program should be flexible with regard to both the schedule of family contact and the goals of the program. The more severely involved child may regress periodically to tube feeding, whereas the child with more competent swallow may regress to restricted food tolerances and need for special feeding techniques. Overall, the goals are to minimize the effect of the fluctuating feeding disorder on parent-child bonding; to assist the parent with feeding strategies that will maintain nutrition and minimize the risk of feeding-related aspiration while encouraging oral feeding whenever possible; to promote acquisition and habituation of oral feeding skills; and to minimize the conditioned aversions to feeding that may result from medical procedures, fatigue, pain, or difficulty with airway protection that have been associated with swallowing (Pressman & Morrison, 1988; Sheppard & Pressman, 1988). Therapeutic strategies include positioning and handling to promote comfortable stable postures; oral sensory experiences during play using toys and swabs that provide a variety of flavors, shapes, and textures; use of pacifier; therapeutic oral feedings of small amounts of preferred foods offered from preferred utensils; analgesics prior to feedings to reduce discomfort (Sheppard & Pressman, 1988); regulation of diet to avoid foods that will cause discomfort; and introduction of new food textures and utensils in therapeutic feedings before they are incorporated into mealtimes (Pressman & Morrison, 1988).

Daily Management of Mealtimes and Ingestion of Oral Medications

The purpose of the daily management program is to facilitate optimum swallow for nutrition, hydration, and oral medications by manipulating the variables that affect adequacy of swallow. These are body posture, bolus characteristics, utensils, bolus presentation, and environmental stresses. Medication preparations are restricted for ease of swallow (Sheppard, 1991). The most commonly used mealtime interventions are appropriate seating, special utensils, and diet restriction for food viscosity and texture (Sheppard, Liou, Hochman, Laroia, & Langlois, 1988). In children with more severe problems, adaptive feeding strategies may

be needed. These may include assistance for maintaining appropriate body postures; restrictions for bolus size and for pacing bolus presentation; and prescribed strategies for placing utensils in, and withdrawing them from, the mouth. Strategies that assist pharyngeal phase swallow may be needed. These include special postures, such as head rotation, chin tuck, and chin down and use of liquid washdown to relieve bolus stasis. Reducing environmental stresses by providing a familiar feeder, moderating noise and distraction, providing music and a communicative environment that allows the child to make known needs and wants, and social verbal reinforcements have been observed to be helpful (Geertsma et al., 1985; Morris, 1981). Oral hygiene following the meal to remove food residuals and maintenance of upright postures to reduce the likelihood of vomiting may also be prescribed (see Table 3–12).

Table 3–12. Components of the mealtime prescription.

Prescription Component	Examples
Environmental restrictions and structure	Low noise level, reduced visual distraction, and familiar music.
Positioning	Chair, adaptive supports, and assistance.
Diet viscosities and textures	Pureed or mashed foods, thickened liquids, and crisp finger foods.
Adaptive utensils	Controlled flow nipples, bottle straw, cut out cup, and shallow bowled spoon.
Feeding techniques	Slow pace, half teaspoon bolus size, spooned liquids, and food placement on tongue body.
Communications strategies	Special signals for child's regulation of feeding speed, food choice, and so on.
	Caregiver response mode and social verbal stimulation.
Behavior management	Praise. Time out. Behavior modification. Preferred food as positive reinforcement.
After meal care	Positioning and oral hygiene. Nonfood rewards.

Drooling in the Child with Dysphagia

Drooling may result from failure in one or more of the component functions involved in control of oral secretions. These failures may result from pharyngeal hyporeflexia; neuromuscular involvement of oral structures and body postural control, especially that of head and neck; oral sensory deficits; and impaired praxis (Blasco & Alaire, 1992; Brodsky, 1992). Related problems that have been associated with drooling are dental caries, gingival infections, malocclusions, side effects of medications, and upper airway obstruction (Brodsky, 1992). Degree of disorder varies from mild, with wetness only on lips, to profuse, with clothing, hands, and objects wet (Crysdale & White, 1989). The full range of treatment options includes medical and dental treatments, oral motor and body postural exercises, behavioral programs, pharmacologic therapy, and surgery (Blasco & Alaire, 1992; Brodsky, 1992).

Appropriate treatment depends on identification of specific contributing causes and the specific component deficits. Figure 3–3 describes a hierarchial treatment plan that addresses the motor issues. Management of related medical and dental issues to the fullest possible extent simplifies the problem of improving the motor competencies needed for control of secretions. Motor control, issues should be addressed in sequence. Oral-pharyngeal reflex reactivity is primary, followed by oral neuromuscular and body postural control, oral sensory deficits, oral motor organization and planning skills (praxis), and finally behavioral issues of habituation. Treatment strategies include enhanced sensory inputs during practice; resisted and assisted movements to improve mobility in cheeks, tongue, mandible, and lips and facilitate maintenance of closed mouth postures; oral motor exercise to enhance coordination of oral structures for containing, transporting, and forming the saliva bolus; and behavioral programs that incorporate feedback and feed forward cuing to habituate control.

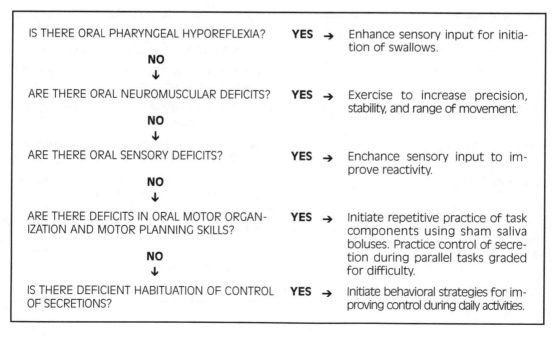

Figure 3–3. Decision tree for treating persistent drooling.

Summary

In developmentally disabled infants and children, the multiple primary and secondary causes of dysphagia complicate its management. The clinical dysphagia evaluation is administered to determine the specific oral, neuromotor, and anatomical causes, the secondary developmental and behavioral issues, and the co-occurring medical and dental issues that may be contributing to the problem. With this information, referrals can be made for further diagnostic testing and interdisciplinary management, and a symptom-specific treatment plan can be developed.

The clinical treatment program includes training and support for the caregiver, therapy for the child to improve swallowing and feeding competencies, and management strategies to meet immediate needs for oral nourishment and ingestion of oral medications. If control of oral secretions is impaired, the program may include oral motor exercises and behavioral strategies to improve underlying motor competencies and increase the frequency and effectiveness of swallow for saliva. Optimally, clinical management of dysphagia should begin with the onset of symptoms. Oral motor exercise, behavioral training, and compensatory strategies can then be administered as needed over time to minimize disruption of development and facilitate achievement of the child's potential feeding and swallowing competencies.

References

Alexander, R. (1987). Oral-motor treatment for infants and young children with cerebral palsy. *Seminars in Speech and Language, 8,* 87–100.

Als, H., Lester, B. M., Tronick, E. Z., & Brazelton, T. B. (1982). Towards a research instrument for the assessment of preterm infants' behavior (APIB): and Manual for the assessment of preterm infants' behavior (APIB). In H. E. Fitzgerald, B. M. Lester, & M. W. Yogman (Eds.), *Theory and Research in Behavioral Pediatrics Vol. 1,* (pp. 35–63). New York: Plenum Press.

Ardran, G. M., Kemp, F. H., & Lind, D. (1958). A cineradiographic study of bottle feeding. *British Journal of Radiology, 31,* 11–22.

Arvedson, J. C., Brodsky, L. (Eds.). (1992) *Pediatric feeding and swallowing disorders: Assessment and management.* San Diego: Singular Publishing Group.

Barnard, K. E. (1981). An ecological approach to parent-child relations. In C. C. Brown (Ed.), *Infants at-risk: Assessment and intervention* (pp. 89–95). New Brunswick, NJ: Johnson & Johnson Baby Products.

Bazyk, S. (1990). Factors associated with the transition to oral feeding in infants fed by nasogastric tubes. *American Journal of Occupational Therapy, 44,* 1070–1078.

Bergen, A. F., Presperin, J., & Tallman, T. (1990). *Positioning for function: Wheelchairs and other assistive technologies.* Valhalla, NY: Valhalla Rehabilitation Publications.

Blackman, J. A., & Nelson, C. L. A. (1987). Rapid induction of oral feedings to tube-fed patients. *Developmental and Behavioral Pediatrics, 8,* 63–67.

Blasco, P. A., Allaire, J. H., and participants of the Consortium on Drooling. (1992). Drooling in the developmentally disabled: Management practices and recommendations. *Developmental Medicine Child Neurology, 34,* 849–862.

Bonanno, P. C. (1971). Swallowing dysfunction after tracheostomy. *Annals of Surgery, 174,* 29–33.

Bramford, O., Taciak, V., & Gewold, I. H. (1992). The relationship between rhythmic swallowing and breathing during suckle feeding in term neonates. *Pediatric Research, 31,* 619–624.

Braun, M. A., & Palmer, M. M. (1985–1986, Winter). A pilot study of oral motor dysfunction in "at-risk" infants. *Physical and Occupational Therapy in Pediatrics, 5,* 13–25.

Brazelton, T. B. (1973). Neonatal Behavioral Assessment Scale. *Clinics in Developmental Medicine* (No. 50). Philadelphia: J. B. Lippincott.

Brodsky, L. (1992). Drooling in children. In J. C. Arvedson, & L. Brodsky (Eds.), *Pediatric feeding and swallowing disorders: Assessment and management* (pp. 389–416). San Diego: Singular Publishing Group.

Bryan, D. W., McLoughlin, L., Pressman, H., & Sheppard, J. J. (1989, October). *A medical model for managing complex dyspha-*

gia in the developmentally disabled. Workshop presented at the annual conference of the American Academy of Cerebral Palsy and Developmental Medicine, San Francisco, CA.

Cameron, J. L., Reynolds, J., & Zuidema, G. D. (1973). Aspiration in patients with tracheostomies. *Surgery, Gynecology and Obstetrics, 136*, 68–70.

Casas, M. J., Kenny, D. J., & McPherson, K. A. (1994). Swallowing/ventilation interactions during oral swallow in normal children and children with cerebral palsy. *Dysphagia, 9*, 40–46.

Case-Smith , J. (1988). An efficacy study of occupational therapy with high-risk neonates. *American Journal of Occupational Therapy, 42*, 499–506.

Cerenko, D., McConnel, F. M. S., & Jackson, R. T. (1989). Quantitative assessment of pharyngeal bolus driving forces. *Otolaryngology — Head and Neck Surgery, 100*, 57–63.

Christensen, J. R. (1989). Developmental approach to pediatric neurogenic dysphagia. *Dysphagia, 3*, 131–134.

Clarren, S. K., Anderson, B., & Wolf, L. S. (1987). Feeding infants with cleft lip, cleft palate or cleft lip and palate. *Cleft Palate Journal, 24*, 244–249.

Cooper, P. J., & Stein, A. (Eds.). (1992). *Feeding problems and eating disorders in children and adolescents*. Chur, England: Harwood.

Crysdale, W. S., & White, A. (1989). Submandibular duct relocation for drooling: A 10-year experience with 194 patients. *Otolaryngology—Head and Neck Surgery, 101*, 87–92.

Davis, N., Glass, R. P., Hayden, P., & Wolf, L. S. (1988, October). *Diagnostic and treatment challenges: Infants with complex feeding, swallowing, breathing disorders*. Workshop presented at the meeting of the American Academy of Cerebral Palsy and Developmental Medicine, Toronto.

Di Scipio, W. J., & Kaslon, K. (1982). Conditioned dysphagia in cleft palate children after pharyngeal flap surgery. *Psychosomatic Medicine, 44*, 247–257.

Di Scipio, W. J., Kaslon, K., & Ruben R. J. (1978). Traumatically acquired conditioned dysphagia in children. *Annals of Otology, 87*, 509–514.

Dowling, S. (1972). Seven infants with esophageal atresia: A developmental study. *Psychoanalytic Study of the Child, 27*, 215–256.

Ekberg, O. (1986). Posture of the head and pharyngeal swallowing. *Acta Radiologica Diagnosis, 27* (Fasc. 6). 691–696.

Farber, S. D. (1982). *Neurorehabilitation: A multisensory approach*. Philadelphia: W. B. Saunders.

Finnie, N. R. (1975). *Handling the young cerebral palsied child at home*. New York: E. P. Dutton.

Geertsma, M. A., Hyams, J. S., Pelletier, J. M., & Reiter, S. (1985). Feeding resistance after parenteral hyperalimentation,. *American Journal of Diseases of Children, 139*, 255–256.

Gisel, E. G. (1991). Effect of food texture on the development of chewing of children between six months and two years of age. *Developmental Medicine and Child Neurology, 33*, 69–79.

Griggs, C. A., Jones, P. M., & Lee, R. E. (1989). Videofluoroscopic investigation of feeding disorders of children with multiple handicap. *Developmental Medicine and Child Neurology, 31*, 303–308.

Groher, M. E. (1992). *Dysphagia diagnosis and management* (2nd ed.). Boston: Butterworth.

Haberman, M. (1988). A mother of intervention. *Nursing Times, 84*, 52–53.

Handon, B. L., Mandell, F., & Russo, D. C. (1986). Feeding induction in children who refuse to eat. *American Journal of Diseases of Children, 140*, 52–54.

Harris, L. I. (1989, April). The effectiveness of a feeding support group as an adjunct to other therapies in an early intervention program. *Zero to Three*, pp. 2, 13–15.

Helfrich-Miller, K. R., Rector, K. L., & Straka, J. A. (1986). Dysphagia: Its treatment in the profoundly retarded patient with cerebral palsy. *Archives of Physical Medicine and Rehabilitation, 67*, 520–525.

Heyman, S., & Respondek, M. (1989). Detection of pulmonary aspiration in children by radionuclide "salivagram". *Journal of Nuclear Medicine, 30*, 697–699.

Hulme, J. B., Shaver, J., Archer, S., Mullette, L., & Eggert, C. (1987). Effects of adaptive seating devices on the eating and drinking of children with multiple handicaps. *American Journal of Occupational Therapy*, *41*, 81–89.

Illingworth, R. S., & Lister, J. (1964). The critical or sensitive period, with special reference to certain feeding problems in infants and children. *Pediatrics*, 65, 839–848.

Imhoff, S. M., & Wigginton, V. M. (1991). Identifying feeding and swallowing problems in infants and young children. *Clinics in Communication Disorders*, *1*, 59–67.

Ingram, T. T. S. (1962). Clinical significance of infantile feeding reflexes. *Developmental Medicine and Child Neurology*, *4*, 159–169.

Jelm, J. M. (1990). *Oral-motor/Feeding Rating Scale*. Tucson, AZ: Therapy Skill Builders.

Jones, P. M. (1989). Feeding disorders in children with multiple handicaps. *Developmental Medicine and Child Neurology*, *31*, 404–406.

Kahrilas, P. J., Dodds, W. J., Dent, J., Logemann, J. A., & Shaker, R. (1988). Upper esophageal sphincter function during deglutition. *Gastroenterology*, *95*, 52–62.

Kaplan, H. I., & Sadock, B. J. (1988). *Synopsis of psychiatry, behavioral sciences, clinical psychiatry* (5th ed.). Baltimore: Williams & Wilkins.

Kenny, D. J., Casas, M. J., & McPherson, K. A. (1989). Correlation of ultrasound imaging of oral swallow with ventilatory alterations in cerebral palsied and normal children: Preliminary observations. *Dysphagia*, *4*, 112–117.

Lazzara, G., Lazarus, C., & Logemann, J. A. (1986). Impact of thermal stimulation on the triggering of the pharyngeal swallow. *Dysphagia*, 1, 73–77.

Larson, K. L., Ayllon, T., & Barrett, D. H. (1987). A behavioral feeding program for failure to thrive infants. *Behaviour Research and Therapy*, *25*, 39–47.

Lewis, M. B., & Pashayan, H. M. (1980). Management of infants with Robin anomaly. *Clinical Pediatrics*, *19*, 519–528.

Limbrock, G. J., Hoyer, H., & Scheying, H. (1990). Drooling, chewing and swallowing dysfunction in children with cerebral palsy:

Treatment according to Castillo-Morales. *Journal of Dentistry for Children*, *57*, 445–451.

Logemann, J. A. (1983). *Evaluation and treatment of swallowing disorders*. San Diego: College-Hill Press.

Logemann, J. A. (1993). Noninvasive approaches to deglutitive aspiration. *Dysphagia*, *8*, 331–333.

Logemann, J. A., Kahrilas, P. J., Kobara, M., & Vakil, N. B. (1989). The benefit of head rotation on pharyngoesophageal dysphagia. *Archives of Physical Medicine and Rehabilitation*, *70*, 767–771.

Markowitz, J. A., Gerry, R. G., & Fleishner, R. (1979). Immediate obturation of neonatal cleft palates. *The Mount Sinai Journal of Medicine*, *46*, 123–129.

Mathew, O. P. (1990). Determinants of milk flow through nipple units: Role of hole size and nipple thickness. *American Journal of Diseases in Childhood*, *144*, 222–224.

Mathisen, B., Skuse, D., Wolke, D., & Reilly, S. (1989). Oral-motor dysfunction and failure to thrive among inner-city infants. *Developmental Medicine and Child Neurology*, *31*, 293–302.

McClannahan, C. (1987). *Feeding and caring for infants and children with special needs*. Rockville, MD: American Occupational, Therapy Associaton.

Morris, S. E. (1981). Communication/interaction development at mealtimes for the multiply handicapped child: Implications for the use of augmentive communication systems. *Language, Speech and Hearing Services in Schools*, *12*, 216–232.

Morris, S. E. (1982). *Pre-speech Assessment Scale: A rating scale for the development of pre-speech behaviors from birth through two years*. Clifton, NJ: J. A. Preston.

Morris, S. E. (1985). Developmental implications for the management of feeding problems in neurologically impaired infants. *Seminars in Speech and Language*, *6*, 293–314.

Morris, S. E. (1987). Therapy for the child with cerebral palsy: Interacting frameworks. *Seminars in Speech and Language*, *8*, 71–86.

Morris, S. E. (1989). Development of oral motor skills in the neurologically impaired child receiving non-oral feedings. *Dysphagia, 3,* 135–154.

Morris, S. E., & Klein, M. D. (1987). *Pre-feeding skills: A comprehensive resource for feeding development.* Tucson, AZ: Therapy Skill Builders.

Mueller, H. A. (1972). Facilitating feeding and prespeech. In P. H. Pearson & C. E. Williams (Eds.), *Physical therapy services in the developmental disabilities* (pp. 283–311). Srinfield, IL: Charles C Thomas.

Myers, E. N., & Stool, E. E. (1985). Complications of tracheotomy. In E. N. Myers, & E. E. Stool, (Eds.), *Tracheotomy* (pp. 54–65). New York: Churchill Livingstone.

Mysak, E. D. (1980). *Neurospeech therapy for the cerebral palsied: A neuroevolutional approach* (3rd ed.). New York: Teachers College Press.

Nelson, C. A., & De Benabib, R. M. (1991). Sensory preparation of the oral-motor area. In M. B. Langley & L. J. Lombardino (Eds.), *Neurodevelopmental strategies for managing communication disorders in children with severe motor dysfunction* (pp. 131–158). Austin, TX: Pro-Ed.

Ottenbacher, K., Dauck, B. S., Gevelinger, M., Grahn, V., & Hassett, C. (1985). Reliability of the Behavioral Assessment Scale of Oral Functions in Feeding. *American Journal of Occupational Therapy, 39,* 436–440.

Palmer, S., & Horn, S. (1978). Feeding problems in children. In S. Palmer & S. Ekvall (Eds.), *Pediatric nutrition in developmental disorders* (pp. 107–129). Springfield, IL: Charles C Thomas.

Palmer, M. M., Crawley, K., & Blanco, I. A. (1993). Neonatal Oral Motor Assessment Scale: A reliability study. *Journal of Perinatology, 8,* 28–35.

Palmer, S., Thompson, R. J., Jr., & Linscheid, T. R. (1975). Applied behavior analysis in the treatment of childhood feeding problems. *Developmental Medicine and Child Neurology, 17,* 333–339.

Passy, V. (1986). Passy-Muir tracheostomy speaking valve. *Otolaryngology—Head and Neck Surgery, 95,* 247–248.

Plaxico, D., & Loughlin, G. (1981). Nasopharyngeal reflux and neonatal apnea. *American Journal of Diseases of Children, 135,* 793–794.

Pipes, P. I., & Holm, V. A. (1980). Feeding children with Down's syndrome. *Journal of the American Dietetic Association, 77,* 277–281.

Pressman, H., & Morrison, S. H. (1988). Dysphagia in the pediatric AIDS population. *Dysphagia, 2,* 166–169.

Pridham, K. F. (1990). Feeding behavior of 6- to 12-month old infants: Assessment and sources of parental information. *Journal of Pediatrics, 117*(2, Part 2), S174–S180.

Reilly, S., & Skuse, D. (1992). Characteristics and management of feeding problems of young children with cerebral palsy. *Developmental Medicine and Child Neurology, 34,* 379–388.

Robbins, J., & Levine, R. (1988). Swallowing after unilateral stroke of the cerebral cortex: Preliminary experience. *Dysphagia, 3,* 11–17.

Rogers, B. T., Arvedson, J., Msall, M., & Demerath, R. R. (1993). Hypoxemia during oral feeding of children with severe cerebral palsy. *Developmental Medicine Child Neurology, 35,* 3–10.

Rogers, B. T., Msall, M., & Shucard, D. (1993). Hypoxemia during oral feedings in adults with dysphagia and severe neurological disabilities. *Dysphagia, 8,* 43–48.

Satter, E. (1990). The feeding relationship: Problems and interventions. *Journal of Pediatrics, 117*(2 , Pt. 2), S181–S189.

Schwartz, R., Moody, L., Yarandi, H., & Anderson, G. C. (1987). A meta-analysis of critical outcome variables in non nutritive sucking in pre term infants. *Nursing Research, 36,* 292–295.

Selley, W. G., & Boxall, J. (1986, May). A new way to treat sucking and swallowing difficulties in babies. *The Lancet,* pp. 1182–1184.

Shaker, K., Milbrath, J., Pen, J., Hogan, W. J., & Campbell, B. H. (1992, October). *Comparison of deglutive vocal cord function in tracheotomized patients and healthy volunteers.* Paper presented to the Dysphagia Research Society, Milwaukee, WI.

Sheppard, J. J. (1964). Cranio-oropharyngeal motor patterns in dysarthria associated with cerebral palsy. *Journal of Speech and Hearing Research*, 7, 373–380.

Sheppard, J. J. (1982). *Dietary skills: Feeding the developmentally disabled client*. Unpublished manuscript.

Sheppard, J. J. (1987). Assessment of oral motor behaviors in cerebral palsy. *Seminars in Speech and Language*, 8, 57–70.

Sheppard, J. J. (1991). Managing dysphagia in mentally retarded adults. *Dysphagia*, 6, 83–87.

Sheppard, J. J., Liou, J., Hochman, R., Laroia, S., & Langlois, D. (1988). Nutritional correlates of dysphagia in individuals institutionalized with mental retardation. *Dysphagia*, 3, 85–89.

Sheppard, J. J., & Mysak, E. D. (1984). Ontogeny of infantile oral reflexes and emerging chewing. *Child Development*, 55, 831–843.

Sheppard, J. J., & Pressman, H. (1988), Dysphagia in infantile cortical hyperostosis (Caffeys' disease): A case study. *Developmental Medicine and Child Neurology*, 30, 111–114.

Simon, B., Fowler, S. M., & Handler, S. D. (1983). Communication development in young children with long-term tracheostomies: Preliminary report. *International Journal of Pediatric Otorhinolaryngology*, 6, 37–50.

Simon, B., & Handler, S. D. (1981). The speech pathologist and management of children with tracheostomies. *Journal of Otolaryngology*, 10, 440–448.

Singer, R. N. (1972). *Readings in motor learning*. Philadelphia: Lea & Febiger.

Stolovitz, P., & Gisel, E. G. (1991). Circumoral movements in response to three different food textures in children 6 months to 2 years of age. *Dysphagia*, 6, 17–25.

Stratton, M. (1981). Behavioral Assessment Scale of Oral Functions in Feeding. *American Journal of Occupational Therapy*, 35, 719–721.

Stroh, K., Robinson, T., & Stroh, G. (1986). A therapeutic feeding programme. I: Theory and practice of feeding. *Developmental Medicine and Child Neurology*, 28, 3–10.

Takagi, Y., & Bosma, J. F. (1960). Disability of oral function in an infant associated with displacement of the tongue: Therapy by feeding in prone position. *Acta Paediatrica*, 49(Suppl. 123), 62–69.

Thornton, H. A. (1985). New infant nursing bottle with angled neck. *Postgraduate Medicine*, 36, 174–177.

Trefler, E. (1984). *Seating for children with cerebral palsy: A resource manual*. Memphis: University of Tennessee Center for the Health Sciences, Rehabilitation Engineering Program.

Tuchman, D. N. (1989). Cough, choke, sputter: The evaluation of the child with dysfunctional swallowing. *Dysphagia*, 3, 111–116.

Vandenberg, K. A. (1990). Nippling management of the sick neonate in the NICU: The disorganized feeder. *Neonatal Network*, 9, 9–16.

Van Dyke, D. C., Mackay, L., & Ziaylek, E. N. (1982). Management of severe feeding dysfunction in children with fetal alcohol syndrome. *Clinical Pediatrics*, 21, 336–339.

Vice, F. L., Heinz, J. M., Giuriati, G., Hood, M., & Bosma, J. F. (1990). Cervical ausculation of suckle feeding in newborn infants. *Developmental Medicine and Child Neurology*, 32, 760–768.

Wolf, L. S., & Glass, R. P. (1992). *Feeding and swallowing disorders in infancy: Assessment and management*. Tucson, AZ: Therapy Skill Builders.

CHAPTER

4

Nutrition Support

KATHLEEN R. WHITE, M.S., R.D.,
SELINA C. MHANGO-MKANDAWIRE, R.D., Ed.D.
AND SUSAN R. ROSENTHAL, M.S., M.D.

CONTENTS

Children with developmental disabilities may have associated nutritional and feeding problems ranging from mild to severe. It is not uncommon for the child with severe developmental disabilities to become marasmic. It was previously believed and accepted that children with cerebral palsy (CP) were thin for age because it was characteristic of the disease (Shapiro, Green, Krick, Allen, & Capote, 1986). However, it is now clear that aggressive nutritional intervention clearly improves weight gain and may increase linear growth as well in children with CP and other developmental disabilities (Patric, Boland, Sloski, & Murray, 1986). Several factors may contribute to poor weight gain in this population, including oral-motor dysfunction, poor dentition, behavior disturbance, or early satiety.

Complicated as the situation is for children with developmental disabilities, their nutritional needs are basically similar to those of other growing children. They require nutrients not only to maintain body functions and activities, but also for growth. Rates of growth change during childhood and are most rapid during the first year of life and at puberty. Children with developmental disabilities may suffer from many other abnormalities and may be further stressed nutritionally, with higher demands for the same nutrients due to their specific disease manifestations. Because not much is known about specific nutrient requirements for children with developmental disabilities we must often extrapolate their needs from adult studies or data on children without developmental disabilities.

This chapter will focus on the specific nutritional demands of children with developmental disabilities and give suggestions for providing optimal nutrition. The degree of malnutrition and feeding problems directly correlate with the type and severity of the child's impairment (see Table 4–1). Children with developmental disabilities are at risk for stunted skeletal growth, poor weight gain, anemia, and dental problems (see Tables 4–2, 4–3).

Vitamin and Mineral Supplementation

Supplementation of specific and/or multiple vitamins and minerals should be made on the basis of biochemical analysis, clinical manifestations, and actual dietary intake. Generally speaking, a child consuming a well varied diet that provides adequate calories typically does not need additional supplements. However children with developmental disabilities do present with nutrient intakes below 70% of Recommended Daily Allowances (RDAs); particularly for vitamins A, C, and D, thiamine, riboflavin, calcium, magnesium, and iron (Wodarski, 1990). There is a large degree of variation among individuals, although total energy intake may be constant. Interestingly, Thommessen, Kuse, Larsen, and Heiberg (1992) found the distribution of calories to be within normal range: fat 33–36% of total energy intake, carbohydrates 46–57%, and protein 12–15%. Despite this, careful attention should be focused on fat intake and percent of essential fatty acids. Children who remain on pureed foods and/or baby foods without adequate whole milk are at risk for inadequate fat consumption because these foods are so low in fat, and parents do not routinely supplement their diets with oil, butter, or margarine.

Medications also can interfere with nutrient intake and absorption. Folate, vitamin D, calcium, cholesterol, and magnesium may all be decreased in these children. Many children have associated seizure disorders for which phenytoin and phenobarbital are prescribed. These medications may interfere with vitamin D metabolism and lead to deficits even with adequate nutrient intakes (see Chapter 16). These drugs also may increase the metabolic requirements for vitamin D because they induce liver enzymes that serve as modulators for conversion of vitamin D to 25 dihydroxycholecalciferol. Folic acid metabolism can also be reduced with seizure medications if the dietary intake is inadequate (Wodarski, 1990). Interestingly hypercholesterolemia has been reported with

Table 4-1. Frequently reported nutrition problems and factors contributing to high nutritional risk in individuals with developmental disabilities.

Syndrome or Disability	Altered Growth Rate/Growth Retardation	Altered Energy Need Needs/Intake	Altered Nutrient Needs Nutrient Deficiencies	Constipation/ Diarrhea	Feeding Problems	Others
Cerebral palsy	X	X	X	X	X	poor appetite orthopedic problems
Epilepsy			X	X		Dilantin-induced hyperplasia of gums drug-nutrient interaction
Muscular dystrophy	X	X		X	X	
Myelomeningocele	X	X	X	X	X	
Cleft lip/palate	x (during infancy)	X	X		X	orthodontic problems
Down syndrome	X	X		X	X	gum disease
Prader-Willi syndrome	X	X		X	X	
PKU and other inherited metabolic disorders		X	X		X	may need specialized nutrients medication
Mental retardation of unknown etiology	X	X		X	X	drug-nutrient interaction
Autism					X	drug-nutrient interaction

Source: From *Journal of the American Dietetic Association.* (1987), *87*(8), 1069–1073, with permission.

Table 4–2. Nutritional problems of children with developmental disabilities and dysphagia.

Marasmus

Hypoproteinemia

Carnitine deficiency

Vitamin deficiencies

    Calcium
    Vitamin C
    Folate
    Vitamin A
    Riboflavin
    Thiamine
    Vitamin D

Iron deficiency

Hypomagnesemia

the use of anticonvulsant medications secondary to induction of cholesterol biosynthesis in the hepatocyte (Wodarski, 1990). Because the cholesterol elevation is a result of increased high density lipoprotein synthesis, the risk of coronary heart disease is not increased. Therefore, a complete lipid profile should be obtained prior to consideration of therapeutic measures.

Calcium status should be monitored because the intake and absorption of calcium may be negatively affected in this population. Calcium supplement preparations are available in various chemical forms such as carbonate, lactate gluconate, citrate, and acetate. The difference is the amount of elemental calcium per dose. For example, calcium carbonate contains approximately 40% elemental calcium; calcium gluconate contains 9% elemental calcium; and calcium lactate contains about 13% elemental calcium. Absorption of these calcium salts varies and is affected by the foods consumed concurrently and the gastric environment (i.e., gastric acidity). It is generally recommended to provide supplemental calcium between meals to avoid its action as a phosphate binder. Additionally, an acidic environment is preferred for optimal absorption (pH < 6.0). Therefore, administering calcium with orange juice or grapefruit juice may be beneficial. Table 4–4 outlines the various calcium supplements and amounts recommended.

Anemia may develop secondary to poor intake or to gastrointestinal (GI) blood loss secondary to gastroesophageal reflux (GER), and esophagitis (see Chapter 12). Hypoproteinemia similarly may develop from GI protein loss secondary to reflux esophagitis, milk protein allergy, and inadequate intake. Protein-calorie malnutrition is a well documented phenomenon in patients with developmental disabilities and oral-motor involvement. Studies of dysphagic adults by Sitzman (1990) demonstrated nutritional deficiencies in this population. There was general weight loss in 80% of the patients, reflecting the chronic character of the dysphagia-induced starvation. Laboratory findings in over 70% of the patients indicated visceral protein depletion suggestive of concomitant acute nutritional depletion. From this study, it may be extrapolated that dysphagic children may experience not only severe weight loss, but also sacrifice normal growth. Veldee and Peth (1992) demonstrated a marked functional decline in a variety of muscles as a result of protein-calorie malnutrition. These changes are accompanied by biochemical alterations within the muscle cells characteristic of an energy-depleted state. In addition, studies of individuals with protein-calorie malnutrition (PCM) have shown a depression in cellular immunity with abnormal T-cell and macrophage function. McLoughlin and colleagues (McLoughlin, Nord, & Oleske, 1987) concluded that "malnutrition in itself has a deleterious ef-

Table 4–3. Specific nutrient deficiencies and their clinical signs.

Type of Deficiency	Clinical Signs
Protein-Calorie Malnutrition	Growth retardation Muscle wasting Apathy Irritability Infection Anemia Low body temperature GI disturbances
Hypoproteinemia	Edema
Iron Deficiency	Anemia, malabsorption, irritability, anorexia, pallor, lethargy
Vitamin Deficiencies	
Vitamin A	Night blindness—Keratomalacia Growth failure
Vitamin D	Rickets
Ascorbic acid (Vitamin C)	Hemorrhage Confusion Sjogren's syndrome Vasomotor instability Impaired iron and folate absorption Arthritis Poor wound healing
Folate	Megaloblastic anemia, stomatitis, glossitis
Thiamine (Vitamin B_1)	Beriberi (neuritis) Edema Cardiac failure Anorexia Restlessness Wernicke's encephalopathy
Riboflavin	Dermatitis Corneal vascularization Growth failure

fect on immune function and may result in defects in cellular immunity."

One of the factors contributing to undernourishment in children with cerebral palsy is reduced food intake and increased energy expenditure (Dietz, 1984). The importance of adequate nutrition in maximizing growth and cognitive potential in this special group of children cannot be overestimated. In 1986, Public Law 99-457 (Isaacs,

Table 4–4. Calcium supplementation.

Age	Product	Dosage
1–6 months	Neo-Calglucon*	1 tsp 3×/day
6 months–3 years	Neo-Calglucon	2 tsp 3×/day
3–5 years	Tums +	1 tablet 3×/day
5–10 years	Tums	2 tablets 3×/day
10 years	Tums	2 tablets 3×/day

*Neo-Calglucon   115 mg. Ca/tsp (5 ml)
 Titralac   400 mg. Ca/tsp
+Tums   500 mg. Ca CHO₃/tablet
 Calcimin   500 mg. Ca/powder packet

Note: Calcium supplementation may be recommended for patients following a milk-free diet for longer than 4–6 weeks. It should be noted that milk is the primary dietary source of Vitamin D (400 I.U./960 cc). In view of the role Vitamin D plays in calcium absorption and metabolism, it may be prudent to supplement with Vitamin D during winter months when exposure to sunlight is minimal and in dark pigmented individuals.

Montagne, & Davis, 1990) was established for nutrition intervention in the public school system for handicapped preschool children. This legislation mandated appropriate and expanded nutrition services for children 3 to 5 years of age. It also enabled a growing number of children with gastrostomy tube feedings to enter school. Follow-up has shown a number of positive results from this intervention (Isaacs, Montagne, & Davis, 1990). These include improved growth parameters, decreased oral feeding sensitivity, increased caloric intake, decreased rumination, decreased feeding time, increased volume of formula fed, positive behavioral changes, and decreased parental-child frustration in children who have taken part in this program.

Nutritional Assessment

Before diet manipulation for children with developmental disabilities is discussed, the importance of nutritional assessment must be stressed (see Table 4–6). Nutritional assessment and intervention in the child with developmental disabilities is one of the roles of a multidisciplinary team. The speech therapist provides essential information regarding feeding skills assessment and behavioral feeding issues. The physician performs a complete history and physical examination of the patient and measures biochemical parameters (see Table 4–5). Information including growth, dentition, physical signs, and symptoms associated with vitamin, mineral, or protein calorie deficiency are noted. In addition, gastrointestinal blood loss is assessed. All the above information is integrated into the nutritional care plan and helps the nutritionist formulate a plan of action. Nutrition assessment is done in a systematic fashion (see Table 4–6).

Measurement of length using a recumbent board is difficult in a child with fixed joint contractures or severe scoliosis. This is especially true of children with spastic quadriplegia who are at particular risk for growth failure. Several alternative methods have been suggested. A recent study by Miller and Koresha (1992) described a

Table 4–5. Biochemical tests commonly used in evaluation of nutritional status.

Albumin

Transferrin

Pre-Albumin

Retinol-Binding Protein

Total Protein

Serum Glucose

Lactose Breath Test

Stool pH

Serum Electrolytes

Complete Blood Count

Serum Ferritin

Iron

TIBC

Stool Hemoccult

Serum Carotene

Cholesterol

Fecal Fat

Vitamin Levels as Indicated

Zinc

Magnesium

---

method to determine height in children with cerebral palsy, scoliosis, or advanced muscular dystrophy. Neither the recumbent board nor arm span (distance from fingertip to fingertip) was felt to be accurate in these children. They developed a method to measure the forearm segment and convert it directly to standing height.

The following formula was used where Y is equal to the forearm length and X is the calculated height:

$$Y = 0.28596X - 2.74377$$

Spender, Cronk, Charnez, and Stallings (1989) suggested using upper arm length and lower leg length in children with cerebral palsy as indicators of linear growth.

Often following an individual child's own growth pattern over time and comparing it with the child's own baseline value as a marker for future growth rate analysis is most useful. Measures of body composition, including muscle mass, body fat, and measures of visceral protein all are used to evaluate new patients with developmental disabilities. Total body fat and muscle mass are estimated using skin fold calipers. However, because alterations in body composition are common in children with developmental disabilities, one must use serial measurements and not standard percentiles when evaluating these children. The mid-arm muscle circumference or limb circumference in children 1 to 4 years of age reflects somatic protein and subcutaneous fat stores. However, in older children it also reflects hypertrophy from overuse of arms rather than legs. Identification of somatic protein (muscle mass) is especially important in protein calorie malnutrition when visceral protein levels are preserved while whole body muscle mass is decreased. It has been reported that children with spastic cerebral palsy have a reduction in body cell mass and an increase in body fat composition (Rice, 1981). This alteration in body composition could be secondary to inactivity, effects of undernutrition, paresis of various major muscles, and poor growth of muscle tissue. Measures of visceral protein include albumin, transferrin, pre-albumin, and retinol binding protein.

The use of fat folds is still the most accurate way of assessing fat stores and fat-free mass in patients with developmental disabilities. Other analytical instruments currently available to measure body fat, in-

Table 4–6. Nutritional assessment.

I. Growth Assessment

   A. Complete growth assessment should include:
      1. Current information

         a. recumbent length (36 months of age) or standing height
         b. weight
         c. head circumference (24 months)
         d. triceps skinfold measurement (>1 year)
         e. mid-upper arm circumference

      2. Background information

         a. as many past growth measurements with age as possible
         b. history of past illness, medications
         c. social history
         d. record of family growth patterns*

   B. Weight: Dietz (1984) highly recommends the use of height per weight as the most accurate way to estimate ideal body weight in children with disabilities. Each child must be assessed as an individual in terms of his or her specific needs. Height per weight is the most accurate way to estimate ideal body weight in preadolescent children with disabilities. Each child must be assessed as an individual in terms of his or her specific needs.

Note: *Measurement alone, without any standard of comparison, limits interpretation of the data.

cluding the Bioelectrical Impedance Analyzer (RJL System) and the Futrex 5000 which measure body fat via electrical conductivity and infrared interactions respectively, are appropriate for use in the pediatric age group.

Energy Requirements

Although intake is often reduced in children with oral motor dysfunction, (Cully & Middleton, 1968; Dietz, 1984; Phelphs, 1951), energy expenditures may actually be increased when expressed per kilogram of lean body mass. Children with athetoid cerebral palsy appear to have increased energy expenditures, probably secondary to chronic muscle activity and contractions (Dietz, 1984).

Once the patient's height and weight are obtained and plotted on a growth chart, at-

tention is focused on the individual growth rate. Separate growth charts are available for children with Down syndrome (Cronk & Crocker, 1988) as these children may appear stunted and obese on standard growth curves. Use of growth velocity charts is indicated to follow growth rates in individual children. In addition to plotting weight for age and height for age, it is essential to plot the individual child's weight versus height to define malnutrition as compared to constitutional short stature or dwarfism. For the normal population, the ideal average weight for height is considered to be the 50th percentile. This indicates adequate and proportionate body fat and muscle mass.

For the child with severe developmental disabilities who is wheelchair bound or has severe gross motor delay, the goal is at least 10th percentile weight for height. At this point the child should be nutritionally stable. A weight for height greater than this may cause difficulties for the child's caregiver in mobilizing the patient. The 25th percentile weight for height is recommended for developmentally disabled children whose activity is less than expected for age, but who are not physically restricted to a wheelchair.

The expected rate of growth for a child with developmental disabilities is difficult to generalize, and it is best to analyze each child on the basis of individual growth patterns. The tendency for children with cerebral palsy to decelerate in the rate of linear growth as they grow older is well established (see Table 4–7). For children with severe cerebral palsy, as much as one third of their reduction in height may be due to limb atrophy and scoliosis (Sanders et al., 1990). A warning sign of failure to thrive in any child is decreasing weight for height.

Often linear growth and head growth are preserved while gains in weight continue to decelerate. It should be noted, however, that children with chronic central nervous system disability often have growth failure that is more pronounced in height than weight. Ruby and Matheny (1962) showed a lag of 12 to 18 months in growth in children with developmental disabilities and a delay in bone age of 19 months to 3 years. These effects were more pronounced in children with athetoid cerebral palsy.

Because of differences in feeding ability, growth potential, physical activity, and health problems the RDA for age is not an appropriate energy measure for these children. Rather, the recommended energy requirements for these children should be based on the RDA for their height age or their weight at the 25th percentile weight for height. In addition, it is important to assess the child's usual intake and compare it to the calculated determination. There may be great variations between the two. If a child is growing appropriately on fewer calories than the estimated value, it is not necessary to increase the child's caloric intake.

If increased caloric intake is desired, an increment of 5% of the usual intake is often sufficient to promote weight gain. Table 4–8 includes recommendations for normal children. Table 4–9 lists requirements for children with developmental disabilities. Because of the use of height age for patients with moderate to severe dysfunction in calculating calories, recommended energy requirements are expressed as calories per centimeter of height.

Table 4–7. Energy expenditure in cerebral palsy.

Group	Number of Subjects	Daily Energy Expenditure (kcal/kg lean body mass)	Height Mean	Age (S.D)
Cerebral Palsy				
Spastic	5	113.7	92.0	(3.6)
Dyskinetic	5	153.8	95.0	(4.7)
Control Group	22	85.6	10.1	(3.7)

Source: Dietz, William. "Nutritional Requirements and Feeding of the Handicapped Child." *Pediatric Nutrition Theory and Practice*, Chapter 28, p. 388, with permission.

Table 4–8. Normal RDA for ages infants through adult.

Category	Age (years)	Average Energy Allowance (kcal)		Average Protein Allowance (g)		
		Per kg*	Per cm*	Per day*	Per kg*	Per cm*
Infants	0.0–0.5	108		13	2.2	
	0.5–1.0	98		14	1.6	
Children	1–3	102		16	1.2	
	4–6	90		24	1.1	
	7–10	70		28	1.0	
Males	11–14	55	16	45	1.0	0.3
	15–18	45	17	59	0.9	0.3
	19–24	40	16	58	0.8	0.3
Females	11–14	47	14	46	1.0	0.3
	15–18	40	13	44	0.8	0.3
	19–24	38	13	46	0.8	0.3

*Figure is rounded.

Source: Adapted from Recommended Dietary Allowances. 10th edition. © 1989 by the National Academy of Sciences. Published by National Academy Press with permission.

The basal metabolic rate (BMR) also may be used to calculate caloric requirements. This is particularly advantageous in the hospitalized patient or child awaiting the initiation of tube feeds. The Mayo Clinic Nomogram is useful for this purpose in patients over 15 kg and 85 cm (see Figure 4–1). If the height is difficult to obtain, needs can also be estimated utilizing the basal metabolic rate and weight (see Table 4–10). The BMR must be adjusted for activity and stress (physical and metabolic) to determine final caloric needs. In practical terms, the needs for calories and protein for developmentally delayed/neurologically impaired children can be estimated using 75 to 80% of RDAs for nondevelopmentally delayed children.

Children with oral motor dysfunction may require extra calories and protein for catch-up growth beyond what is normally recommended (see Table 4–11). Failure to thrive is a common problem in the population. Nutritional demands may be further increased by recurrent pulmonary infections secondary to GER and aspiration.

To increase calories, the formula may be concentrated, modular supplements added, or both (see Tables 4–12, 4–13). The method of concentrating formula should be in small increments (i.e., 2 cals/oz up to approximately 26 to 28 cal/oz by concentration). Once this level is achieved it is generally advised to add fat or carbohydrate to increase calories further. Although it is possible to increase concentration up to 30 cal/oz this may not be well tolerated in younger infants and children or those with compromised intestinal or renal function or children who are osmotically sensitive (i.e., very sensitive to increased osmolar load). Decreasing the amount of free water via a concentration of the formula with decreased water or increased liquid or powder concentrate can

Table 4–9. Recommended energy requirements for children with developmental disabilities.

Developmental Disability	Guide for Caloric Intake			
	(kcal/kg)	(kcal/lb)	(kcal/cm)	(kcal/in.)
Normal				
Infant 0–0.5 year	115	52	-	-
Infant 0.5–1 year	105	48	-	-
Toddler 1–3 years	100	45	14.4	36.6
Preschool 4–6 years	85	39	14.5	36.8
Down Syndrome				
Boys	-	-	16.1	40.9
Girls	-	-	14.3	36.3
Prader-Willi Syndrome				
For maintenance	-	-	10–11	26.7
For weight loss	-	-	8.5	21.6
Spina Bifida				
For weight loss*	-	-	7.0	17.8
Cerebral Palsy				
5–11 years, mild/moderate activity	-	-	13.9	35.3
5–11 years, limited activity	-	-	11.1	28.2

*Generally recommended to be 50 percent of the caloric requirements of a normal child.
Source: From Lifshitz, F., Finch, N. M., & Lifshitz, J. Z. (1991). The handicapped child, *Children's Nutrition* (p. 389). Boston, MA: Jones & Bartlett, with permission.

cause hypernatremia and dehydration, particularly in children with compromised renal function and extra-renal losses, including vomiting, fever, and diarrhea. In addition, renal solute load is increased, and this may be a problem in premature infants and children with limited fluid intake and renal problems. The addition of carbohydrate or fat to the formula will add calories without affecting the renal solute load but will not add protein, vitamins or minerals. Therefore, the use of carbohydrate or fat modular supplements alone may dilute the intake of vitamins or minerals as well as protein and overall nutritional quality of the formula. If the volume of formula consumed is appropriate, this concern is lessened. The use of carbohydrate will increase the osmolality slightly and may be contraindicated in

patients with pulmonary disease who retain carbon dioxide. The metabolism of carbohydrates is associated with a large by-product of carbon dioxide that may interfere with respiration or weaning the patient off mechanical ventilation.

Although the feeding process is slow and often frustrating in these children and poor posture alignment and oral hypersensitivity often cause further problems, oral feeding skills may still be enhanced. Thommessen, Rus, Kuse, Larsen, and Heiberg (1992) studied a group of children between the ages of 1 and 16 years with multiple developmental disabilities to determine what feeding problems they had and the effect these problems had on energy intake. The study revealed several feeding practices among caregivers:

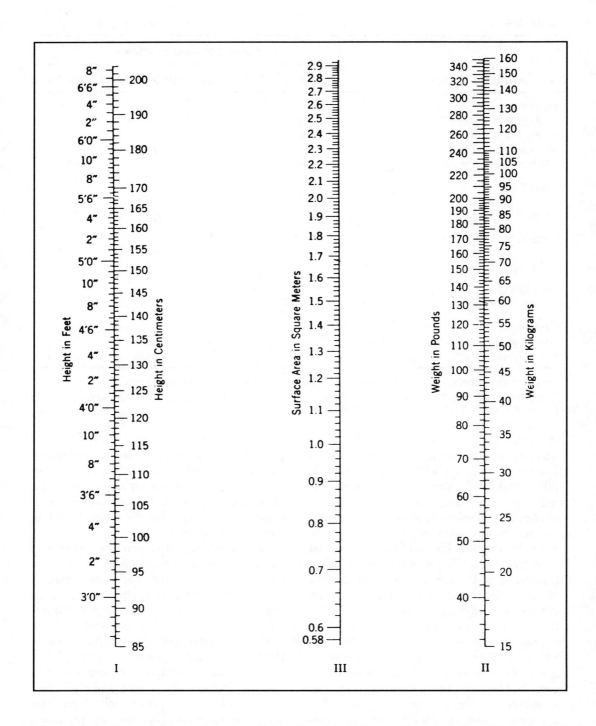

Figure 4–1. Mayo Clinic Nomogram. From Pike R.L. & Brown M.L:, *Nutrition: An Integrated Approach*. 2nd ed. New York: John Wiley & Sons, 1975 p. 829, with permission.

Table 4–10. Basal metabolic rates for infants and children.

| Age 1 wk to 10 mo | | Age 11 to 36 mo | | | Age 3 to 16 yr | | |
Weight (kg)	Metabolic Rate (kcal/hr) Male or Female	Weight (kg)	Metabolic Rate (kcal/hr) Male	Female	Weight (kg)	Metabolic Rate (kcal/hr) Male	Female
3.5	8.4	9.0	22.0	21.2	15	35.8	33.3
4.0	9.5	9.5	22.8	22.0	20	39.7	37.4
4.5	10.5	10.0	23.6	22.8	25	43.6	41.5
5.0	11.6	10.5	24.4	23.6	30	47.5	45.5
5.5	12.7	11.0	25.2	24.4	35	51.3	49.6
6.0	13.8	11.5	26.0	25.2	40	55.2	53.7
6.5	14.9	12.0	26.8	26.0	45	59.1	57.8
7.0	16.0	12.5	27.6	26.9	50	63.0	61.9
7.5	17.1	13.0	28.4	27.7	55	66.9	66.0
8.0	18.2	13.5	29.2	28.5	60	70.8	70.0
8.5	19.3	14.0	30.0	29.3	65	74.7	74.0
9.0	20.4	14.5	30.8	30.1	70	78.6	78.1
9.5	21.4	15.0	31.6	30.9	75	82.5	82.2
10.0	22.5	15.5	32.4	31.7			
10.5	23.6	16.0	33.2	32.6			
11.0	24.7	16.5	34.0	33.4			

Source: From Altman, P. L., & Dittner, D. S. (Eds), Metabolism, 1968, Bethesda, MD: Federation of American Societies for Experimental Biology, with permission.

Table 4–11. Estimating energy and protein needs for catch-up growth.

Kcal/kg = Ideal Weight for Height X RDA kcal/kg Weight Age
            Actual Weight

Gms Pro/kg = Ideal Weight for Height X RDA gms Pro/kg Weight Age
              Actual Weight

1. Plot the child's height and weight on the NCHG growth charts.

2. Determine at what age the present weight would be at the fiftieth percentile (weight age).

3. Determine recommended calories for weight age.

4. Determine the ideal weight (fiftieth percentile) for the child's present age.

5. Multiply the value obtained in (3) by the value obtained in (4).

6. Divide the value obtained in (5) by actual weight.

Note: Guidelines are used to estimate catch-up growth requirements; precise individual needs will vary and be mediated by medical status and diagnosis. A gradual progression toward "catch-up growth" needs is recommended to prevent metabolic stress from caloric overload.

Table 4–12. Dilution and concentration of formula.

Generally, feeding preparations are available in ready-feed, liquid concentrate, and/or powdered form which can be prepared according to individual needs.

Standard Dilution

Infant formula	0.67 cal/cc or 20 cal/oz
Enteral feeding preparation	1.10 cal/cc or 30 cal/oz

Increasing Caloric Density

When necessary caloric density of a feeding preparation may be increased by:
1. adding *carbohydrate* (i.e., polycose, dextrose, karo syrup)
2. adding *fat* (i.e., corn oil, MCT)
3. increasing concentration of formula base or any combination of the above.

Note: Formula orders should specify desired method of caloric increase.

Example: 25 cal/oz by polycose
25 cal/oz by concentration
25 cal/oz by polycose (2 cal/oz)
and MCT Oil (3 cal/oz)

The method used to increase caloric density is dependent on individual needs and tolerance. Regardless, increases should be made *slowly* (i.e., 2–3 cal/oz/day) *altering one ingredient* (i.e., polycose, MCT Oil) at a time.

Feeding preparations containing amino acids, peptides, mono and/or disaccharides may not be well tolerated by osmotically sensitive patients. These patients should be slowly fed small volumes of dilute formula and progressed as tolerated. *Do not increase* both *volume* and *caloric density* in any single 24-hour period.

It is important to note that:
1. Increasing caloric density of a feeding will also increase osmolality, the extent of which is dependent on ingredients used, i.e. dextrose versus polycose.
2. Increasing formula concentration will also increase renal solute load while decreasing free water available for excretion. To estimate renal solute load allow:
4 mOsm/gm Protein provided in a liter of formula
1 mOsm/mEq of Na^+, K^+, and Cl^-

Estimated Normal Fluid Requirements[1]

Based on Body Size (ml/Kg)		Based on Energy Intake (ml/kcal)	
Infants	100–120	Infants	1.5
1–10 yrs.	60–80	Adults	1.0
11–18 yrs.	41–55		
> 18 yrs.	20–30		

Decreasing Caloric Density

Similac 13 can be ordered when dilute regular formula is desired for short-term use with acute diarrhea. Formulas should always be diluted with sterile water, *not* 5 or 10% glucose or electrolyte solutions (which also contain glucose). Half and 3/4 strengths can be ordered from the Milk Lab in routine ordering time frames.

Source: From Howard & Herbold. *Nutrition in Clinical Care*, New York, McGraw-Hill, 1982, p. 155, with permission.

Table 4–13. Commonly used supplements.

Product	Food Source	Kcal /gm	kcal	CHO gm	PRO gm	Fat gm	Na+ mEq	mOgm/Kg in 5% dilution	Indications for Use Rationale
				Content/Tbsp.					
Polycose (Ross)	hydrolysed corn starch, glucose polymer 1,4 linkage	3.75	30	7.5	-	-	.4	65	Low osmolarity; easily combined with a variety of foods, relatively tasteless.
Moducal (Mead Johnson)	hydrolysed corn starch, glucose polymers, small amts. glucose, maltose, isomaltose	3.8	30	7.6	-	-	.2	27.6	See comments above. Lower sodium content rarely a significant consideration. Requires special order/not routinely stocked.
Dextrose	D glucose powder anhydrous	3.8	46	11.9	-	-	-	276	High osmolarity; CHO source in disaccharide intolerance; availability may be a problem for home use.
Casec (Mead Johnson)	calcium caseinate	3.6	17	-	4	-	.3	low	Easily combined with formula and/or pureed foods monitor all protein sources. 75 mg. calcium/tbsp.
Rice Cereal	rice flour, barley malt flour, soya lecithin, soya oil	3.8	9	1.8	.2	.1	-	very low	Used to thicken formula, easily combined with fruit and/or pureed foods. 11 mg. iron/tbsp.

(continued)

Table 4-13 *(continued)*.

Product	Food Source	Content/Tbsp. Kcal /gm	kcal /ml kcal	Content/Tbsp. (15 ml) CHO gm	PRO gm	Fat gm	Na+ mEq	mOgm/Kg in 5% dilution	Indications for Use Rationale
MCT Oil (Mead Johnson)	fractionated coconut oil, primarily C_8-C_{10} saturated fatty acids	7.67	115	-	-	13.8	-	low	Of use with low pancreatic lipase; low bile salts; defective fat absorption and transport.
Corn Oil	-	8.4	126	-	-	14	-	very low	Excellent source of lineolic acid; easily combined with a variety of foods readily available.
Lipomul (Upjohn)	polysorbate 80, glyceride phosphates, sodium saccharin	6.0	91	.1	-	10	.3	low	Easily combined with a variety of foods; availability may be a problem for home use.

References: Bowes & Church, *Food Values of Portions Commonly Used*, 1980; Ross Products Handbook, 1981; Mead Johnson, *Adult Nutritional Handbook*, 1981

Source: From Queen, P., & Gallagher, L. (1987). *Pediatric Nutrition Handbook*. Boston, MA: Boston Children's Hospital, with permission.

1. Many parents of children in this group delayed the initiation of self feeding in their children. There was also prolonged use of pureed foods up to 6 years of age.
2. Approximately 50% of parents reported that they felt their child had chewing or swallowing difficulty and they continued using pureed foods even though food with more texture may have been tolerated.
3. Some parents fed their children pureed food because it was easier and quicker than food with more texture. Approximately 33% of parents were afraid to feed solid or semisolid foods.

The study also found that the presence of oral motor dysfunction and prolonged assisted feeding did have a significant effect on the children's nutrient intake.

When progressing from semisolid to solid foods, there is a logical progression of consistency (see Chapter 3). The texture indicated is based on the child's developmental readiness and oral skills. However, it is generally agreed that the introduction of higher texture foods is beneficial (see Table 4–14).

Encouragement of self-feeding with the use of utensils and finger feeding is recommended when the child is able. Liquids may require thickening for ease of swallowing and increased fluid intake (see Table 4–15).

A study was done by Stanek, Hensley, and Van Riper (1992) to assess factors affecting the use of food and commercial agents to thicken liquid for individuals with swallowing disorders. They concluded that bread crumbs, tofu, and cracker crumbs were the least effective agents to thicken liquids. Pudding (instant) and applesauce worked well to increase viscosity; however, they also increased the volume of food required for consumption which further compromised fluid intake. Nutra-thick™, Thickit™, and Thick 'N

Table 4–14. Benefits of higher texture foods in children with developmental disabilities.

Stimulation of salivary flow
Improvement in oral muscle tone
Decreased oral hypersensitivity
Strengthening of chewing and swallowing skills
Increased variety of foods
Lesser incidence of carotenemia*
Increased fiber intake
Improved feeding experience

*Many baby foods are carrot based and pureed consistency increased the absorption of betacarotene.

Easy™ produced excellent viscosity at a low level and added an average of 37 cal/serving.

Some children may find it easier to consume formula or milk rather than solid foods of varying textures. Parents also find that this expedites the feeding session and more importantly, provides a reliable source of nutrition compared to the struggle with self- or assisted spoon feeding. Many formulas available can provide close to 100% of the RDAs for age. Thus it is reassuring to both the parent and the health care provider. Formula also has benefits for children who are making a transition from one level of feeding to the next. For example, if a child is on thickened pureed foods and the speech therapist feels the child is displaying vertical jaw movement and chewing; ground foods will be initiated. The initial phase of this transition can be difficult and lengthy and alter the overall intake until the child has adjusted. At this time formulas such as Pediasure, Ensure, Sustacal, and Nutren would be advantageous. Otherwise, there is no reason that an older child without oral mechanical

Table 4–15. Thickening agents.

Thickit (Milana Foods, Division of DiaFoods)

Thicken Up (Sandoz)

Nutra-thick (Menu Magic)

Classic Instant Food Thickener (Sysco)

Baby cereal

Pureed fruits added to juices

Oatbran

Dehydrated potato flakes

Bread crumbs

---

problems should be on a liquid diet providing 80–100% of calories.

One needs to consider the long-term effects of not allowing the child to progress beyond the point of pureed food or assisted feeds when he or she may be capable of it. Parents and caretakers might assume that the child is at his or her highest level, but if the child is not challenged appropriately, actual "potential" may not surface.

Tube Feedings

In severe cases of undernutrition or specific conditions that complicate oral feeding, the health care team may need to consider alternate means of nutritional support. This can be provided either through enteral route (via tube feeds) or parenteral route (via intravenous nutrition). However, with a functioning gut the first line of treatment is tube feedings. In this section tube feedings will be addressed in reference to indications, equipment, type of tube feeding, advantages, and selection of formulas.

Indications

In general the criteria for tube feedings include one or more of the following:

- Weight/height <5%
- Prolonged feeding times
- GI abnormality/malabsorption
- Failure to thrive with oral supplements
- Upper airway obstruction, esophageal atresia
- Oral motor dysfunction, dysphagia

The decision on the feeding tube or route of administration (nasogastric, nasoduodenal, nasojejunal, gastrostomy, or jejunostomy) will depend on the anticipated duration of tube feeding, physiology of the GI tract, risk of aspiration, and whether surgery is an option (see Chapter 5). It is generally recommended that the child be evaluated by a pediatric gastroenterologist prior to initiation of gastrostomy tube feeds to rule out gastroesophageal reflux. This is usually done using a pH probe to measure to degree of gastric acid backwash into the lower esophageal area. Introduction of a tube into and beyond the lower esophageal sphincter alone can increase the patient's susceptibility to reflux. The patient may require surgical correction to minimize the risk of aspiration with tube feedings. This is then followed by surgical placement of gastrostomy tube. A noninvasive gastrostomy tube placement, referred to as a PEG (percutaneous endoscopic gastrostomy), is the nonsurgical placement of a feeding tube. This method is rapidly replacing the use of surgical gastrostomies in many centers (see Chapters 12 and 13).

Equipment

The tube feeding apparatus includes some or all of the following: feeding pump, formula bag, feeding tube, connecting tube and formula. Feeding tubes used in the 1950s and 1960s, consisting of polyvinyl chloride (PVC) material, have been replaced by silicone or polyurethane. The newer materials do not require frequent feeding changes, because they are resistant to decomposition by digestive secretions and low pH medium. Silicone tubing is softer, more flexible, and has a smaller lumen than PVC; therefore, it is more susceptible to collapse, rupturing, and stretching. Polyurethane tubing is stronger and has a larger lumen and thinner walls. The size of the tube is identified by the *outer lumen diameter*, not the inner lumen where the formula is infused. The size is referred to in French units ranging from 5–16 Fr. units. The higher the number the larger the diameter. However, because the polyurethane tube has a larger lumen, the same French unit in a silicone tube will be *smaller* inside; therefore, selection of French units alone is insufficient. The narrower lumen in silicone tubing may cause problems with kinks, occlusions, and so on. Likewise, the larger lumen tubes may allow for decreased resistance with viscous formulas or blenderized feeds, *but* they may also cause GI irritation and trauma such as partial obstruction. In the pediatric population, the 5 or 8 French tubes work well in infants and small-for-age children up to 1½ years. The larger sized (10, 12) French tubes are appropriate for older children.

In general, polyurethane tubes are used for nasogastric tube feeds. Nasoduodenal and nasojejunal feeds often require different tubing to secure positioning of the tube transpylorically. Such a tube is the silastic tube which has a weighted tungsten tip (3, 5, 7 grams) in the form of pellet, powder, or segments. Placement of any tube should be verified by chest x-ray or roentgenogram. Nasoduodenal and nasojejunal tubes are indicated in patients with delayed gastric emptying and GER. However, long-term maintenance of these tubes is difficult, and these patients generally require placement of a percutaneous endoscopic gastrostomy.

Nasogastric and Nasoduodenal Tube Feeding

If the child requires short-term nutritional rehabilitation (less than 3 months), nasogastric tube feeding would be indicated. Nasogastric tube feedings are often used at night while the child is sleeping, but they are also used for infants and children during the day either through continuous drip or bolus feeds. Once the patient reaches the goal weight between 10–25th percentile weight/height and nutritional status has improved, cessation of the tube feedings can be considered. This should only be done if the patient can sustain adequate oral intake to maintain the desired weight. Nasogastric tube feedings are contraindicated with GER, delayed gastric emptying, intractable vomiting, and long-term nutritional support.

Gastrostomy Tube Feedings

Gastrostomy tube feedings are indicated for long-term nutritional support to provide 50 to 100% of caloric needs. It is also possible that some children with developmental disabilities may require tube feeding intermittently, depending on oral intake, illnesses, and other problems.

Advantages

Several studies have been conducted to illustrate the potential benefits of tube feedings. One such study demonstrated improved weight gain with increased wt/ht ratio after 1 year of tube feeding. However only limited gains in height growth velocity were achieved. Therefore, tube feeding does not eliminate growth retardation but does improve weight gain, nutritional status, and immune competence. It appears that early intervention has a greater impact on height growth than later intervention as demonstrated by research conducted by Sanders et al. (1990), who found that the children showed an improved height curve if enteral feeds were started within 1 year of CNS insult. However, the older group of children (>8 years) who were severely malnourished did not respond with increase in height percentiles yet there was some improvement in weight. Rempel, Colwell, and Nelson (1988) reported that 33% of their CP patient population showed an improvement in height curve if enteral feeds were started before 2 years of age.

Selection of Formulas

A vast array of formulas that meet the nutrient needs of most children is commercially available. Exactly which formula to select will be determined by the child's developmental age, nutritional needs, food allergies, and gastrointestinal function. The osmolality of the formula, route of delivery, cost, and volume restriction (see Chapter 5) also need to be considered.

Infant formulas are adapted to meet the needs of infants below 1 year of age but can be used beyond 1 year of age, if necessary. For example, a $1\frac{1}{2}$-year-old child who has the weight age of a 9-month-old and has been on limited solids can be maintained on infant formula until her weight reaches that of a 1-year-old. Specific nutrient deficiencies are inherent in soy formulas when they are used in children older than 1 year of age. Some nutrients which are deficient include calcium, zinc, vitamin A, vitamin D, and iron. However, there is a formula marketed for children between the ages of 1–6 years by Ross Pharmaceutical called Pediasure. It is a higher calorie formula (1 cal/cc) with higher calcium, taurine, and iron than infant formulas and lower sodium, potassium, and chloride phosphate than adult formulas.

Adult formulas should be used cautiously in children younger than 1 year of age. The main concerns are increased electrolyte and protein load and specific nutrient inadequacies. Some elemental formulas (which are made for adults) are extremely low in fat which limits the intake of essential fats for the growing child.

Many adult formulas also are low in folic acid and B vitamins. When small volumes of adult formula are infused over a 24-hour period (<1–1.5 liters), this problem becomes particularly important. If malabsorption is not a concern, intact nutrient formulas (polymeric formulas) can be delivered via all routes. Elemental or semi-elemental formulas with free amino acids or small peptides and hydrolyzed fats or primarily medium chain triglycerides are indicated in malabsorption and for transpyloric feeds.

The use of whey-based formulas for children with spastic quadriplegia has been proposed in a recent study (Fried et al., 1992). It was hypothesized that whey protein was superior to hydrolysate because of increased gastric emptying with whey-based formula. Although only 9 patients with CP were studied, whey predominant formulas may play some role in patients with increased gastric emptying time. Whey predominant formulas, including Peptamen, Enfamil, and PM 60/40, may decrease the risk of aspiration.

Blenderized feedings are used less often than commercial formulas because of convenience and cost. Some families prefer preparing the child's formula from the foods of a typical family meal. Psychologically, the parents are comforted by knowing that the child is being fed the "real thing" with a recipe of pureed table foods or baby foods along with formula, milk, or water as a base to liquify. The calories are brought close to 1 cal/cc. The only concern is the viscosity of the formulas which may limit the use of nocturnal continuous drip feeds.

Most blenderized feeds need to be infused with syringe and bolus volume. The following case study illustrates the principles of gastrostomy feedings in a child with developmental disabilities.

Case Study

P.W. is a 16-month-old male with microcephaly, moderate developmental delay, a seizure disorder, and poor weight gain.

He presented to the GI clinic at 16 months of age with severe growth retardation, feeding difficulties, refusal to take liquids, and lengthy feeding times. He is followed at an Early Intervention Program where a variety of feeding strategies have been explored to enhance his feeding skills. These include specific relaxation techniques, positional feeding, oral stimulation, and facilitation techniques. He has a positive gag reflex. He tolerates pureed and baby foods but has extreme difficulty coordinating suck-swallow for liquids. His mother has been using a syringe to provide minimal amounts of fluids.

In August 1989 a nasogastric feeding tube was attempted; however, he choked and gagged severely. No history of vomiting with oral feeds has been reported in the past. Thickened liquids were attempted to increase fluid intake. These attempts were unsuccessful in promoting weight.

Due to P.W.'s significant failure to thrive and inability to consume adequate calories by mouth, it was determined that a gastrostomy tube feeding was necessary for long-term nutrition support. Guidelines were given to enhance calories of pureed foods with polycose until his admission for aggressive nutritional rehabilitation.

Anthropometric measurements and dietary analysis:

weight: 6.8 kg 2.5 S.D. below the 5th percentile

height: 75 cm 3rd percentile

Dietary analysis of 3-day food record reflected an average intake of 480 calories (71 cal/kg), 1.4 gram protein/kg and 60 cc fluid/kg. In view of developmental disability the preferred method of calculating calories is utilizing the basal metabolic rate as follows:

BMR $\times$ 24 $\times$ activity factor $\times$ stress factor

15.56 cal/hr $\times$ 24 $\times$ 1.2 $\times$ 1.3 = 583 calories or 85 cal/kg

The differential between usual intake and required intake is 103 calories. The usual suggestion is to make increments by 5% above usual intake every 24 hours (i.e., 25 kcal per day) until 100 calories added to intake.

Polycose was added to the pureed and baby foods by adding 1 tablespoon per meal and 1 tablespoon to juice which provided 92 calories.

Summary

The use of tube feedings provides a reliable source of nutrition for developmentally disabled children, and they do promote weight gain. However, they are not without complications. The greatest benefit may be in the facilitation of care. Caregivers report improvement in the child's disposition and ease in feeding. The nutritional status also improves with decreased incidence of illnesses and hospitalizations and improved well being.

References

Cronk, C., & Crocker, A. (1988). Growth charts for children with Down syndrome: 1 month to 18 years of age. *Pediatrics, 81*(1), 102–115.

Cully, W. J., & Middleton, T. D. (1968). Calorie requirements of mentally retarded children with and without motor dysfunction. *Journal of Pediatrics, 75*, 380–384.

Dietz, W. H. (1984). Nutritional requirements and feeding of the handicapped child. In R. Grand, J. Sutphen, & W. H. Dietz, *Pediatric nutrition: Theory and practice* (pp. 387–392). Butterworth.

Fried, M. D., Khoshoo, V., Secker, D. J. et al. (1992). Decrease in gastric emptying time and episodes of regurgitation in children with spastic quadraplegia fed a whey-based formula. *Journal of Pediatrics, 120,* 569–572.

Isaacs, J. S., Montagne, M. J., & Davis, B. (1990). Transitioning the child fed by gastrostomy into school. *Journal of the American Dietetic Association, 90*(7), 982–985.

Lifshitz, F., Finch, N. M., & Lifshitz, J. Z. (1991). The handicapped child. *Children's nutrition* (pp. 383–398). Boston, MA: Jones and Bartlett Publishers.

McLoughlin, L. C., Nord, K. S., Oleske, M. J., & Connor, E. (1987). Severe gastrointestinal involvement in children with acquired immunodeficiency syndrome. *Journal of Pediatrics, Gastroenterology, and Nutrition, 6,* 517–24.

Miller, F., & Koresha, K. (1992). Height measures of patients with neuromuscular disease and contractures. *Developmental Medicine and Child Neurology, 34,* 55–60.

Patric, J., Boland, M., Sloski, D., & Murray, G. E. (1986). Rapid correction of wasting in children with cerebral palsy. *Developmental Medicine and Child Neurology, 28,* 734–739.

Phelphs, W. M. (1951). Dieting requirements in cerebral palsy. *Journal of the American Diabetic Association, 27,* 869–870.

Queen, P., & Gallagher, L. (1987). Pediatric nutrition handbook. Boston Children's Hospital, Department of Nutrition and Food Service.

Rempel, G., Colwell, S., & Nelson, R. (1988). Growth in children with cerebral palsy fed via gastrostomy. *Pediatrics, 82*(6), 857–862.

Rice, B. L. (1981, September/October). Nutritional problems of developmentally disabled children. *Pediatric Nursing,* 15–18.

Ruby, D. O., & Matheny, W. D. (1962). Comments on growth of cerebral palsied children. *Journal of the American Dietetic Association, 40,* 525–527.

Sanders, K., Cox, K., Cannon, R., Blanchard, D., Pitcher, J., Papathakis, P, Varella, L., & Maughan, R. (1990). Growth response to enteral feeding by children with cerebral palsy. *Journal of Parenteral and Enteral Nutrition, 4*(1), 23-26.

Shapiro, B., Green, P., Krick, J., Allen, D., & Capote, A. Growth of severely impaired children: Neurological vs nutritional factors. *Developmental Medicine and Child Neurology, 28,* 729–733.

Sitzman, M. D. (1990). Nutritional support of the dysphagic patient: Methods, risks and complications of therapy. *Journal of Parental and Enteral Nutrition, 14,* 60–65.

Spender, Q. W., Cronk, C. E., Charnez, E. B., & Stallings, V. A. (1989). Assessment of linear growth of children with cerebral palsy: Use of alternative measures to height or length. *Developmental Medicine and Child Neurology, 31,* 206–214.

Stanek, K., Hensley, C., & Van Riper, C. (1992). Factors affecting use of food and commercial agents to thicker liquids for individuals with swallowing disorders. *Journal of the American Dietetic Association, 92*(4), 488–490.

Thommessen, M., Rus, G., Kuse, B., Larsen, S., & Heiberg, S. (1992). Energy and nutrient intakes of disabled children: Do feeding problems make a difference? *Journal of the American Diabetic Association, 91,* 1522–1525.

Veldee, M., & Peth, L. (1992). Can protein calorie malnutrition cause dysphagia? *Dysphagia, 7,* 86–101.

Wodarski, L. A. (1990). An interdisciplinary nutrition assessment and intervention protocol for children with disabilities. *Journal of the American Diabetic Association, 90*(1), 1563–1568.

CHAPTER

5

Nutritional Support for the Child with AIDS

SELINA C. MHANGO-MKANDAWIRE, R.D., ED.D.

CONTENTS

Children with AIDS develop neurologic complications leading to developmental disabilities. Dysphagia may result, both from neurologic and infectious complications of human immunodeficiency virus infection (HIV). By supporting optimal nutritional status, diet management can attempt to support growth, prevent weight loss, minimize protein depletion, and improve responses to treatment of opportunistic infection. The child's nutritional therapy must be suited to each change in his or her disease state (see Chapter 6).

Generally, many children with AIDS may appear in good nutritional status. However, the process of educating both the child and family must begin immediately. Portion size, protein intake, and caloric requirements are all discussed. Nutritional status and immune status are interrelated, and AIDS and malnutrition are often linked. The Task Force on Nutrition Support in AIDS (Winick, 1989) stated that: individuals with protein calorie malnutrition (PCM) and other nutrient deficiencies show a depression in cellular immunity with abnormal T-cell and macrophage function. Malnutrition has a deleterious effect on immune function and may cause defects in cellular immunity, neutrophil function, and secretory IgA response (McLoughlin, 1988). Therefore, nutritional support is a vital factor in managing children with AIDS (Bentler & Stanish, 1987), as the immune deficit in AIDS may be secondary to both malnutrition and the AIDS virus itself (Raiten, 1990) (see Table 5–1).

Nutritional assessment for children with AIDS is similar to that for any other child (see Chapter 4). The most important problem in pediatric AIDS patients is failure to thrive (Bentler, 1992). This has been well described in children with HIV infection without secondary infection, as well as in children with AIDS. (Wilkinson & Greenwald, 1988) Most children with AIDS require extra calories and protein for catch-up growth (see Chapter 4). Specific nutrient deficits in zinc, selenium, and folate have been described as well (Raiten, 1990) (see Table 5–2). Nutrient needs are further increased for disease-associated manifestations such as fever and diarrhea.

Nutritional Support for Infants 0–1 Year Old

Nutritional management for the age group 1 month to 1 year must be monitored closely because of the rapid growth and frequent fluctuations in weight. The main food intake at this age is infant formula. The role of breast-feeding is controversial. The risk of transmission is felt to be low; however, three cases of HIV contracted from cell-free breast milk of infected mothers have been reported (Bentler, 1992). The World Health Organization recommends breast-feeding when there are no appropriate available alternatives (World Health Organization, 1987).

In one study (Blanche et al., 1989), 27% of babies born to HIV seropositive mothers were found to develop manifestations of HIV or AIDS by 18 months of age. Each child has to be treated as an individual. An appropriate formula is determined according to individual symptoms. Regular cow's milk formula is recommended if tolerated. We routinely recommend the use of iron-fortified formula because this population is at high risk for anemia. Currently recommended milk formulas include:

Enfamil with Iron (Mead Johnson)

Similac with Iron (Ross Laboratories)

SMA (Wyeth Laboratories)

Often the volume of formula necessary to provide optimum amounts of calories and protein is difficult for the sick infant to tolerate. In these cases, the caloric density of the formula should be increased to 24 to

Table 5–1. Immunological changes associated with AIDS and protein-energy malnutrition.

Immunological Systems	Changes in AIDS	Protein-energy Malnutrition
Cellular Immunity		
T cells	Decreased (++)	Decreased (++)
Helper T cells	Decreased (+++)	Decreased (++)
Helper:suppressor T-cell ratio	Inverted	Inverted
Delayed cutaneous hypersensitivity	Anergy (+)	Anergy (++)
Immature T cells	Increased (++)	Increased (++)
Lymphokine production	Decreased (+)	Decreased (+)
Cytotoxic T cells	Decreased (+)	?
Alloreactivity	Decreased	?
Helper T-cell activity	Decreased (+++)	Decreased (+)
Humoral Immunity		
Serum immunoglobulins	Increased (++)	Increased (++)
Immune complexes in serum	Present (+++)	Present
Primary antibody response	Diminished (++)	Diminished (+)
Circulating immunoglobulin secreting B cells	Increased (+++)	Increased (++)
Antibody affinity	Decreased (++)	Decreased (++)

Source: From Raiten, D. (1990). *Nutrition and HIV infection: A review and evaluation of the extant knowledge of the relationship between nutrition and HIV infection.* (Report Number 223-88-2124), p. 44. Prepared for the Food, Safety, and Applied Nutrition Food and Drug Administration, Department of Health and Human Services, Washington, DC, with permission.

Note: + = Mild, ++ = Moderate, +++ = Severe, ? = No information reported.

Table 5–2. Changes in measures of nutritional status in AIDS.

Nutrient	Measures
Protein	Serum albumin ↓ Serum retinol-binding protein ↓ Serum total protein ↑ Total iron-binding capacity↓
Amino acids	Most serum amino acids ↓
Lipids	Serum triglycerides ↑ Serum fatty acids ↓ Serum cholesterol normal ↓
Folate	Folate in CNS ↓ Serum and erythrocyte folate ↓
Vitamin B12	Serum cobalamin ↓
Vitamin B6	
Zinc	Serum zinc ↓ Zinc-thymulin ↓ Zinc taste test ↓
Selenium	Plasma or serum selenium ↓ Erythrocyte selenium ↓ Cardiac selenium ↓
Copper	Serum copper normal
Iron	Serum ferritin normal Serum iron ↓ Hemoglobin ↓

Source: From Raiten, D. (1990). *Nutrition and HIV infection: A review and evaluation of the extant knowledge of the relationship between nutrition and HIV infection* (Report No. 223-88-2124), p. 26. Prepared for the Food, Safety and Applied Nutrition Food and Drug Administration, Department of Health and Human Services, Washington, DC.

30 cal/oz either by concentration of the formula or addition of modular nutrient supplements (see Chapter 4). There are several high-calorie infant formulas on the market, but their distribution is limited to hospitals only:

Similac with Iron	24	cal/oz
Similac	27	cal/oz
Enfamil with Iron	24	cal/oz
SMA	24	cal/oz
SMA	27	cal/oz

Recommended daily food intake for infants is listed in Table 5–3. Introduction of solids should start at 4 to 6 months; however, the child with developmental disabilities and AIDS may need to be maintained

Table 5-3. Recommended daily food intake for infants.

Food	0–4 months	5–6 months	7–9 months	10–12 months
Beverages	Formula or breast milk	Formula or breast milk	Formula or breast milk	Formula, cows or breast milk
Bread			Zweiback toast, crackers	Enriched bread or toast, crackers
Cereal		Fortified infant rice cereal	Fortified infant cereal, cooked cereal	Enriched dry or cooked cereal
Egg			Egg yolk	Yolk—small amount of white
Fat			Butter and margarine	Margarine
Fruit and fruit juices		Strained, cooked fruit, fruit juices	Cooked fruit, junior fruit, mashed banana, fruit juices	Cooked fruit, banana peeled fresh fruit, fruit juices
Meat, poultry fish, cheese			Strained or pureed meat, cottage cheese, finely chopped meat	Chopped meat, flaked fish, cheese
Soup			Soup made with cooked meat and vegetables	Meat soup
Vegetables		Strained vegetables	Chopped Vegetables, potatoes	Cooked vegetables some raw, according to ability to chew
Desserts		Gelatin	Gelatin, plain, cakes, and cookies (soft)	Plain cakes, cookies (soft), custard

Source: From Mkandawire, S. C. M. (1991). Nutrition and pediatric AIDS. Report of the Subcommittee on the Nutritional Impact of HIV infection in children, American Academy of Pediatrics, (FDA Report No. 223-86-2117), p. 59.

Note:
0–4 months: 100% infant formula[1] or breast milk.
5–6 months: – 90% of total calories should be derived from breast milk or baby formula.
7–9 months: 70–80% of total calories should be from breast milk or formula.
10–2 months: 50–60% of total calories should be from breast milk or formula.
Above 12 months child may switch to whole cow's milk supplying 50% of total calories.

[1]Breast feeding is discouraged in HIV infected mothers because the HIV has been isolated in breast milk of HIV+ mothers.

on formula until able to accept spoon feedings (Pressman & Morrison, 1988).

Lactose intolerance secondary to chronic malnutrition or chronic gastrointestinal infection is common. These infants may require a soy-based formula or the addition of Lactaid® to their formula. Other special formulas are also available (see Table 5–4).

Nutritional Support of Pediatric AIDS Patients Aged 1–18 Years

Nutrient intake should be based on a *balanced diet* that provides adequate nutrients from meats, milk, fruit, and vegetables, as well as starches. It should be emphasized that, due to lack of specific

Table 5–4. Formulas appropriate for infants with diarrhea and/or malabsorption.

Etiology of Diarrhea	Formula Product	Rationale for Use
Lactose intolerance	Pediasure	Lactose free
	Prosobee	Soy protein, sucrose free
	Isomil	Soy protein
	Nursoy	Soy protein, corn oil free
	Lactofree	Soy protein
Chronic persistent	Same as above	
	Nutramigen	Casein hydrolysate
		Lactose free
		Corn syrup solids
	Alimentum	Casein hydrolysate
		Lactose free
		Contains sucrose
Milk protein allergy	Soy-based formula	
	Nutramigen	
	Alimentum	
Intractable diarrhea	Pregestamil	Pre-digested formula
		Casein hydrolysate
		Corn syrup solids
		58% MCT oil
	MJ 3232A	Predigested formula
		Casein hydrolysate
		Mono and disaccharide free
		87% MCT oil
Fat malabsorption	Portagen	Fat is 88% MCT oil
	Lipisorb	86% MCT oil
		Lactose free

Source: Adapted from Children's Hospital of New Jersey Pediatric Outpatient Nutrition Services Manual, Newark, NJ.

knowledge about nutritional needs of children with AIDS, nutritional support has been based on a symptomatic approach. When these children are feeling well, they should be encouraged to eat a high calorie, high protein balanced diet.

Nutritional Management of the Asymptomatic HIV Infected Child

This section is devoted to the stable child with AIDS who is not yet experiencing any acute illness or symptoms. Most children with AIDS have difficulty gaining weight and may lose it very easily. Because of this, the goal is to help the child maintain and gain weight and prevent weight loss. The usual diet for a stable child with AIDS is 100 to 150% of the recommended daily intake, depending on individual child needs. The goal is to provide a diet well balanced in meat, milk, fruit, vegetables, and starches. Food intake is outlined according to age. Table 5–5 contains the recommended daily food intake for children aged 1 to 18 years. Following this plan should ensure that the child eats adequate calories and nutrients for growth. High calorie nutritious supplements are recommended to increase calories (see Table 5–6). The methods described use food found in the home. The ingredients will vary according to the appetite and individual tolerance of the patient. The best results are often obtained if caloric intake is increased gradually. Foods may be added to meals, used as between meal feedings, or taken as bedtime snacks.

If the stable child with developmental disabilities and AIDS aged 1 to 18 years is well fed using the four food groups and supplemented with high calorie snacks, there is no reason the child needs to be maintained on an expensive formula to achieve a high calorie intake. It should be emphasized that food intake by the oral route utilizing table foods in the home is the goal for the nutritionist.

The Infant and Child with AIDS Experiencing Acute Diarrhea

Diarrhea with secondary nutrient malabsorption in infants and children with AIDS is very common. The formulas in Table 5–4 are recommended for these children.

A clear liquid diet is often used initially in a child with acute diarrhea. If diarrhea persists however, a more complete nutritional source such as a specialized formula must be considered.

Clear Liquid Diet

Purpose

The purpose of a clear liquid diet is to provide a readily absorbed source of fluids with an extremely small amount of residue (see Tables 5–7 and 5–8). Commercially prepared, low-residue or chemically defined formula diets are used to provide adequate nutrients when absorption is a long-term problem (see Table 5–4).

Adequacy

The clear liquid diet is inadequate in all nutrients.

Lactose Free Diet

Purpose

The level of restriction is adjusted to the individual child. This diet excludes all foods that contain lactose. In children with chronic diarrhea, the gastrointestinal tract (GI) may lack the enzyme lactase. Lactase helps digest the sugar (lactose) found in milk and milk products. Although some children may eat food with reduced lactose load (i.e., cheese and yogurt) without problems, others cannot tolerate foods that contain any lactose. The level of restriction is adjusted to the individual child's needs (see Tables 5–9 and 5–10).

Table 5-5. Recommended daily food intake for children 1 to 18 years old.

Foods	Servings Per Day	Average Size Servings for Age					
		1 yr.	2–3 yrs.	4–5 yrs.	6–9 yrs.	10–12 yrs.	13–18 yrs.
Milk and Cheese	4	1/2 cup	1/2–3/4 cup	3/4 cup	3/4–1 cup	1 cup	1 cup
Meat Group	3 or more	2 tbsp.	2 tbsp.	4 tbsp.	2–4 oz.	3–4 oz.	4 oz. or more
Fruits and Vegetables							
Vitamin C Source	1 or more	1/3 cup	1/2 cup	1/2 cup	1/2 cup	1/2 cup	1/2 cup or more
Vitamin A Source	1 or more	2 tbsp.	3 tbsp.	4 tbsp.	1/4 cup	1/3 cup	1/2 cup
Other Vegetables	2	2 tbsp.	3 tbsp.	1/4 cup	1/3 cup	1/2 cup	3/4 cup
and Fruits		1/4 cup	1/3 cup	1/2 cup	1 medium	1 medium	1 medium to large
Cereals and Breads	4 or more						
Whole grain or enriched bread		1/2 slice	1 slice	1½ slices	1–2 slices	2 slices	2 or more slices
Cereal		1/4 cup	1/3 cup	1/2 cup	1/2 cup	3/4 cup	1 cup or more
Fats	3	1 tsp.	1 tsp.	1 tsp.	1 tsp.	1 tsp. or more	1 tsp. or more
Desserts	2	1/4 cup Simple dessert	1/3 cup Simple dessert	1/3 cup Simple dessert	1/2 cup	1/2 cup	1/2 cup or more

Source: From Mkandawire, S. C. M. (1985). *Diet Guidelines for Children with AIDS*, p. 5. Children's Hospital of New Jersey, Newark, NJ. Copyright registration number TX2290070.

Table 5–6. Suggestions for increasing calories.

1. To add 500 calories, select one of the following:

    a. 1 pint half milk and half cream
    b. 1 pint milk, 1½ slices bread, 1 tsp. butter or margarine
    c. 8 oz. hot chocolate, 4 butter cookies
    d. 6 oz. milk, 1 egg, 1 cup buttered vegetables, and 3 slices bread
    e. 1 cup cooked or 1½ cups dry cereal, 8 oz. milk, 1 banana, and 1½ tbsp. sugar
    f. 2 slices bread, 2 oz. meat, 2 tsp. butter, and ½ cup ice cream

2. To add 1000 calories, select two of the above groups or one of the following:

    a. Three 6 oz. glasses eggnog, malted milk, or other milk nourishment; 3 tbsp. jelly and 3 tsp. butter or margarine and 2 slices of bread
    b. 4 slices bread, 3 tsp. butter or margarine, 1 cup vegetable, 1 egg, 1 pint of milk, and 2 tbsp. sugar or jelly
    c. Four servings of instant breakfast—distribute throughout the day

Table 5–7. Clear liquid diet.

Foods	Allowed	Not Allowed
Beverages	Weak tea, carbonated beverages, soda, Citrotein (high calorie protein supplement)	Milk, cream, milk drinks
Dessert	Plain gelatin dessert, water ices, popsicles, high protein jello	All others
Fruit Juices	Apple, cranberry & grape juice, fruit punch	All others
Soup	Fat-free bouillon (chicken or beef) or fat-free broth, high protein beef or chicken broths	
Sweets	Sugars, honey, syrups, hard candy	All others

Source: From Mkandawire, S. C. M. (1985). *Diet guidelines for children with AIDS*, p. 7. Children's Hospital of New Jersey, Newark, NJ. Copyright registration number TX2290070.

Because of increased demands for protein and calories in children with AIDS and developmental disabilities, the child may need to eat 5 to 6 times a day. Consistency and texture have to be changed according to individual taste and tolerance.

Adequacy

This diet is not sufficient in Vitamin D, calcium, and riboflavin. A daily multiple vitamin is needed to supplement the diet, and a calcium supplement may be prescribed by the health care provider (see Chapter 4).

Table 5–8. Suggested meal plan for clear liquid diet.

Meal	Foods
Breakfast	Apple Juice (¹/₂ cup)
	Jello (¹/₂ cup)
	Weak Tea (1 cup)
	Sugar (1 tsp.)
Morning Snack (10 a.m.)	Apple Juice (¹/₂ cup)
Lunch	Broth (1 cup)
	Grape Juice (¹/₂ cup)
	Fruit Ice (¹/₂ cup)
	Weak Tea (1 cup)
	Sugar (1 tsp.)
Afternoon Snack (3 p.m.)	Grape Juice (¹/₂cup)
Dinner	Broth (1 cup)
	Cranberry Juice (1 cup)
	Fruit Ice (¹/₂ cup)
	Jello (¹/₂ cup)
	Weak Tea (1 cup)
	Sugar (1 tsp.)

Source: From Mkandawire, S. C. M. (1985). *Diet guidelines for children with AIDS*, p. 6. Children's Hospital of New Jersey, Newark, NJ, with permission. Copyright registration number TX2290070.

Nutritional Support for the Child with AIDS Experiencing Thrush and/or Dysphagia

A study done by Pressman and Morrison (1988) revealed that 45% of children with AIDS had dysphagia ranging from mild to severe. Oral thrush in the pediatric AIDS population has been known to extend into the esophagus and cause fever, poor appetite, weight loss, and vomiting. A diet that is generally acceptable for these children is pureed-bland. Children with pediatric AIDS and dysphagia tolerate semisolid foods with the consistency and smooth texture of a pudding. A speech therapist is vital to the health care team for determining appropriate positioning of the child and evaluating swallowing problems.

Thrush is caused by *Candida albicans*. It can affect the mouth, throat, esophagus, and make eating so painful that providing adequate nutritional intake becomes extremely difficult (see Table 5–11). Some parents find that warm soup before a soft meal helps the child eat food without much irritation. Other parents use ice pops to numb the child's irritated mouth. Diet for each child should be individualized according to food preferences (see Table 5–12).

Bland Pureed Diet for the Child with Thrush, Herpes, and Dysphagia

The pureed-bland diet is bland and mechanically soft to reduce irritation. Citrus

Table 5–9. Lactose-free diet.

Foods	Allowed	Not Allowed
Beverages	Weak tea, carbonated	Instant coffee, powdered soft drink mix
Milk	Soy bean milk, lactose-free formulas (e.g., Prosobee) lactose-free nutrient supplement (e.g., Sustacal, Ensure, Resource, etc.)	Milk and milk products: whole, skimmed, dried, evaporated, condensed; buttermilk, yogurt, ice cream, malted milk, cocoa, sherbet, Ovaltine, hot chocolate
Soup	Broth, bouillon, broth-based soups	Cream soups, commercial soups that contain milk products
Fruit and juices	All fresh, canned or frozen that are not processed with milk	Any canned or frozen processed lactose
Meat, fish, poultry	Plain beef, lamb, veal, pork, ham, fish, shellfish, poultry, lentils, peanut butter	Creamed or breaded meat, fish, poultry, sausage, frankfurters, cold cuts containing dry milk solids. Peanut butter containing milk fillers
Eggs	All except those prepared with milk	Any that are prepared with milk
Cheese	None	All
Vegetables	All fresh, frozen, canned prepared without milk or milk products	Any processed with lactose, creamed, breaded, or buttered vegetables
Potatoes and substitutes	White and sweet potatoes, yams, macaroni, spaghetti, rice, noodles, all prepared without milk or milk products	Those prepared with milk or milk products. Frozen french fries if processed with lactose. Instant potatoes
Breads and Cereals	Any that do not contain milk and milk products: French and Italian bread, low sodium bread, cereals containing no milk, milk products, or lactose	Any products containing milk products of lactose: commercially baked goods and mixes, some dry cereals, snack foods (Read labels carefully.)
Fats	Margarines and dressing made without milk products. Shortening bacon, water-based gravies, olives, nuts	Margarines or dressing containing milk products or lactose. Butter, cream cheese
Desserts	Water and fruit ices, gelatin, and desserts made without milk products. High protein jello	Ice cream, sherbets, custard, puddings, commercial cakes, pies, cookies, and mixes if they contain milk
Condiments and others	Soy sauce, sugar, jellies, marmalades, corn syrup, baker's cocoa, honey, pure sugar candies, salt, pepper, pure spices, pickles, herbs, catsup, mustard, hard candy, lollipops	Cream candies, milk chocolate, caramels, peppermint, butterscotch, any that contain milk products or lactose

Source: From Mkandawire, S. C. M. (1985). *Diet guidelines for children with AIDS*, p. 9–10. Children's Hospital of New Jersey, Newark, NJ, with permission. Copyright registration number TX2290070.

Table 5–10. Suggested meal plan for lactose-free diet.

Meal	Foods
Breakfast	Apple juice (1/2 cup) Farina (1/2 cup) Soft cooked egg (1) Margarine (1 tsp. or more)
Lunch	Grape Juice (1/2 cup) Broiled Chicken (1–2 oz.) Rice (1/2 cup) Spinach (1/2 cup) Lettuce and tomato (Dressing) Pineapple slices (2) Margarine (1 tsp. or more)
Afternoon snack (3 p.m.)	Apple juice (1/2 cup) Crackers and peanut butter (3)
Dinner	Apple juice (1/2 cup) Roast beef (1–2 oz.) Mashed potatoes (1/2 cup) Carrots (1/2 cup) Pear Halves (2) French Bread (1 slice) Margarine (1 tsp.)
8 p.m. or bedtime	Meat (1–2 oz.) sandwich on 1 slice of bread Juice (1/2 cup)

Source: From Mkandawire, S. C. M. (1985). *Diet guidelines for children with AIDS*, p. 8. Children's Hospital of New Jersey, Newark, NJ, with permission. Copyright registration number TX2290070.

and pineapple juices are eliminated unless the child can tolerate these juices (see Tables 5–13 and 5–14). The goal of this diet is to provide high calorie, low volume foods designed to reduce chemical and physical irritation. It also reduces the effort needed to chew and swallow. This diet generally progresses from full liquid to solid food. The diet consists of six small daily feedings taken at a frequency of every 3 to 4 hours. Food is served at room temperature. For the child who has difficulty swallowing liquids, the consistency of the food will need to be adjusted accordingly. Products such as Thickit™, jello powder, or baby dry cereal may be used to thicken the liquid food to enhance safe swallowing (see Chapter 4). Thickeners generally add to the caloric density of the food, and are therefore advantageous for the child's overall nutritional care. For children who tolerate semisolid foods, the most well-accepted is pudding consistency.

Nutrition Support for the Child with AIDS and Fever

It is generally accepted that caloric needs increase by 7% for every degree Fahrenheit above normal temperature in a febrile child (Bentler & Stanish, 1987). Fever predisposes children as well as adults to higher energy expenditure (labored breathing has a

Table 5-11. Oral and esophageal manifestations of AIDS that interfere with food intake.

Condition or Lesion	Location	Signs and Symptoms
Candidiasis	Oral or esophageal	Pain, dysphagia (difficulty swallowing), odynophagia (painful swallowing), dysguesia (impairment in sense of taste), nausea, esophagitis, decreased salivation
Herpes simplex virus	Oral or esophageal	Dysphagia, odynophagia, esophagitis
Human papilloma virus	Oral	Oral warts, papillomas, condylomata and focal epithelia, hyperplasia
Herpes zoster	Oral	Unilateral pain, vesicular eruption
Cytomegalovirus	Oral or esophageal	Dysphagia, odynophagia (rare), esophagitis
Hairy Leukoplakia	Oral	Usually asymptomatic
Cryptosporidiosis	Esophageal	Dysphagia
Premature progressive periodontitis	Oral	Irregular, generalized bone destruction
Gingivitis	Oral	Halitosis, bleeding gums
Nonspecific esophageal ulcers	Esophageal	Odynophagia

Source: From Raiten, D. (1990). *Nutrition and HIV infection: A review and evaluation of the extant knowledge of the relationship between nutrition and HIV infection,* Report No. 223-88-2124, p. 35. Prepared for the Food, Safety, and Applied Nutrition Food and Drug Administration, Department of Health and Human Services, Washington, DC, with permission.

Table 5–12. Some suggestions to relieve oral discomfort when feeding by mouth.

Condition	Acidic Foods/ Beverages	Temperature	Texture/ Consistency	Consistency
Mouth pain, sores	Avoid citrus pineapple	Avoid extremes	Nonabrasive easy to swallow foods	Spices and salt may not be tolerated
Dulled taste Sensation	Provide acids to breakdown mucus	Provide extremes to stimulate appetite	Variety of textures	Provide as tolerated to stimulate appetite
Partial esophageal obstruction	Avoid open lesions	N.A.	Adjust for mechanical soft or liquid as tolerated	Avoid hot spices on open lesions
Swallowing dysfunction	N.A.	Provide extremes (hot or cold) to stimulate	Avoid thin liquids Avoid true solids Provide food or food combinations resulting in cohesive bolus Avoid sticky foods Avoid slippery foods	Provide to stimulate mouth sensation

Source: From Winick, J. (1989). Task Force on Nutrition Support in AIDS: Guidelines for nutrition support in AIDS. *Nutrition*, 5(1), 39, with permission.

similar effect on energy use, although the amount of energy needed is generally up to 150% of the RDA). For example, if a child's caloric needs were 900 cals per day and the child had a fever of 5° Fahrenheit above normal body temperature, the child's caloric needs would increase by (7% of 900) 63 × 5 = 315. The child's total caloric needs would therefore be 315 cals + 900 cals = 1215 kcals per day. The 315 additional calories are to compensate for increased body temperature which increases energy use.

Enteral Formulas

When adequate nutrient intake cannot be achieved by the oral route, a commercial nu-

tritional supplement may be used to increase protein, calories, vitamins, and minerals. At present, there are no special formulas for pediatric AIDS patients. For the infant, either milk formula or specialized infant formulas are used (see Table 5–4). Pediasure® (Ross Laboratories) is a nutritionally complete formula designed to meet the nutrient needs of children aged 1 to 6 years. It is lactose-free, but otherwise unsuitable for children with severe malabsorption. Because of its cost and individual taste preference, adult formulations are also utilized. Excellent formulations are available for children with and without malabsorption (see Tables 5–15, 5–16, 5–17, and 5–18). When adult formulas are used, caution must be taken to ensure vitamin and

Table 5–13. Bland-pureed diet.

Foods	Allowed	Not Allowed
Milk	Milk, plain yogurt with soft fruit	Chocolate milk and yogurt with hard fruits or nuts
Soup	Soup, strained cream soup, strained vegetable soup	Broth, bouillon cube
Fruits, juices, and beverages	Pureed or strained fruits (e.g., applesauce, apricot nectar, etc.). Ripe banana Fruit juices except those not allowed. Milk, ginger ale, 7-Up, orange soda	Fresh fruits, citrus and pineapple juices. Coke, Pepsi with caffeine
Meats	Pureed or cooked until very tender. Fish without bones	Fried meats, tough meats, etc.
Eggs	Soft-boiled, scrambled, etc.	Fried eggs
Cheese	Cottage cheese, American cheeses, Swiss cheese	Hard cheese, cheeses with seeds, etc.
Vegetables	Pureed or strained vegetables, mashed yellow squash	Raw vegetables, hard cooked vegetables
Potatoes	Mashed white and sweet potatoes	All others
Breads and Cereals	Refined cooked cereal, bread, plain muffins	All others
Fats	Butter, margarine, oil, mayonnaise	All others
Desserts	Custard, jello, plain pudding	Chocolate
Seasoning	Salt	All spices (e.g., hot black pepper, hot sauce, vinegar, chili powder)

Source: Mkandawire, S. C. M. (1985). *Diet guidelines for children with AIDS*, pp. 11–12. Children's Hospital of New Jersey, Newark, NJ, with permission. Copyright registration number TX2290070.

mineral adequacy. "The major problem with the use of adult formulation . . . is that the vitamin and mineral intake may be inadequate when provided in small pediatric volumes" (Grand, Sutphen, & Dietz, 1987). Therefore, we recommend a multiple vitamin and mineral supplement for children in this age group who are taking adult formulas. The major deciding factor in choosing an enteral supplement for the child without malabsorption is how well the child likes the product. One method that has been successful for determining the individual child's preference is to hold taste panels using the different products. Children are able to identify a preference for a specific product so that when the need arises to provide the child with nutritional supplementation, prescriptions can be written for their favorite product. Many of these enteral formulas may be taken by mouth to supplement meals and if necessary to replace meals.

Table 5–14. Sample menu for bland-pureed diet.

Meal	Foods
Breakfast	Apple juice ($1/2$ cup) Cream of Wheat (1 cup) Soft boiled egg (1) Slice of bread (1) Weak tea with sugar
Morning Snack	Milk ($1/2$ cup, made from $1/2$ cream and $1/2$ milk) Graham crackers (2)
Lunch and Dinner	Cream soup (1 cup, pureed or soft cooked meat) Mashed potatoes ($1/2$ cup) Pureed carrots ($1/2$ cup) Custard ($1/2$ cup)
Afternoon Snack	Jello with whipped cream ($1/2$ cup) Vanilla milk snack (1 cup)
Bedtime	Vanilla milk shake (1 cup)

Source: From Mkandawire, S. C. M. (1985). *Diet guidelines for children with AIDS*, p. 11. Children's Hospital of New Jersey, Newark, NJ, with permission. Copyright registration number TX2290070.

Enteral formulas may be increased in caloric density by using a modular nutrient supplement (see Chapter 4). Case Study 1 illustrates some of these principles in an infant.

Case Study 1

KF is a 12-month-old Black HIV+ male born at 22 weeks gestation to an 18-year-old cocaine-abusing mother. The baby has gastroesophageal reflux (GER) as well as short bowel syndrome secondary to an ileal resection following necrotizing enterocolitis. He had long-term parenteral nutrition in the neonatal nursery and developed cholelithiasis. In addition, his problems include bronchopulmonary dysplasia, retinopathy of prematurity, and a seizure disorder. He is developmentally delayed, and hearing and vision are impaired.

Nutritional Assessment

WT: 6.05 kg < 5%

HT: 66.2 cm

WT/HT: < 5%

Ideal Body Weight = 7.5 kg (WT/HT at the 50th percentile)

Caloric Needs = 120 cal/kg/day (based on RDA for weight/age)

Ideal Calories for KF = 120 × 7.5
                      = 900 cal/Day

Actual Caloric Intake = 314–400 cal/Day (based on 24-hour recall)

Level of Malnutrition (see Table 5–19):

$$\frac{\text{Actual Weight} \times 100}{\text{Ideal Weight}}$$

Table 5-15. Standard meal replacement formulas.

	PediaSure (Ross)	Ensure (Ross)	Sustacal (Mead Johnson)	Newtrition (Knight Medical)	Entera (Fresenius)
Cal/ml	1	1.06	1.0	1.06	1.06
Protein g/dl	3	3.7	6.1	3.6	3.8
Source	Na caseinate Low lactose whey	Na & Ca caseinate Soy protein isolate	Ca & Na caseinate Soy protein isolate	Ca & Na caseinate Soy protein isolate	Ca & Na caseinate Soy protein isolate
% Cal	12%	14%	24%	14%	15%
Fat g/dl	4.9	3.7	2.3	4	3.4
Source	Safflower, soy & MCT oil	Corn oil	Soy oil	Corn oil	Sunflower & MCT oil
% Cal	44%	31.5%	21%	34%	30%
Carbohydrate g/dl	11	14.5	14	14	13.8
Source	Hydrolyzed corn starch Sucrose	Corn syrup Sucrose	Sucrose Corn syrup	Sucrose Maltodextrin Glucose solids	Maltodextrin Sucrose
% Cal	44%	54.5%	55%	52%	55%
Osmolality	325	470	620–700	450	420
Na (mEq/L)	16.5	37	41	26	35
K (mEq/L)	33.5	40	54	26	34
Ca (mg/L)	970	528	1010	600	800
P (mg/L)	800	528	950	600	640
Ca/P ratio	1.2:1	1:1	1:1	1:1	1.25:1
Volume to meet the USRDA	1100	1887	1080	1665	1892
Form	Liquid/Flavored	Liquid/flavored	Liquid/flavored	Liquid/flavored	Liquid/flavored

(Continued)

Table 5–15. *(Continued)*

	Nutrapak (Corpak)	Resource (Sandoz)	Nutren 1.0 (Clintec)	Meritene (Sandoz)	Carnation Instant Breakfast mixed with 8 oz. whole milk (Clintec)
Cal/ml	1.06	1.06	1.0	1	1.05
Protein g/dl	3.7	3.7	4	5.8	5.7
Source	Na & Ca caseinate Soy protein isolate	Na & Ca caseinate Soy protein isolate	Ca caseinate	Skim milk Na caseinate	Nonfat milk Soy protein Na caseinate
% Cal	14%	14%	16%	24%	22%
Fat g/dl	3.7	3.7	3.8	3.2	3.08
Source	Corn oil	Corn oil	Corn & MCT oil	Corn oil	Milkfat
% Cal	31.5%	31.5%	33%	30%	26%
Carbohydrate g/dl	14.5	14.5	12.7	11	13.4
Source	Corn syrup solids Sucrose	Maltodextrin Sucrose	Maltodextrin Corn syrup & sucrose	Corn syrup solids Sucrose Lacrose	Sucrose, corn syrup solids & lactose
% Cal	54.5%	54.5%	51%	46%	51%
Osmolality	450	430	340	505	700
Na (mEq/L)	37	30	22	38	42
K (mEq/L)	40	30	32	41	71
Ca (mg/L)	530	550	500	1200	1845
P (mg/L)	530	550	500	1200	1533
Ca/P ratio	1:1	1:1	1:1	1:1	1.2:1
Volume to meet the USRDA	1892	1893	2000	1250	1060
Form	Liquid/flavored	Liquid/flavored Powdered	Liquid/flavored	Liquid/flavored Powdered	Liquid/flavored

(Continued)

Table 5-15. *(Continued)*

	Osmolite (Ross)	Isocal (Mead Johnson)	Newtriton Isotonic (Knight Medical)	Entralife (Corpak)	Attain (Sherwood Medical)
Cal/ml	**1.06**	1.06	1.6	1.0	1
Protein g/dl	**3.7**	3.4	3.6	3.5	4
Source	**Na & Ca caseinate Soy protein isolate**	Na & Ca caseinate Soy protein isolate	Na & Ca caseinate Soy protein isolate	Na & Ca caseinate	Na & Ca caseinate
% Cal	**14%**	13%	13.5%	14%	16%
Fat g/dl	**3.8**	4.4	3.6	3.5	4
Source	**MCT, corn & soy oil**	Soy & MCT oil	Corn & MCT oil	Corn & MCT oil	Corn oil
% Cal	**31.4%**	37%	30.5	31.4%	36%
Carbohydrate g/dl	**14.5**	13.3	14.8	13.6	12
Source	**Hydrolyzed cornstarch**	Maltodextrin	Maltodextrin	Maltodextrin	Maltodextrin
% Cal	**54.6%**	50%	56%	54.6%	48%
Osmolality	**300**	300	300	300	300
Na (mEq/L)	**28**	23	26	26	30
K (mEq/L)	**26**	34	26	25	29
Ca (mg/L)	**528**	630	600	500	625
P (mg/L)	**528**	530	600	500	625
Ca/P ratio	**1:1**	1.1:1	1:1	1:1	1:1
Volume to meet the USRDA	**1887**	1890	1900	2000	1600
Form	**Liquid/unflavored**	Liquid/unflavored	Liquid/unflavored	Liquid/unflavored	Liquid/unflavored

Source: From Hendricks, K., & Walker, W. (1990). *Manual of pediatric nutrition* (2nd ed.). p. 94, 95, 96. Philadelphia: B. C. Decker, with permission.

Table 5-16. Meal replacement formulas with fiber.

	Jevity (Ross)	Profiber (Sherwood)	Newtrition Isofiber (Knightic Medical)	Enrich (Ross)	Sustacal with Fiber (Mead Johnson)	Vitaneed (Sherwood)	Compleat (Sandoz)
Cal/ml	1.06	1.06	1.2	1.1	1.06	1	1.07
Protein g/dl	4.4	4	5	4	4.6	4	4.3
Source	Na & Ca caseinate	Na & Ca caseinate	Casein Soy protein isolate	Na & Ca caseinate Soy protein isolate	Na & Ca caseinate Soy protein isolate	Pureed beef, Ca & Na caseinate	Pureed beef Nonfat milk
% Cal	17%	16%	17%	14.5%	17%	16%	16%
Fat g/dl	3.7	4	3.7	3.7	3.5	4	4.3
Source	MCT, corn & soy oil	Corn oil	Corn & MCT oil	Corn oil	Corn oil	Pureed beef Corn oil	Pureed beef Corn oil
% Cal	30%	36%	30%	30.5%	30%	36%	36%
Carbohydrate g/dl	15.2	13.2	16	16.2	14	12.8	12.8
Source	Hydrolyzed cornstarch soy polysaccharide	Hydrolyzed cornstarch	Maltodextrin	Hydrolyzed cornstarch Sucrose	Maltodextrin Sucrose	Pureed green beans, peaches, carrots Maltodextrin	Cereal solids, pureed beans, peas, peaches, Maltodextrin
% Cal	53%	48%	53%	55%	53%	48%	48%
Osmolality	310	300	310	480	480	300	405
Na (mEq/L)	40.5	32	36	37	31	30	56.5
K (mEq/L)	40	32	32	40	36	32	36
Ca (mg/L)	910	667	847	719	845	667	670
P (mg/L)	758	667	847	719	704	667	1300
Ca/P ratio	1.2:1	1:1	1:1	1:1	1.2:1	1:1	1:5
Volume to meet the USRDA	1321	1500	1250	1391	1420	1500	1500
Form	Liquid/ unflavored	Liquid/ unflavored	Liquid/ unflavored	Liquid/ flavored	Liquid/ flavored	Liquid	Liquid/ blenderized
Features/ indications	14.4 g fiber/L	12 g fiber/L	14 g fiber/L	14.4 g fiber/L	5.9 g fiber/L	6 g fiber/L	

Source: From Hendricks, K., & Walker, W. (1990). *Manual of pediatric nutrition* (2nd ed.), p. 97. Philadelphia: B. C. Decker, with permission.

Table 5-17. Meal replacement formulas with high protein-caloric density.

	Ensure Plus (Ross)	Sustacal HC (Mead Johnson)	Resource Plus (Sandoz)	Nutren 1.5 (Clintec)	Comply (Sherwood)	TraumaCal (Mead Johnson)
Cal/ml	1.5	1.5	1.25	1.5	1.5	1.5
Protein g/dl	5.5	6.1	5.5	6	6	8.3
Source	Na & Ca caseinate Soy protein isolate	Na & Ca caseinate	Na & Ca caseinate Soy protein isolate	Caseinate	Na & Ca caseinate	Na & Ca caseinate
% Cal	14.7%	16%	14.7%	16%	16%	22%
Fat g/dl	5.3	5.8	5.3	6.7	6	6.8
Source	Corn oil	Corn oil	Corn oil	MCT & corn oil	Corn oil	Soy & MCT oil
% Cal	32%	34%	32	39%	36%	40%
Carbohydrate g/dl	20	19	208	17	18	14.3
Source	Corn syrup Sucrose	Corn syrup solids Sucrose	Maltodextrin Sucrose	Maltodextrin Corn syrup	Hydrolyzed corn starch	Corn syrup Sucrose
% Cal	53%	50%	53.3%	45%	48%	38%
Osmolality	690	650	600	420–600	410	490
Na (mEq/L)	50	36	39	33	48	51
K (mEq/L)	54	38	45	49	47	36
Ca (mg/L)	706	850	634	761	1000	750
P (mg/L)	706	850	634	761	1000	750
Ca/P ratio	1:1	1:1	1	1:1	1:1	1:1
Volume to meet the USRDA	1420	1200	1600	1333	1000	2000
Form	Liquid/flavored	Liquid/flavored	Liquid/flavored	Liquid/flavored	Liquid/unflavored or flavored	Liquid/flavored

(Continued)

Table 5–17. *(Continued)*

	Ensure HN (Ross)	Entralife HN (Corpak)	Isocal HN (Mead Johnson)	Isocal HCN (Mead Johnson)	Ensure Plus HN (Ross)	Isosource (Sandoz)
Cal/ml	1.06	1	1.06	2	1.5	1.2
Protein g/dl	4.4	4.2	4.4	7.5	6.3	4.3
Source	Na & Ca caseinate Soy protein isolate	Na & Ca caseinate	Na & Ca caseinate Soy protein isolate	Na & Ca caseinate	Na & Ca caseinate	Na & Ca caseinate
% Cal	16.7%	16.7%	17%	15%	16.7%	14%
Fat g/dl	3.55	3.4	4.5	10.2	5	4.2
Source	Corn oil	Corn & MCT oil	Soy & MCT oil	Soy & MCT oil	Corn oil	MCT & Canola oil
% Cal	30%	30.4%	36%	45%	30%	30%
Carbohydrate g/dl	14.1	13.3	12.4	20	20	16.5
Source	Corn syrup Sucrose	Maltodextrin	Maltodextrin	Corn syrup	Hydrolyzed corn starch Sucrose	Maltodextrin
% Cal	53.2%	52.9%	47%	40%	53.3%	56%
Osmolality	470	300	300	690	650	390
Na (mEq/L)	40.5	40	40.5	35	51.5	31.3
K (mEq/L)	40	32	41	43	47	43
Ca (mg/L)	756	800	850	761	1059	680
P (mg/L)	756	800	850	761	1059	680
Ca/P ratio	1:1	1:1	1:1	1:1	1:1	1:1
Volume to meet the USRDA	1321	1250	1500	1000	947	1500
Form	Liquid/Flavored	Liquid/unflavored	Liquid/unflavored	Liquid/flavored	Liquid/flavored High nitrogen	Liquid/flavored

(Continued)

Table 5-17. *(Continued)*

	Magnacal (Sherwood)	Nutren 2.0 (Clintec)	Pulmocare (Ross)	Osmolite HN (Ross)	Isosource HN (Sandoz)	TwoCal HN (Ross)
Cal/ml	2	2	1.5	1.06	1.2	2
Protein g/dl	7	8	6	4.4	5.3	8.4
Source	Na & Ca caseinate	Casein	Na & Ca caseinate	Na & Ca caseinate Soy Protein isolate	Na & Ca caseinate	Na & Ca caseinate
% Cal	14%	16.%	16.7%	16.7%	17%	16.7%
Fat g/dl	8	10.6	9.2	3.7	4.2	9.1
Source	Soy oil	Corn & MCT oil	Corn oil	MCT, corn & soy oil	MCT & canola oil	Corn & MCT oil
% Cal	36%	45%	55.2%	30%	30%	40%
Carbohydrate g/dl	25	19.6	10.6	14.1	15.5	21.7
Source	Maltodextrin Sucrose	Maltodextrin Corn syrup	Sucrose Hydrolyzed cornstarch	Glucose polymers	Maltodextrin	Hydrolyzed cornstarch Sucrose
% Cal	50%	39%	28.1%	53.3%	53%	43%
Osmolality	590	800	520	300	390	690
Na (mEq/L)	43.5	43	57	40.5	31.3	46
K (mEq/L)	32	64	49	40.3	44	59.5
Ca (mg/L)	1000	1000	1057	758	680	1057
P (mg/L)	1000	1000	1057	758	680	1057
Ca/P ratio	1:1	1:1	1:1	1:1	1:1	1:1
Volume to meet the USRDA	1000	1000	947	1321	1500	947
Form	Liquid/flavored	Liquid/flavored	Liquid/flavored High fat formulaftion for dietary management of respiratory insufficiency	Liquid/unflavored	Liquid/flavored	Liquid/flavored

Source: From Hendricks, K., & Walker, W. (1990). *Manual of pediatric nutrition* (2nd ed.), p. 98, 99, 99, 100. Philadelphia: B. C. Decker, with permission.

Table 5–18. Meal replacement formulas with semi-elemental modifications.

	Criticare (Mead Johnson)	Peptamen (Clintec)	Tolerex (Norwich Eaton)	Vivonex T.E.N. (Norwich Eaton)	Pepti-2000 (Sherwood)	Vital HN (Ross)
Cal/ml	1.06	1	1	1	1	1
Protein g/dl	3.8	4	2.1	3.8	4	4.2
Source	Hydrolyzed casein	Hydrolyzed whey	Free amino acids	Free amino acids	Hydrolyzed lactalbumen	Partially hydrolyzed whey, meat, soy & free amino acids
% Cal	14%	16%	8.2%	15.3%	16%	16.7%
Fat g/dl	0.5	3.9	.15	.28	1	1.08
Source	Safflower & soy oil	MCT & safflower oil	Safflower oil	Safflower oil	MCT & corn oil	Safflower & MCT oil
% Cal	3%	33%	1.3%	2.5%	8.5%	9.40%
Carbohydrate g/dl	22	12.7	22.6	20.6	19	18.5
Source	Maltodextrin Modified corn starch	Maltodextrin Starch	Glucose Oligosaccharides	Maltodextrin	Maltodextrin	Sucrose Hydrolyzed corn starch
% Cal	83%	51%	90.5%	82%	75.5%	73.9%
Osmolality	650	260	550	630	490	500
Na (mEq/L)	27	22	20	20	30	20
K (mEq/L)	34	32	30	20	30	34
Ca (mg/L)	530	600	550	500	625	667
P (mg/L)	530	500	550	500	625	667
Ca/P ratio	1:1	1.2:1	1:1	1:1	1:1	1:1
Volume to meet the USRDA	1890	2000	1800	2000	1600	1500
Form	Liquid/unflavored	Liquid/flavored	Powdered/unflavored	Powdered/unflavored	Liquid/unflavored	Powdered/flavored

(Continued)

Table 5–18. *(Continued)*

	Reabilan (O'Brien)	Reabilan HN (O'Brien)
Cal/ml	1	1.33
Protein g/dl	3.15	5.8
Source	Whey peptides & casein peptides	Whey peptides & casein peptides
% Cal	12.5%	17.5%
Fat g/dl	4.3	5.7
Source	MCT, oenothera biennis & soy oil	MCT, oenothera biennis & soy oil
% Cal	35%	35%
Carbohydrate g/dl	13.1	15.7
Source	Maltodextrin & tapioca starch	Maltodextrin & tapioca starch
% Cal	52.5%	47.5%
Osmolality	350	490
Na (mEq/L)	30.4	43
K (mEq/L)	32	42
Ca (mg/L)	499	450
P (mg/L)	499	501
Ca/P ratio	1:1	1:8
Volume to meet the USRDA	2250	1875
Form	Liquid/unflavored	Liquid/unflavored

Source: From Hendricks, K., & Walker, W. (1990). *Manual of pediatric nutrition* (2nd ed.), p. 101, 102. Philadelphia: B. C. Decker, with permission.

Table 5–19. Method for determining levels of malnutrition.

$$\left(\frac{\text{Actual Weight}}{\text{Ideal Body Weight}}\right) \times 100$$

90–100%	Well Nourished
80–89%	Mild Malnutrition
70–79%	Moderate Malnutrition
<70%	Severe Malnutrition

Source: From Mkandawire, S. C. M. (1991). Unpublished doctoral dissertation: An investigation of protein-energy malnutrition in Malawi with special reference to children in the age group infancy to five years. Columbia University Teachers College, New York. Publisher, U.M.I. Dissertation Information Service, 300 N. Zeeb Road, Ann Arbor, Michigan 48106.

$$\frac{6.05 \ (\text{KF's actual weight})}{7.05 \ (\text{KF's ideal body weight})} = 80\% \text{ of I.B.W.}$$

Recommendations

Patient is currently taking 24 oz. of Pregestimil 20 cal/oz. His caregiver was instructed to gradually increase the concentration to 30 calories/ounce by the following method:

1. Pregestimil   12 scoops   480 cal
   Polycose   4 Tbsp   92 cal
   Add enough water to bring to 24 oz.
                            = 24 cal/oz.
2. Pregestimil   12 scoops   480 cal
   Polycose   4 Tbsp   92 cal
   MCT Oil   6 cc   48 cal
                            = 26 cal/oz.
3. Pregestimil   14 scoops   560 cal
   Polycose   4 Tbsp   92 cal
   MCT Oil   9 cc   64 cal
                            = 30 cal/oz.

This provides about 120 cal/kg which should meet needs for normal growth rate. For catch-up growth, patient would require closer to 135 cal/kg/day. This balance could be met with pureed foods, or an additional 90 cal/day.

Other goals include:

1. Promote hyperplasia of remaining small bowel through enteral feeding.
2. Minimize GER by encouraging proper positioning during and after feedings, using predigested formula and thickened feedings.
3. Promote growth and healing of lung tissue providing high protein and calories.

Drug/Nutrient Interactions

When anorexia, nausea, vomiting, glossitis, diarrhea, constipation, mouth sores, and taste changes interfere with the nutrient intake of a child with AIDS, the role of the drugs the child is on must be investigated (see Table 5–20). Occasionally, therapeutic manipulation will alleviate some of the child's symptoms.

The Role of Tube Feeding in Pediatric AIDS Patients

In the child with chronic inadequate oral intake accompanied by poor weight gain and a functional gastrointestinal tract, tube feedings may be appropriate. Nasogastric tubes, gastrostomy tubes, and jejunal tubes may be selected (see Table 5–21). A blenderized feeding such as Compleat Modified, made by Sandoz Nutrition, is an isotonic lactose-free formula that is thin enough not to clog the small feeding tubes which are commonly used in young children (see Table 5–14). Generally, the formulas used for tube feedings are not palatable. Some efficient caregivers may manage blenderizing food in the house under sanitary conditions. This practice is generally not recommended for the AIDS patient because of risk of contamination. The Women, Infants and Children (W.I.C.) food

Table 5-20. Possible side effects and or nutritional interactions of some drugs used in the treatment of AIDS and AIDS-related infections.

Drug	Use	Possible Side Effects or Nutritional Interactions
Antiviral		
Azidothymidine	HIV infection, hairy leukoplakia, cytomegalovirus, Epstein-Barr virus	Severe megaloblastic anemia (nonnutritional), nausea, dysguesia, edema of tongue and lips, mouth ulcers, constipation, reduced serum Vitamin B12
Bromopirimine	RNA and DNA viruses, Kaposi's sarcoma	Nausea, vomiting, fatigue, diarrhea
Acyclovir	Herpes simplex	Diarrhea, nausea, vomiting, fatigue, sore throat, dysguesia, nephrotoxicity
Ganciclovir	Cytomegalovirus, herpes viruses, retinitis	Nausea, anorexia
Dextran sulfate	HIV	Poor wound healing
Foscarnet	Cytomegalovirus, hepatitis B, herpes viruses, visna lentivirus	Renal dysfunction, anemia, nausea, headache, fatigue, neurologic impairment, calcium imbalance, hyperphosphatemia
Interferon	Cytomegalovirus, hepatitis B, respiratory infections, Kaposi's sarcoma	Flu-like symptoms, CNS disturbances, thrombocytopenia, leukopenia, depression, weakness
Suramin	Murine leukemia, sarcoma virus, avian myoblastosis virus	Gastrointestinal symptoms, dyspnea, reversible inhibition of hemoglobin synthesis
Rifabutin	*Mycobacterium avium-intracellulare*	Possible liver dysfunction, dysguesia, headache, anorexia, fatigue; absorption decreased when given with food
Sulfadiazine	*Toxoplasma gondii*	Nausea, vomiting, anorexia, diarrhea

(Continued)

Table 5-20. *(Continued)*

Drug	Use	Possible Side Effects or Nutritional Interactions
Antifungal		
Amphotericin	Cryptococcal meningitis	Possible decreased potassium and magnesium levels, weight loss, anorexia, nausea, vomiting, diarrhea, severe nephrotoxicity
Ketoconazole	Esophageal and oral candidiasis cryptococcal meningitis	Possible nausea, vomiting, abdominal pain, decreased sodium; should not be given with antacids because it needs acidic environment for absorption
Nystatin	Candidiasis	Diarrhea, nausea, vomiting, fever, gastrointestinal distress
Antibacterial		
Trimethoprim sulfamethoxazole	*Pneumocystis carinii* pneumonia	Pancreatitis, anorexia, glucose intolerance, possible folate deficiency, glossitis, stomatitis
Trimetrexate	*Pneumocystis carinii* pneumonia	Mucositis
Antiparasitic		
Pentamidine	*Pneumocystis carinii* pneumonia	Nephrotoxicity, nausea, vomiting, hypoglycemia, pancreatitis, folate deficiency, dysguesia, possible diabetes
Spiramycin	Cryptosporidiosis	Nausea, vomiting, diarrhea, acute colitis

Source: From Raiten, D. (1990). *Nutrition and HIV infection: A review and evaluation of the relationship between nutrition and HIV infection,* Report Number 223-88-2124, p. 36. Prepared for the Food, Safety, and Applied Nutrition Food and Drug Administration, Department of Health and Human Services, Washington, DC, with permission.

Table 5–21. Delivery site of enteral alimentation.

Delivery Site	Advantages	Disadvantages or Complications	Advancement[1]	Contraindications
Gastric				
Nasogastric	Surgery at Nasogastric: not required	Nasal, esophageal, or tracheal irritation	Increase concentration, then volume	Vomiting, delayed gastric emptying, reflux
Gastrostomy	More stable Allows patient more mobility	Local skin care required, Risk of intra-abdominal leak with peritonitis		
Jejunal	Bypasses stomach and pylorus, helpful with delayed gastric emptying or gastroesophageal reflux Decreases risk of aspiration Can be used immediately post-operative	Requires continuous infusion. Requires "elemental" formula. Risk of perforation. Change in small intestinal flora. Tube displacement	Increase volume daily until fluid requirements met, then increase concentration	Distention
Cervical esophagoscopy	Avoids abdominal surgery Easily replaced if accidently removed	Risk of stricture or esophagitis	As above	Obstruction esophagitis. stricture; after certain radiation treatments of esophagus

Source: From Walker, W., & Hendricks, K. (1985). Enteral nutrition—Support of the pediatric patient. *Manual of pediatric nutrition*, p. 77. Philadelphia: W. B. Saunders, with permission.
[1]Volume should be increased first if discontinuation of IV is desired.

supplement program and Medicaid provide funding for most of the enteral formulas.

Tube Feeding for the Child with a Poorly Functioning Gastrointestinal Tract

Elemental Formulas

Some patients may need to use products that are partially or completely hydrolyzed due to malabsorption. Products included in this group are: Tolerex, T.EN., Criticare HN, and Peptamen, made by Sandoz Nutrition, Mead Johnson, and Carnation, respectively. These products are very useful in children with intractable diarrhea (see Table 5–18).

Tube Feedings in Children Under 1 Year of Age

Children in this age group may utilize the different infant formulas mentioned earlier. If gastrostomy tube feedings are utilized, polymeric formulas may be used. For jejunal feedings, an elemental infant formula, such as Pregestimil, is utilized. As expressed by Bentler (1992) continuous tube feedings seem to be, in general, better tolerated than bolus feedings (see Chapter 4). For many patients with AIDS, lactose-free formulas seem to be tolerated best because of lactose intolerance and subsequent diarrhea. Even though some pediatric patients with AIDS have aggressive nutrition support, failure to thrive remains a continuing problem. Whether an underlying metabolic derangement is contributory or causative has not been delineated (Raiten, 1990). Tube feeding at any age may be initiated when nutrient intake is less than 80% of the ideal caloric intake. A child may be taken off tube feedings when the total oral intake exceeds 80% of ideal caloric needs. The delivery site of enteral alimentation must be individualized (see Table 5–21).

Nutrition Management of the Child who is Receiving Continuous Gastrostomy Feedings at Home.

Over the past several years, more complicated cases of chronically ill children have been managed in the home. Nutritionists will choose the appropriate type of formula for the child and instruct and direct the home care team in proper management of the feedings as well. Case Study 2 illustrates how a child who was initially on bolus feeding was changed to continuous tube feeds at home.

Case Study 2

Patient was referred for nutrition evaluation specifically to address the following issues:

1. Feeding schedule and amounts taken. The caregiver wished to modify the feeding time to (a) include the pump that will eventually replace bolus feedings, (b) schedule feedings to promote appropriate diet tolerance by KC as well as fit in KC's foster mother's existing schedule, and (c) ensure that feeding will be done safely in the home.
2. Caloric adequacy.
3. Nutritional status.
4. Identify the necessary services and other support systems for mom to ensure continued proper feeding management.

Present Feeding Schedule

1. Mom states that KC is fed Compleat Modified mixed with 2 tablespoons of polycose via gastrostomy tube at the following times:

Time	Amount	Total Calories
7–7:30 a.m.	7 oz.	256
10–10:30 a.m.	7 oz.	256
1–1:30 p.m.	7 oz.	256

4–4:30 p.m.	7 oz.	256
7–7:30 p.m.	7 oz.	256
10–10:30 p.m.	7 oz.	256

KC is also given ad-lib Sustacal HC in a bottle (8 oz. high calorie Sustacal = 360 calories). Total calories taken in a day by KC on a good day as estimated from recall by foster mother = *2,034 kcals*.

Growth

KC's growth statistics are:

Weight 26 lbs. < 5%; Length 40"< 5%

Ideal body wt/ht = ~ 35 lbs. = 15.9 kg.

Age = 7 years

Nutrient Adequacy

To initiate weight gain, KC has to take about 1600 to 2000 kcals per day. At present, she is reported to take about 2000 cals/day. However, whether she is actually ingesting this amount and whether, in addition, she is malabsorbing nutrients is not clear.

Nutritional Status

Patient is in poor nutritional status and aggressive nutrition intervention is in order. Considering ≥ 90% of IBW (as per wt/ht) as *well nourished*, KC is < 60% of her IBW, which classifies her as *severely malnourished* (see Table 5–19).

Modification of Feedings

The patient was placed on continuous feeds with Compleat Modified formula. To encourage most of her nutritional intake to be taken care of in the home, an infusion pump was recommended to enhance night feedings at tolerable speed and amount of formula.

Feeding Schedule

Goal for KC's nutritional management is: 108–130 cc/hr. = 1260 cc formula to be infused over 10 hours.

Feeding may begin at 8 p.m. and cease at 6 a.m. if infusion during sleep poses no problems such as vomiting.

KC'S Rate of Hourly Infusion

Day	Rate	Duration
Day I	30–40 ml/hr.	8 hours
Day II	50–60 ml/hr.	8 hours
Day III	70–80 ml/hr.	8 hours
Day IV	90–100 ml/hr.	8 hours
Day V	110–120 ml/hr.	8 hours
Day VI	125–130 ml/hr.	10 hours

Note: 125 ml/hr. is best tolerated in most children KC's age. *Time and Content of Feeding:* Start feeding at 4 p.m. Formula concentration to **remain the same** to avoid confusion on the part of the caregiver.

KC's caregiver was given the name and telephone number of a home infusion company. Such companies normally give instruction to the caregiver on delivery of the infusion pump. The physician's verbal request is adequate. The company then mails all the paperwork to be signed by the medical doctor on the care team. The pump is infused through the night. It should be checked about twice a night for any problems once everything is running smoothly. The child should be weighed weekly in the home. Caring for the formula should be done according to the following method.

Caring for Formula

1. Replace formula every 8 hours.
2. Infusion sets should be changed every 24 hours to decrease risk of bacterial contamination.
3. The feeding tube must be irrigated with 5 to 10 cc water through the pump to clear the tube and prevent clogging after each feeding.

The child should be weighed weekly in the home. Caring for the formula should be done according to the following method.

Total Parenteral Nutrition (TPN)

If caloric needs cannot be met because of severe diarrhea, fluid restriction, ileus, or intolerance to oral feedings, TPN will be utilized. TPN should be considered for children with AIDS and severe malnutrition only if using the enteral route is not possible. Total parenteral nutrition is administered by a central venous catheter. Although central line infections may be a problem (Wilkinson & Greenwald, 1988), this appears to vary with the institution. Oral feeding is maintained along with TPN so the child still maintains chewing and swallowing skills.

Case Study 3

JS is a little boy with cryptosporidium infection and chronic weight loss. On his most recent admission, it was decided that he would be placed on total parenteral nutrition (TPN). Calculations were made based on JS's age, height, and weight at discharge: age - 5 years, Ht. - 97.5 cm (< 5%), Wt. - 15 kg (< 5%). The following was calculated: Ideal Body Weight = 19.5 kg.

$$\text{cal/kg/day} = \frac{90 \text{ cal/kg/day} \times 19.5 \text{ kg}}{15 \text{ kg}}$$
$$= 117 \text{ cal/kg/day}$$

Total cals required per day = 1755

Protein requirement/kg/day:
$$\frac{1.1 \text{ gm/kg/day} \times 19/5 \text{ kg}}{15 \text{ kg}}$$
$$= 1.43 \text{ gm of protein/kg/day}$$

Total protein required per day = 22 grams

Because of increased protein needs, however, protein was increased to 10% of calories or 33 gm per day.

Note that actual calories provided may be reduced by 25% because digestion is not required. Therefore, the goal is about 1300 cal via TPN. The dextrose concentration was generally increased to 20% in 1500 cc and fat was provided via 150 cc of 20% intralipid. The amino acid concentration necessary to supply about 33 grams of protein was 2.2%. The above provides 1320 cal, 2.2 gm protein/kg, and 2 gm fat/kg.

Summary

Follow-up on all pediatric patients with AIDS is vital. However, sometimes constraints, particularly personnel shortages, do not allow proper follow-up to ensure diet compliance. The sequence of nutritional management should be as follows: First, exhaust all ways to improve nutritional intake orally and encourage use of food which is readily available in the home. Use high calorie and high protein foods, as well as nutritional supplements to boost total caloric intake. Second, all feedings must be tailored to secondary disease manifestation (e.g., lactose intolerance, thrush, and malabsorption). Third, tube feeding may be considered if oral intake is not maintained. Finally, total or partial parenteral nutrition support is used in situations where enteral nutrition has failed or is not appropriate. Although nutrition does not provide a cure for AIDS, it does contribute to a better quality of life for these children.

Acknowledgment

The author is very grateful to editor Susan Rosenthal, M.D., for reorganizing Chapter 5 beyond the call of duty of an editor and also for contributing special tables that greatly enhanced this chapter.

References

Bentler, M. M. (1992). Pediatric acquired immunodeficiency syndrome. In S. Ekval's (Ed.), *Pediatric Nutrition in Chronic and Developmental Disease/Disorders*. New York: Oxford University Press.

Bentler, M., & Stanish, M. (1987). Nutrition support of the pediatric AIDS patient. *Journal of the American Dietetic Association*, 87, 488.

Blanche, S., Rouzioux, C., Moscato, M.L., Veber, F., Mayaux, Jacomet., C., Tricoire, J., Deville, A., Firtion, G., de Crepy, A., Doward, D., Robin, N., Courpotin, C., Ciraru-Vigneron, N., le Derst, F., Griscill G., & the HIV Infection in Newborn French Collaborative Study Group. (1989). A prospective study of infants born to women seropositive for human immunodeficiency virus type HIV Infection in Newborns French Collaborative Study Group. *New England Journal of Medicine*, *320*, 1643–1648.

Children's Hospital of New Jersey outpatient nutrition service manual. Newark, NJ: R. Meike-Taylor & S. C. M. Mkandawire.

Grand, R. J., Sutphen, J. L., & Dietz, W. H., Jr. (1987). *Pediatric nutrition theory and practice*. Boston: Butterworth.

Hendricks, K., & Walker, W. (1990). *Pediatric nutrition* (2nd ed). Philadelphia: B. C. Decker.

McLoughlin, L. C. (1988). Nutrition and gastrointestinal disease in acquired immunodeficiency syndrome. *Topics in Clinical Nutrition*, *3*, 72–76.

Mkandawire, S. C. M. (1985). *Diet guidelines for children with AIDS*. Newark: Children's Hospital of New Jersey.

Mkandawire, S. C. M. (1991). *An investigation of protein energy malnutrition in Malawi with special reference to children in the age group of infancy to five years*. Doctoral dissertation, Columbia University Teachers College, New York. Publisher: U. M. I. Dissertations Service, 300 N. Zeeb Road, Ann Arbor, Michigan, 48106.

Mkandawire, S. C. M. (1991). Nutrition and pediatric AIDS. Report of the Subcommittee on the Nutritional Impact of HIV Infection in Children (FDA Report No. 223-86-2117). *The American Academy of Pediatrics*, Illinois.

Pressman, H., & Morrison, S. H. (1988). Dysphagia in the pediatric aids population. *Dysphagia*, *2*, 166.

Raiten, D. J. (1990). *Nutrition and HIV infection: A review and evaluation of the extant knowledge of the relationship between nutrition and HIV infection* (Report No. 223-88-2124). Prepared for the Food Safety and Applied Nutrition Food and Drug Administration, Department of Health and Human Services, Washington, DC.

Walker, W., & Hendricks, K. (1985). Enteral nutrition—support of the pediatric patient. *Manual of pediatric nutrition* (p. 77). Philadelphia: W. B. Saunders.

Wilkinson, J. D., & Greenwald, B. M. (1988). The acquired immunodeficiency syndrome: Impact on the pediatric intensive care unit. *Critical Care Clinics*, *4*, 831–844.

Winick, J. (1989). Nutrition: An international journal of applied and basic nutritional science. Task force on nutrition support in AIDS: Guidelines for nutrition support in AIDS. *Nutrition*, *5*(1), 39.

World Health Organization. (1987). Breast-feeding/breast milk and human immunodeficiency virus (HIV). *Weekly Epidemiology Records*, *62*(33), 245–246.

CHAPTER

6

Dysphagia in Children with AIDS

HILDA PRESSMAN, M.A.

CONTENTS

There were 3,471 cases of Acquired Immune Deficiency Syndrome (AIDS) in children under the age of 13, reported to the Centers for Disease Control (CDC) as of December 31, 1991. Adolescents are counted in the adult statistics and comprise an-other significant group of patients. It is estimated that three times as many children are positive for the Human Immuno-deficiency Virus (HIV+) and will develop AIDS within 5 to 7 years. The period during which patients are living with the disease is becoming longer as the result of the use of antiviral drugs and supportive care and AIDS is now being considered a chronic illness (Connor & McSherry, 1991). Up to one third of the children have neurological complications and display developmental delay (Schmitt, Seeger, Kreuz, Enenkel, & Jacobi, 1991). Dysphagia is a frequent finding in children with AIDS. It is seen both in those who have neurological impairment and those who are neurologically intact. For this latter group the dysphagia is related to other aspects of their illness, which will be detailed below.

In a study of 55 patients who were referred for evaluation, Pressman and Morrison (1988) found that 25 of the children (45%) had dysphagic symptoms at some point in their illness. Some of the children were HIV+. The majority had AIDS at varying levels of severity. Of those who had dysphagia symptoms, 11 fell into the mild-to-moderate category (able to be maintained on oral feeding but evidenced difficulty with specific consistencies, insufficient intake to meet caloric needs, increased feeding time, and/or inability to progress from bottle to purees or from purees to chewables as appropriate for age), and 14 were severely impaired (unable to be maintained on oral feedings without intervention). In a second study, Pressman (1992) followed a cohort of 96 children over a 2-year period. Again, the majority of the children had AIDS at varying levels of illness, while some of the children remained HIV+ but did not meet the criteria for AIDS. These children were seen for baseline assessment and then every 6 months unless evaluations were requested sooner. Of these children, 20 (20.8%) evidenced dysphagia.

Children who are positive for the Human Immunodeficiency Virus (HIV) are deemed to have AIDS when they meet guidelines set by the CDC (Centers for Disease Control, 1987) including Lymphoid Interstitial Pneumonitis (LIP), progressive encephalopathy,

wasting syndrome, opportunistic infections such as esophageal candidiasis and pneumocystis carinii pneumonia (PCP), or recurrent serious bacterial infections. There are many variations of the virus within each individual, and the virus affects multiple body organ systems. Current medication, including antiretroviral treatment, are at best moderately helpful and are thought to prolong the period in which the individual is HIV+ but does not have AIDS.

HIV is transmitted by blood exchange or sexual contact. Children who are at risk are those born to intravenous drug abusers (IVDAs) or female sexual partners of IVDAs or bisexual men, recipients of blood products, and victims of sexual abuse. Perinatal transmission (during pregnancy or delivery) accounts for 80% of the cases of pediatric AIDS (Rogers, 1988). Children who acquire the disease from their mothers are thought to acquire it in utero (50%) or perinatally (50%) because of exposure to blood during birth. The virus can also be passed in breast milk and so breast-feeding is not recommended for these youngsters.

Diagnosis by serology is difficult, at best. Utilizing the more conventional tests, all children born to a woman who is HIV+ will test positive until 18 months of age because these tests reflect the mother's antibodies. Only 25–30% of the children, however, will actually be HIV+ (Connor & McSherry, 1991). Newer tests are being developed which are able to test children by 4 months of age and may even be able to test them in the first 6 weeks of life. One third of the children are symptomatic in the first year of life and 50–60% are symptomatic by the second year.

Etiologies Of Dysphagia in AIDS

Neurological

Dysphagia in children with AIDS may have multiple etiologies. Most commonly, these are neurological and may be divided primarily into two categories, static encephalopathy (SE) and progressive encephalopathy (PE). Children with static encephalopathy evidence developmental delay involving nonprogressive motor deficits, microcephaly, and seizure disorder. The etiologies of their disorder are the same as for other children with developmental disability, including complications of prematurity, intrauterine exposure to toxins and infectious agents, genetic factors, and head trauma. Children with AIDS, however, are more difficult to manage because of their chronic illness. In one study of 159 HIV-infected children, 14% had SE. These children may go on to develop PE as part of the progression of their disease (Mintz, 1992).

Children with progressive encephalopathy demonstrate neurological deterioration due to direct brain infection with HIV. The method of transmission is unclear, although the virus is found in cerebrospinal fluid (Epstein et al., 1987). PE has been noted in up to 75% of pediatric patients with AIDS and indicates a poor prognosis once it is present (Mintz, 1992). The clinical hallmarks are loss or plateau of developmental milestones, progressive motor dysfunction, impaired brain growth, and generalized weakness with pyramidal tract signs (Mintz, Epstein, & Koenigsberger, 1989).

The reported symptoms include dysphagia, gait ataxia, weakness, spasticity, and global loss of language and motor milestones. In older children with PE, spastic quadriparesis of varying severity and pseudobulbar palsy including dysphagia, dysarthria, and perioral hyperreflexia are seen. Significant apathy is noted as the disease progresses (Table 6–1).

Other neurological manifestations of AIDS include stroke, and mass lesions of the central nervous system (CNS). Although stroke is rare, it is a significant problem when it does occur. One youngster was able to be maintained on oral feedings after his first stroke but required gastrostomy following subsequent strokes because of severe oral preparatory phase dysphagia for consistencies other than liquids and aspiration of even thick liquids, documented on Modified Barium Study.

CNS lymphoma is seen primarily in infants and young children, whereas Toxoplasma gondii abscesses are rare in the young and more commonly seen in older children, adolescents, and adults. The lesions may present with focal neurologic deficits or focal seizures (Table 6–2). One youngster with lymphoma initially presented with anomia and no evidence of dysphagia; however, significant dysphagia was seen postoperatively.

Odynophagia

A very common cause of refusal of feedings and of dysphagia is odynophagia, or pain on swallowing. Older children and adults describe this as a burning or constricting feeling which may be severe enough to cause a fear of eating secondary to the pain.

TABLE 6–1. Clinical hallmarks of progressive encephalopathy in children with AIDS.

Loss or plateau of developmental milestones

Progressive motor dysfunction

Impaired brain growth

Generalized weakness with pyramidal tract signs

Dysphagia

Dysarthria

Gait ataxia

Weakness

Spasticity

Global loss of language and motor milestones

TABLE 6–2. Neurological causes of dysphagia in children with AIDS.

Static encephalopathy

Progressive encephalopathy

Stroke

CNS lymphoma

Toxoplasma gondii abscesses

Odynophagia is usually associated with esophageal mucosal damage which may be viewed on x-ray, but is always identified with endoscopy. It is associated with a number of infections, most commonly Candida esophagitis or thrush. Infants presenting with Candida esophagitis may hungrily take the bottle and then begin to cry after 1–2 sucks. This will happen on repeated trials, and they may require hospitalization because of total refusal of feedings. Oral thrush usually presents first and is cleared more easily than esophageal thrush which requires more prolonged treatment (Raufman, 1988). Rapid symptomatic relief is provided with medication. In adult patients, it is even recommended that treatment be given based on symptoms and that radiologic or endoscopic confirmation only be carried out for nonresponders (Raufman, 1988). Unlike other causes of debilitation in AIDS, this one is very treatable.

Other causes of odynophagia may include mycobacterial esophagitis, herpes simplex gingivostomatitis, CMV esophagitis and rarely cryptosporidiosis (Table 6–3) (Laine, Bonacini, Sattler, Young, & Sherrod, 1992). Decompensation of feeding skills is often seen secondary to the pain. Delayed introduction of timely feeding experiences may occur in these children because of the pain, their chronic illness, and their developmental delay.

Gastrointestinal Manifestations

Gastrointestinal (GI) disorders have a significant effect on the patients desire for and ability to handle oral feedings. Presenting symptoms may include abdominal pain, distention, anorexia, diarrhea, GI bleeding, oropharyngeal or esophageal ulcerations, and failure to thrive which may be associated with malabsorption (Table 6–4). Chronic diarrhea and wasting frequently occur without any proven infection (McLoughlin, 1988). Opportunistic infections affect the GI tract including Mycobacterium avium-intracellulare (MAIC), Cytomegalovirus (CMV), and Cryptosporidium and may cause esophageal and colonic ulcers. Treatment often involves long-term use of medication. Lymphoma may cause gastric outlet obstruction, but this is rare in children. If absorption is a problem, nasogastric (NG) or gastrostomy tube (GT) feedings may need to be pumped slowly over a long period of time, rather than given as bolus feedings. Total Parenteral Nutrition (TPN) may become necessary. Malnutrition may actually cause changes in the gastrointestinal mucosa and create further problems (McLoughlin, Nord, Joshi, Oleske, & Connor, 1987).

Complications of AIDS and Dysphagia That Compromise Nutritional Status

Patients with dysphagia are at risk for further nutritional compromise secondary to their poor intake. Additionally, however, infections, fever, and increased respiratory rate related to lung disease increase caloric needs. Malnutrition may affect muscles, including the heart and respiratory muscles, affecting the ability to clear secretions and aerate the lungs (Pressman & Morrison, 1988). They are at risk for aspiration

TABLE 6–3. Causes of odynophagia in children with AIDS.

Candida esophagitis—thrush
Mycobacterial esophagitis
Herpes simplex gingivostomatitis
CMV esophagitis
Cryptosporidiosis

pneumonia because of their neurological disorder, poor ability to fight infection, and the chronic lung changes that are often seen. Additionally, patients with dysphagia are known to have decompensation of feeding skills when they are ill, and these children are ill more often.

Social isolation is a significant factor for children with dysphagia. In many homes in the United States, mealtime is the only time the family is together. A child who is being maintained on TPN or is receiving continuous GT feedings may not be able to participate in mealtime.

With progressive encephalopathy, children are at risk for fatigue with eating. The oral preparatory phase becomes prolonged and hand-to-mouth coordination becomes impaired. Depression is known to decrease appetite, and these children are certainly at risk for depression because of their prolonged hospitalization and loss of friends and relatives. Anorexia may present as part of the disease process, related to odynophagia or as a side effect of the medication (Table 6–5).

Many of the children have tachypnea and/or tachycardia or bradycardia. Caregivers often report limited intake, especially for bottle-fed babies. The effort expended for maintenance of respiratory and cardiac function is too great and may not allow for the additional energy expenditure necessary when coordinating sucking, swallowing, and breathing. Full oral feeding may not be feasible for these children until the respiratory and/or cardiac issues are brought under control.

The degree of dysphagia varies with the child's overall condition and often improves significantly with medical treatment. During the more acute phases, however, inpatient admission may be necessary to maintain adequate nutrition and hydration

Presenting Complaints

There are several presentations which may indicate dysphagia in the child with AIDS. Caregivers often report coughing on food or liquid; and evaluation may, in fact, reveal aspiration that is specific to consistency or position. Reactive airway disease and right upper lobe pneumonia must also be suspect. Slow feeding is a common complaint in neurologically impaired children with AIDS, whether they have static or progressive encephalopathy. The oral preparatory phase is often impaired, affecting sucking in young children and chewing and bolus formation in older children. The child with failure to thrive may have dysphagia as a component of the problem, and this should always be considered in the differential diagnosis.

TABLE 6–4. Gastrointestinal manifestations of AIDS and drug side effects.

Abdominal pain
Distention
Anorexia
Diarrhea
GI bleeding
Oropharyngeal or esophageal ulcerations
Failure to thrive

TABLE 6–5. Consequences of dysphagia in pediatric AIDS.

Further nutritional compromise

Aspiration pneumonia

Social isolation

Fatigue with eating

Depression

Anorexia

Gagging on solids is frequently seen and is usually related to deprivation of timely experiences. The first year of life is critical for the introduction of a variety of food types. This becomes a problem, however, in children with AIDS. As a result of their frequent illness and developmental delay, caregivers, including physicians, often do not introduce age-appropriate foods. Hypersensitivity and oral defensiveness may develop secondary to the lack of experience with a variety of foods. Additionally, young children with severe motor impairment may not experience normal oral exploration of fingers and toys.

On examination, all phases of dysphagia are found. Oral preparatory, oral initiation, and pharyngeal phases of swallow are affected secondary to developmental delay and neurological impairment. When esophageal phase is affected, it is usually related to infection.

Intervention Issues

Nutrition must be the primary issue. The goals of the therapy program are to achieve functional feeding skills, and compensatory strategies may be the most useful. It is important to take the caregivers' needs into consideration. Small frequent feedings may play havoc with other household demands. Often, other members of the household are also ill with AIDS and may have a limited ability to follow through on very demanding schedules. The goal of improving skills may be inappropriate in the presence of progressive encephalopathy, and treatment may be solely palliative. Although the goals may differ, the assessment and therapy techniques are the same as those for any other child with developmental delay and are detailed in Chapters 4 and 5.

When children are on continuous NG or GT feedings, it is important to advance them to bolus tube feedings before attempting oral feeding. If the GI tract cannot tolerate bolus feedings, then full oral feedings may not be a realistic goal. If malabsorption is an issue, alternatives may include continuous NG or GT feedings at night with PO feeding during the day in an effort to approximate some hunger-satiation cycle while achieving adequate caloric intake and absorption. TPN may be necessary in cases of severe malabsorption. Small amounts are then offered by mouth to maintain oral skills, avoid oral defensiveness, and maintain function of any villi in the GI tract that may be working. Children on TPN, however, are not hungry. For the child who is fed orally, food supplements may be necessary to achieve adequate caloric intake. For further information see Chapters 4 and 5.

In children with progressive encephalopathy, the oral preparatory phase becomes prolonged as their disease progresses. It may become necessary to move backwards from solid foods to soft-to-chew foods and eventually to a pureed diet. It is important that the length of the meal be kept to 30 minutes because excessive calories are burned if the meal exceeds this time period, and the child will not gain weight even if he or she eats the full meal. Aspiration is a less common finding in children with progressive neurological disease.

If hand-to-mouth coordination has deteriorated, then self-feeding may also lead to prolonged feeding time, and the patient may tire to the point where only small amounts are able to be taken. In these cases, the caregiver should be encouraged to feed the child all or part of the meal. Children who are in the process of becoming more independent may resist being fed, and a compromise may be necessary. This may involve the child self-feeding while the caregiver offers additional amounts with a second spoon or provides hand over hand assistance.

The families of these children have a great deal of difficulty coping with the deterioration of feeding skills. They are often resistent to feeding the child or using pureed foods as this is considered a major step backward and evidence of the progression of the child's illness. Careful questioning of the family will usually point up the fact that the child has already shown a preference for soft foods such as macaroni and cheese or puddings. The children rarely have a negative reaction to the necessary changes in their diets because eating becomes less effortful for them with appropriately chosen foods. Additionally, many have become apathetic at this point in their illness.

In children with gastroenterological, cardiac, and respiratory complications, medical treatment is primary. The dysphagic symptoms do not respond to treatment until medical intervention is successful. Surgical intervention may be necessary if gastrointestinal blockage is present. Oral and esophageal thrush are responsive to drugs such as Ketaconozol® and Fluconozole® and rapid symptomatic relief is seen, usually within 24 to 48 hours. Esophageal symptoms may require long-term use of the medication. CMV esophagitis is responsive to Ganciclovir® or Foscarnet®, which again must be used on a long-term basis. Acyclovir® is used to treat herpes gingivostomatitis. For chronic pain, the use of mild analgesics 20 minutes prior to feeding often improves acceptance of food. Cardiac and respiratory problems may respond to medications. The

use of oxygen by nasal canula, during feeding, may need to be considered. If oxygen is used regularly, increasing the flow during feedings may be useful. As these conditions wax and wane, the degree of dysphagia will also vary.

The medical treatments themselves, however, may cause additional difficulties. The drugs most commonly used to treat AIDS, including Trimethoprim-Sulfa (Bactrim®), Ketaconozole®, and Fluconozole®, all have side effects of nausea and vomiting. Additionally, Ranitidine®, which is used to treat esophagitis, and Ketaconozole® change the pH level and increase reflux which may have a significant effect on the acceptance of foods. Most of the children take multiple medications throughout the day. Problems are seen with acceptance of some of the medications because of taste. Appetite is certainly affected by the repeated administration of medication and the liquids or solids that must be given in order for the patient to swallow the medication. In older children, pills may be given by placing the solid pill in the center of a spoonful of jello or pudding and having the child swallow the pill as part of the bolus.

Odynophagia is usually responsive to medical treatment. For children with prolonged or intermittent odynophagia, food consistency, texture, and level of acidity must be taken into consideration. Smooth cold foods such as pudding and ice cream are well tolerated. Strong flavors and acidic foods such as ketchup and foods which have sharp edges such as potato chips may have to be avoided.

The use of antiretroviral drugs such as azidothymidine (AZT), and the dideoxynucleosides (DDI and DDC) often bring improvement in neurological function and in related dysphagic symptoms. The problem has been that each has a limited duration of response, and the child may have to be switched from one to the other to maintain any level of improvement. The degree of dysphagia will fluctuate with the level of neurological function and with improvement in other areas such as respiratory and gastrointestinal function.

Case Studies

CB, a 10-month-old youngster with both developmental delay and progressive encephalopathy, was seen in the Early Intervention Program. On the day she was observed, she was noted to be coughing on both purees and liquids. Her mother also reported similar behavior at home, but on an inconsistent basis. After consultation with the nurse and physician on her team, a Modified Barium Study (MBS) was planned.

Before this could be done, she presented to the emergency room with moderate-severe respiratory distress. Nasal flaring, tachycardia, rales, rhonchi, and minimal wheezing in both lung fields were noted and she was admitted. Weight on admission was below the 5th percentile.

On examination, she was able to manage her bottle with a somewhat weak but still productive suck. Attempts to offer purees were unsuccessful. She did not close her lips to remove the bolus from the spoon, and a severe tongue thrust was seen. Oral transit time was prolonged for the purees. Coughing was noted 2 minutes after the feeding. A modified barium swallow was completed with CB seated upright in the Tumble Form® seat. She was given purees by spoon, thick and then thin liquid by oral gavage. (See Chapter 9 for details of the MBS.) She was found to have poor oral transport of all consistencies, but a normal swallow. As her respiratory status improved, with medication, her coughing disappeared and she resumed her intake of purees. Nutritional consultation increased the number of calories per ounce in her formula. Discharge recommendations included upright positioning for feeding, limiting meals to 30 minutes, offering purees by spoon and liquids by nipple, monitoring of respiratory status, and outpatient followup in the Early Intervention Program.

EA was a 9-year-old who had been followed in the clinic for 5 years. She had a bilateral sensorineural hearing loss, unrelated to AIDS, for which she wore hearing aids. Speech and language were delayed secondary to her hearing loss. EA had a seizure disorder which was under control with medication and had a history of PCP pneumonia and reactive airway disease which was controlled by Ventolin®.

The neurologist's note indicated that she had pseudobulbar syndrome which included oromotor discoordination, pyramidal tract signs, and frontal lobe behavior as well as progressive encephalopathy and CMV encephalitis. On Computed Tomography (CT) scan, she was found to have accelerated atrophy and was described as having the brain of a 50-year-old.

She was admitted because of coughing, vomiting, and diarrhea with a weight loss of 2 kg in the preceding 3 months. Oral examination was unremarkable. She was fed by her father because of hand tremors that affected scooping and hand-to-mouth coordination. She was found to have adequate chewing skills and oral transport for solids; however, her father had to remind her to swallow, often reminding her twice for each bolus. She was watching TV and talking with food in her mouth and had poor attention to task. Fluids were managed by straw without difficulty.

A modified barium study was completed to rule out microaspiration as a contributing factor to her reactive airway disease. She was seated in an upright position and fed a cookie, pureed fruit, and liquid. Rapid oral transport was noted with no evidence of laryngeal penetration or tracheal aspiration. The impression was that oral transport was competent when she was attending to the task of eating.

Recommendations were for supervision at mealtimes, and an Occupational Therapy consultation was requested to assist in hand-to-mouth coordination.

Summary

Children with AIDS present ongoing illness over a long period of time. Many are developmentally delayed because of the neurological manifestations of their illness or because of prenatal and perinatal events. The illness affects multiple systems which impact on adequacy of feeding. It is essential, therefore, that these children be treated by a multidisciplinary team. The degree of illness varies and requires multiple reassessments to deal with the specific areas of difficulty at any given time. Children with AIDS are living for progressively longer periods of time and present unique challenges to the professionals who are charged with their care.

REFERENCES

Centers for Disease Control. (1987). Revision of the CDC surveillance case definition for acquired immunodeficiency syndrome. *Morbidity and Mortality Weekly Report, 36,* S-6.

Connor, E. & McSherry, G. (1991). Antiviral treatment of Human Immunodeficiency Virus infection in children. *Seminars in Pediatric Infectious Diseases, 2*(4), 285–300.

Epstein, L. G., Goudsmit, J., Paul, D. A., Morrison, S. H., Conner, E. M., Oleske, J. M., & Holland, B. (1987). Expression of Human Immunodeficiency Virus in cerebrospinal fluid of children with progressive encephalopathy *Annals of Neurology, 21*(4), 397–401.

Laine, L., Bonacini, M., Sattler, F., Young, T., & Sherrod, A. (1992). Cytomegalovirus and candida esophagitis in patients with AIDS. *Journal of Acquired Immune Deficiency Syndromes, 5*(6), 605–609.

McLoughlin, L. C. (1988). Nutrition and gastrointestinal disease in acquired immunodeficiency syndrome. *Topics in Clinical Nutrition, 3*(4), 72–76.

McLoughlin, L. C., Nord, K. S., Joshi, V. V., Oleske, J. M., & Connor, E. M. (1987). Severe gastrointestinal involvement in children with the acquired immunodeficiency syndrome. *Journal of Pediatric Gastroenterology and Nutrition, 6*(4), 517–524.

Mintz, M. (1992). Neurological abnormalities. In R. Yogev & E. Connor (Eds.), *Management of HIV infection in infants and children* (pp. 247–285). St. Louis: Mosby Year Book.

Mintz, M., Epstein, L. G., & Koenigsberger, M. R. (1989). Neurological manifestations of acquired immunodeficiency syndrome in children. *International Pediatrics, 4*(2), 161–171.

Pressman, H. (1992). Communication disorders and dysphagia in Pediatric AIDS. *ASHA,* 45–47.

Pressman, H. & Morrison, S. H. (1988). Dysphagia in the pediatric AIDS population. *Dysphagia, 2,* 166–169.

Raufman, J. P. (1988). Odynophagia/dysphagia in AIDS. *Gastroenterological Clinics of North America, 17*(3), 599–614.

Rogers, M. F. (1988). Pediatric HIV infection: Epidemiology, etiopathogenesis and transmission. *Pediatric Annals, 17,* 324–330.

Schmitt, B., Seeger, J., Kreuz, W., Enenkel, S., & Jacobi, G. (1991). Central nervous system involvement of children with HIV infection. *Developmental Medicine and Child Neurology, 33,* 535–540.

CHAPTER

7

Behavior Aspects of Feeding Disorders

JULIANA RASIC LACHENMEYER, Ph.D.

───── CONTENTS ─────

This chapter will focus on the behavioral aspects of eating problems in children with developmental disabilities. Children with eating problems can be categorized into (a) those whose poor eating has led to problems in rate of growth and therefore are at risk for problems in neurological development and failure to thrive and (b) those whose rate of growth is unaffected. The dis-

tinction between organic and nonorganic feeding problems as well as organic and nonorganic risk factors for eating problems will be briefly reviewed. An argument will be made for the need for empirically derived categories of feeding problems based on etiology, course, and treatment outcome (Lachenmeyer, 1991). The primary focus of the chapter will be on assessment and treatment of these problems with some additional attention on special issues in tube-fed children.

Failure to Thrive

Children whose rate of growth has been affected by their eating history clearly present a more serious and immediate challenge than children whose eating behavior affects family interactions but not their growth. Failure to thrive (FTT) is a syndrome used to describe infants and children who show weight loss or difficulties in gaining weight with an overall weight below the third percentile for the appropriate age group (Roberts & Maddux, 1982). Although all children who fail to thrive do not have developmental disabilities, many do. The developmental disabilities may be a result of inadequate nutritional intake, or the inadequate nutritional intake may be due to developmental disabilities. The developmental disabilities and the poor growth may be a result of a third set of variables. Additionally, a child's level of functioning will influence the type of intervention as well as the rate of progress that is attained. Developmental disabilities combined with parental personalities influence parental perceptions and caregiver-child interactions.

FTT may be categorized as organic or nonorganic in etiology. According to Bithoney and Rathburn (1983), Organic Failure To Thrive (OFTT) is a growth symptom of all serious pediatric illnesses, the common factor being the medical illness of malnutrition; Nonorganic Failure To Thrive (NOFTT) is a failure of growth without any diagnosable organic cause.

Factors Associated with Failure to Thrive

Although children with developmental disabilities and dysphagia suffer from OFTT, anxiety and stressors associated with their feeding behavior may cause complications that are seen in NOFTT as well. Many experts still appear to be working from a psychoanalytic view and cite an anxiety-ridden, disturbed mother-child relationship as the core pathology underlying FTT. Roberts and Maddux (1982) in their review discuss the traditional conceptualization of FTT as mothers who have unmet dependency needs because of their own experience of inadequate mothering and who therefore look to the infant for fulfillment of their own needs. The mother attributes intent to the child's behavior and interprets it as a rejection or anger toward herself. Talbot, Sobel, Burke, Lindemann, and Kaufman (1947) refer to NOFTT as maternally induced failure of the mother-child bond formation. Nutritional and developmental characteristics are seen as secondary to the maternal pathology. NOFTT has also been used interchangeably with maternal neglect (Fitch, Cadet, & Goldson, 1976; Koel, 1969). However, studies that discuss neglect do not assess neglect independently of the NOFTT diagnosis. Chatoor et al. (1985) attempt to categorize FTT children who have clear neurological deficits along dimensions of maternal psychopathology. The primary difficulty with this orientation is that it makes no attempt to look at child characteristics, therefore treatment is not related to child assessment and is not empirically determined. In addition, it can lead to blaming the caregiver especially the mother.

Hypothetically, a caregiver's psychological impairment or reaction to psychosocial stressors could lead to poor relationships with her or his children. Whether this is either necessary or sufficient for any psychological disorder in the child is unclear. It has not been empirically demonstrated that such a chain of events is causally implicated in NOFTT. The best that empirical evidence shows is that a caregiver's psychological difficulties, stress, and an impaired mother-child relationship are associated with NOFTT. A poor mother-child relationship may be a result of either NOFTT or OFTT.

An alternative explanation to the psychoanalytic one of maternal pathology is an interactional point of view. Sameroff and Chandler (1975) in a seminal article on the impact of early learning on later development argue for an explanatory model that involves empirical observations of caregiver characteristics, child characteristics, and interactions between caregiver and child. They point out that the interaction is always in process, with both the child and the environment undergoing continual restructuring. The authors suggest that in the course of normal development there are correcting influences. Therefore, if early negative factors have an enduring effect, this is because there are enduring negative influences rather than because of discrete negative events at specific points in development.

Because behavior is generally conceived of as multidetermined (in this case the many factors are child variables, caregiver variables, and their interaction), it is important to look at factors that are associated with NOFTT and OFTT. Child characteristics such as temperament, health and physical status, neurodevelopmental and cognitive developmental variables all play a role in both eliciting behaviors from caregivers and in the child's responses to caregivers. They also influence a caregiver's perception of the child which, in turn, affects her or his behavior toward the child. In a study that looked at maternal perception of temperament, Kotelchuck (1977) found that NOFTT children were perceived as having a distinct temperament: highly reactive but slow. Parent-child interactions in children with developmental disabilities and dysphagia may similarly be influenced by the parents' perception of the child's temperament. Whether these differences

represent an accurate view of the child or a distortion or selective perception on the part of the mother, they directly influence maternal behavior and thereby indirectly influence the child.

In terms of health and physical status, FTT children are by definition small. Because of uncertainty about their size and health, frequent doctor's visits are made. The uncertainty about the child's health affects caregivers' handling of these children. Infants who are malnourished and those who are premature have less vigorous sucking (Gryboski, 1969). Lester and Zeskind (1978) found that high-risk infants needed more pain stimulation to cry, had longer latency of response to pain, shorter cry bursts, and higher pitched cries than did low-risk infants. This may mean that a caregiver will respond less quickly to the child's needs as well as receive less satisfaction from an infant who is not very responsive.

Neurodevelopmental difficulties are seen as resulting from FTT. Although this may be the case, often there is a more complex, circular interaction. Gross or even subtle neurodevelopmental difficulties can cause problems with feeding. Consequent growth difficulties can cause neurodevelopmental problems. In the literature little consideration is given to how these subtle neurodevelopmental effects on feeding mechanisms lead to secondary psychosocial stressors. Additionally, children with FTT show marked delays in cognitive development (Dowling, 1972; Ferhold & Provence, 1976; Fitch et al., 1976; Gordon, 1979; Kotelchuck, 1980).

Maternal factors that have been associated with FTT include lack of nutritional information, improper feeding techniques, unrealistic expectations especially in relation to feeding, misreading of child needs, neglect, and psychosocial stressors such as low socioeconomic status and isolation (Kotelchuck, 1980). Organic risk factors that have been associated with FTT including minor congenital anomalies, neurological conditions including developmental disabilities, maternal cigarette smoking and or poor nutrition during pregnancy, prematurity at birth, perinatal complications, and many ongoing or previous physical illnesses.

Empirically Derived Categoriesof FTT

Lachenmeyer (1987) has argued for the need for empirically derived categories of FTT. Clearly, FTT is not homogeneous. It is defined primarily by the lack of adequate nutrition and consequent poor growth. Within this broad syndrome there are some for whom there is a medical cure (e.g., medication for reflux). For many, despite the various etiologies, there is no medical cure. Lachenmeyer (1991) empirically derived the following categories of FTT based on a sample of 40 children over several years:

1. The child who is simply a difficult eater; this child may or may not have growth related problems.
2. The child whose feeding problem has a medical etiology for which there is medical treatment (e.g., reflux).
3. The child with neurodevelopmental problems who may have low tone oromotor difficulties or sensitivities.
4. The child with medical and or neurodevelopmental difficulties that do not directly explain the poor nutritional intake.
5. The child who has developed a conditioned dysphagia: a conditioned aversive response that leads to food avoidance (e.g., history of vomiting, choking or gagging).
6. The child who because of medical problems has a history of nonoral feeding, and who, therefore, may not have

learned to associate oral feeding with pleasure and may not be aware of hunger and satiety cues.
7. The child whose primary caregiver is not adequately responsive to the child's nutritional needs due to pathology, ignorance of appropriate feeding behavior or psychosocial stressors.
8. The child who initiates demands for food less often because a caregiver is less responsive.
9. The child with multiple physical and cognitive problems.

Caregivers may be instrumental in maintaining the above problems although not in initiating them. This is an important distinction. Caregivers must not be made to feel responsible for their child's feeding problem. However, it should be clear that they are in the best position to do something about it.

Assessment

Assessment is related to treatment of the feeding behavior and is ongoing. Medical assessment precedes behavioral assessment and should include a history that lists all major medical illnesses past and present. The initial focus is to determine if there are any existing medical conditions under developmental disabilities and dysphagia that are contributing to the poor nutritional intake and can be treated medically. When the behavioral component is of such prominence or complexity that psychological intervention is deemed necessary, a behavioral psychologist with expertise in feeding disorders should be consulted.

Following the initial telephone contact and prior to the behavioral assessment, the primary caregiver should be asked to keep a Daily Food Intake Diary. This is the primary assessment tool and should include the time of food intake, the behaviors associated with intake, and the quantity. A food intake diary defines and delineates the problem. It is the basis on which interventions are made. It is also a baseline against which to measure progress so that both the therapist and the caregiver can not only gauge where they should go, but also see how far they have come.

A diary that includes family routines is also important and can be requested at or following the first meeting. Often, when there are feeding problems, attempts to feed are made throughout the day and affect all aspects of the family life and interactions. Knowing what daily routines are like gives specific information about the impact of feeding attempts, activities that the child enjoys, parenting styles, and the degree of social support that a caregiver has. Food diaries and knowledge of daily routines are the basis for specific therapeutic interventions. It is useful to keep this information in a notebook in which the therapist adds positive comments on achievements as well as specific recommendations. These are then recorded so that the caregiver can be reminded in between sessions.

If, once treatment has been started, a caregiver reports that she or he is unable to do any successful feeding, observation of the feeding behavior may be necessary. If the child is very young, feeding in the office could be attempted. For an older child (2 1/2 years and older), a home visit would be preferable. Such observations can provide the therapist with valuable information: the child's initial reaction to food when presented, the caregiver's reaction to food refusal, and the child's behavior that precedes a caregiver's terminating the feeding attempt. Additionally, these sessions allow the therapist to coach the caregiver and even to model feeding behavior.

If one is parenting a child who has difficulty eating, regardless of etiology, the care-giver-child interaction is affected. The perceived etiology can also affect the relationship. For example, if the child has a developmental disability and has had a medical complication, the caregiver will act differently than if eating problems are solely attributed to being stubborn or being angry at the caregiver. What the caregivers perceive as the cause of the child's eating refusal must be addressed. Additionally, observation of the caregiver and child together will give information about the extent to which and the ways in which the eating behavior has affected their relationship. It can also provide information about the extent to which the social or nonfeeding interactions affect the feeding behavior. From these observations and from parental report should come a record of problematic interactions other than feeding: the problematic behavior, what precedes the behavior, and how the caregiver handles it. Parental perception of lack of control over a child in any one area influences the perceptions of child behavior in other areas. A child who refuses food may be seen as a powerful, willful child who then controls the family in other ways.

Assessment should be problem focused and continuous. The data obtained from eating diaries and observations are the basis for treatment recommendations as well as the means by which the success of the treatment is evaluated. These records also provide support for caregivers during the difficult day-in and day-out feeding. Having ongoing records can show caregivers how far they have come and what progress has been made.

Treatment

Issues in the treatment of eating problems in children with developmental disabilities are in some ways similar to those in the treatment of children without these handicapping conditions. Priority is placed on the use of rewards, with negative consequences possibly following later. With both groups an attempt is made to minimize disruptive noncompliant behavior. There are two broad areas in which a child's level of cognitive and language functioning can influence a treatment plan: the child's characteristics themselves and the attribution the caregiver makes about the child's functioning.

A child with developmental disabilities may take more trials to learn appropriate behavior. Additionally, rewards should be set at the level at which the child is functioning. Higher functioning and verbal children will learn to generalize faster across situations, and their behavior is more likely to come under verbal control. In the author's clinical experience, caregivers of children with developmental disabilities tend to attribute noncompliance to the child's disability. The implication is that if the child only understood he or she would comply. This leads to an inconsistent approach to the child, with the caregiver sometimes seeing the child as unable to "control himself" and at other times as manipulative. The psychologist has to help the caregiver delineate the contribution of the disability to the child's eating behavior.

Sessions usually involve the therapist, the primary caregiver, and the child. It is advisable to have periodic meetings with both caregivers and to establish this from the onset so that a less involved caregiver feels committed to the treatment and has some understanding of what is involved. However, the more frequent sessions may include only the primary caregiver so that specific recommendations can be made. Direct feedback may be given to the caregiver carrying out the treatment plan. When the child is seen, neurodevelopmental, cognitive, and behavioral functioning can be assessed. Treatment may be done with or without the child present. There

are certain conditions in which the child may be included in the treatment sessions: if subtleties of the caregiver-child interaction need to be assessed, observations of feeding behavior are needed, and/or therapist modeling of feeding or social interactions is part of the intervention. If the child is present, an attempt should be made to have the child feel that he or she is earning some reward or control through improved eating behavior. Usually, parents will see what the therapist is doing and support him or her in this endeavor. If the child can understand the specific behavioral recommendations being made, it is preferable that the child not be in the room when these recommendations are made.

Family Interventions

There are some global interventions that do not directly involve eating behavior. The caregiver should be given a possible explanation for organic reasons why her child is not eating. For example, a child with developmental disabilities, dysphagia, and gastrointestinal reflux (GER) who is receiving most of her nutrition through nighttime continuous feedings and daytime bolus feedings may not experience hunger and, possibly, does not know hunger and satiety cues. It is important to avoid blaming the caregivers and to strongly and actively negate any notions that they are to blame. The caregiver should be made to feel that she or he, in fact, can do something about this problem.

Expectations as to how long it will be before there is significant improvement should be addressed. The caregiver should be told that success will mean hard work on her part, and that she can expect slow but steady progress. There may be occasional setbacks if the child becomes ill with a flu or cold. However, once the behavior has been learned it will be relearned more easily. In order to see rapid improvement, sessions should be at least twice a week. When this is not possible, telephone calls between sessions are useful. If one is in touch with the caregiver only once a week, initial progress may be too long in coming. Also, if the caregiver has had minor successes, she will benefit from immediate feedback.

As mentioned earlier, attempting to feed a child who refuses significant quantities of food is very difficult on a day-to-day or meal-to-meal basis. It is crucial that the caregiver have some social support and, when possible, someone to share the feeding responsibilities. The caregiver should also have available to her other activities such as recreation or work. If the caregiver has time for activities that do not directly involve the child, the primary caregiver will be more effective at carrying out the specific strategies that will improve the child's eating. Someone whose whole sense of self is based on whether and how much the child eats will have a difficult time carrying out specific recommendations.

A "matter of fact" attitude toward the child will make a caregiver more effective. Caregivers can be assisted with this if they are reminded that the child's medical and nutritional needs are being met. Expressing feelings of anger and frustration to the child are not likely to help the feeding interactions. They may cloud the caregiver's judgment as to what is working and what further changes should be made in the treatment plan. The caregiver benefits from discussions of her feelings and thoughts.

If caregivers feel they have no control over a child with eating difficulties, they will attribute the inconsistent eating to a child's mood. In fact, they often have more control than they think. This can be pointed out to them in questions related to their daily routines. Such questions tell the therapist what caregivers do in these situations. Caregivers may increase control through use of age-appropriate contingencies. Sometimes changes

in tone and manner can often accomplish the same end.

Lastly, if nonoral feedings are to be considered, this should be presented to the caregivers as a realistic possibility rather than a threat to be feared. Whenever possible, nonoral feedings should only supplement oral feeding. Most tube feedings affect hunger, and therefore tube feedings must be adjusted as oral intake is increased. It is difficult to maintain a balance in which the child receives enough nourishment by tube to maintain or increase weight and still undertakes increasing amounts of oral intake (see Chapter 4).

Feeding Interventions

Initial goals must be set based on medical priorities such as weight gain. Specific behavioral recommendations will vary based on the specific goals. If weight gain or maintenance is the goal, then high caloric intake will be the focus (see Chapter 4). Introduction of different types of food may have to be postponed. Increase in quantity or variety of oral foods may be a goal, in which case, the choice would be to go with foods that have the highest probability of being eaten. For a child who had a previous history of good eating, one would reintroduce favorite foods from the past or foods of similar taste and texture to those the child presently eats. Increase in the variety of oral foods would presume that the current caloric intake is adequate. In this case, highly pleasurable foods might follow the tasting of less pleasurable foods.

A discrimination should be made between feeding times in which the focus is on caloric intake and social eating during which a child sits with family and/or peers and is allowed to play with food. A time limit (30–40 minutes) should be set for feedings. This clearly differentiates feeding times from nonfeeding times and allows a focus on food during times when intake must occur. Other times should be ones in which the primary caregiver and child have pleasurable interactions. Frequent (approximately 4) and small meals are desirable with set feeding times, although preferred foods may be available as snacks. Feeding should occur in areas of minimal distraction. During this time feeding behavior should be reinforced and nonfeeding behavior should be ignored. This represents a departure from using cajoling to make a child eat. Rewards must be achievable. Rewarding the level of eating that occurred prior to the intervention is therefore most effective at the outset. Caregivers have to understand that a child is to be rewarded for what he or she is eating, not punished for what he or she should be eating. Once there has been an acceptance of the child's current eating behavior, then the criteria for rewards can be gradually changed. This usually means increases in the quantity and variety of foods eaten. The behaviors to be rewarded, as well as the rewards used, are empirically determined for each child. They are based on an evaluation of eating patterns as presented in the eating diary. Eventually, the child should be rewarded for eating different foods and for greater amounts. Some children hold food in their mouths. So, rewards may be made contingent on swallowing.

The kinds of rewards available depend on the child's age and developmental level. At least one reward should be achievable at each sitting; the criteria should be individually based on what the child currently achieves. For an older child with a mental or chronological age of 3 years and older, daily or weekly rewards should also be available. After some eating has been established through rewards, negatives may also be introduced. Time out may be used following disruptive behavior (Handen, Mandell, & Russo, 1986). The child who is exhibiting refusal behavior or cannot be contained may be put in time out for a period of time. Feeding should not be resumed until the next feeding time. A child with a mental age 3 years or older may be released from the eating situation after a certain amount of food has been eaten. The amount should be one that the child has previously eaten. It is always preferable to use positive rewards first. Negative contingencies such as strong brief reprimands may be introduced following gagging or vomiting behavior. If a child exhibits vomiting behavior, food may be reintroduced immediately following a Time Out. The implementation of negative contingencies should be done matter-of-factly with little negative affect.

Caregivers are often concerned about generalizing and maintaining the improved feeding behaviors once rewards are discontinued. Although the behavioral literature suggests that this is an area of concern, the studies cited usually compare behavior change in tightly controlled settings to behavior in completely different settings. In terms of feeding behavior, changes accomplished in a hospital or therapy setting must be generalized to the home in which there is less structure and support. Inpatient feeding programs should spend considerable time planning the maintenance and increase in feeding behavior once the child has gone home. This can be accomplished by making sure that the primary caregiver has gained the necessary skills and confidence to continue the feeding program and that a behavioral psychologist with experience in feeding and parenting issues is available. Because inpatient treatment is not likely to continue until a relatively normal eating pattern has been established, the psychologist can plan with the caregiver what further steps need to be taken and assist the caregiver in carrying them out. In home-bound based programs, generalization is less of a concern (see Chapter 16).

Issues In Weaning from Tube Feeding

Children who are tube fed, as a group, have a history of medical problems and feeding problems that were severe enough to necessitate nonoral feeding. These children have been fed noncontingent on determinations of hunger and often are, or have become, unaware of sensations of hunger and satiety. Additionally, because of medical procedures and then probable unsuccessful attempts at feeding, food and interactions surrounding food have become unpleasant, if not aversive. These children usually experience more enduring eating problems due to the complexity and severity of their problems. When oral feedings are reintroduced, even the most competent caregivers often have difficulty with their slow progress and occasional setbacks due to routine childhood illnesses.

The primary consideration in weaning from tube feeding is sufficient nutritional intake to lead to continual growth. Children are usually fed either during the night or during the day or a combination of both. Although continuous night feedings have the advantage of being less obtrusive in family life, and therefore less likely to lead to power struggles, day feedings are preferable. They more closely approximate a normal eating schedule and can follow oral feedings. The amount given by tube should be contingent on the amount taken orally. If nighttime feedings are not used, the child is more likely to be hungry and to respond to behavior rewards.

Due to the difficult and frustrating time caregivers of these children have had, they are often likely to suggest "pulling the tube out" before it is nutritionally indicated. For a child who has had a long-standing feeding problem, abrupt termination of tube feeding usually leads to more rapid weight loss. It is important in these children to reduce the caloric intake by tube slowly and thereby allow for increased hunger and increased oral intake. Generally, a reduction of intake given by tube of 25% of total calories at a time is recommended. This does not have to be preceded by a comparable increase in amount of oral intake. However, the oral feeding should be well enough established that one would expect some increase following the reduction in tube feeding.

Summary

Children with developmental disabilities and feeding problems are not a homogeneous group. Etiologies include behavioral, neurodevelopmental, and cognitive. The caregiver-child interactions, both feeding and social, are shaped by the medical and family history. A medical problem can, over time through various interactions, become behavioral. Many feeding problems that are medical in origin must also be treated by working on the caregiver-child interaction. What is needed is an empirically based approach to etiology and treatment. It is important not to blame the caregiver and to enlist support. The therapist makes the recommendations and trains the caregiver to carry them out.

References

Bithoney, W. B., & Rathbun, J. M. (1983). Failure to thrive. In W. B. Levine, A. C. Carey, A. Crocker, & R. J. Gross (Eds.), *Developmental behavioral pediatrics,* 557–572. Philadelphia: W. B. Saunders.

Chatoor, I., Dickson, L., Shaefer, F., & Egan, J. (1985). A developmental classification of feeding disorders associated with failure to thrive: Diagnosis and treatment. In D. Drotar (Ed.), *New directions in failure to thrive: Implications for research and practice* (pp. 844–850). New York: Plenum Press.

Dowling, S. (1972). Seven infants with esophageal atresia: A developmental study. *Psychoanalytic Study of the Child, 27,* 215–256.

Ferhold, J., & Provence, S. (1976). Diagnosis and treatment of an infant with psycho-physiological vomiting. *Psychoanalytic Study of the Child, 31,* 439–459.

Fitch, M. F., Cadet, R. V., & Goldson, E. (1976). Cognitive development of abused and failure to thrive children. *Pediatric Psychology, 1,* 32–37.

Gordon, A. H., & Jameson, J. C. (1979). Infant-mother attachment in patients with non-organic failure to thrive syndrome. *Journal of the American Academy of Child Psychiatry, 18*(2), 251–259.

Gryboski, J. D. (1969). Suck and swallow in the premature infant. *Pediatrics, 43,* 96–102.

Handen, B. L., Mandell, F. & Russo, D. C. (1986). Feeding induction in failure to thrive children. *American Journal of Diseases of Children, 140,* 52–59.

Koel, B. S. (1969). Failure to thrive and fatal injury as a continuum. American *Journal of Diseases of Children, 118,* 565–567.

Kotelchuck, M. (1977). *Child abuse: Prediction and misclassification.* Presented at the Conference on Prediction of Child Abuse, Wilmington, DE.

Kotelchuck, C. M. (1980). Nonorganic failure to thrive: The status of interactional and environmental etiologic theories. In B. Camp (Ed.), *Advances in behavioral pediatrics* (pp. 24–51). Greenwich: JAI Press.

Lachenmeyer, J. R. (1987). Failure to thrive: A critical review. In B. Lahey & A. Kazdin (Eds.), *Advances in clinical child psychology* (pp. 335–337). New York: Plenum Press.

Lachenmeyer, J. R. (1991). *Empirically derived categories of failure to thrive.* Unpublished manuscript.

Leonard, M., Rhymes, J. P., & Solnit, A. J. (1966). Failure to thrive in infants. American *Journal of Diseases of Children, 111,* 600–612,

Lester, B. M., & Zeskind, P. S. (1978). The organization of crying in the infant-at-risk. In T. Field (Ed.), *The high risk newborn* (pp. 301–317). New York: Spectrum.

Roberts, M. C. & Maddux, J. E. (1982). A psychosocial conceptualization on non-organic failure to thrive. *Journal of Clinical Child Psychology, 11*(3), 216–223.

Sameroff, A., & Chandler, M. (1975). Reproductive risks and the continuum of caretaker casualty. In. F. D. Horowitz (Ed.), *Review of childhood developmental research* (pp. 187–197). Chicago: University of Chicago Press.

Talbot, N. B., Sobel, E. H., Burke, B. S., Lindemann, E., & Kaufman, S. B. (1947). Dwarfism in healthy children. *New England Journal of Medicine, 236,* 783–793.

The Influence of Posture and Positioning on Oral Motor Development and Dysphagia

ELAINE K. WOODS, M.A., P.T.

CONTENTS

The development of oral motor skills parallels and is closely tied to overall physical development. To attain optimum swallowing and eating skills, a child must have good head and trunk control permitting oral-pharyngeal and facial structures to move independently from the rest of the body (Mueller 1975, cited in Ottenbacher, Bundy, & Short, 1983). The child with abnormal neuromotor development often exhibits developmental delays in many areas. These include difficulties with the retention of primitive reflexes and postural and tonal imbalances that affect all stages of oral-pharyngeal function and development.

Abnormal oral development is often detected at an early age. Poor sucking causes disturbances of the highly coordinated rhythmical interplay that exists between sucking, swallowing, and breathing and is often the first sign of neuromuscular developmental problems. A child dominated by primitive reflexes has poor body alignment which affects oral-pharyngeal function (Farber, 1982). As with primitive postural reflexes, primitive and exaggerated oral reflexes may persist, resulting in disordered feeding behaviors. These disorders have a significant impact on overall medical status, health, and growth and continue to interfere with function as the child grows older (Scherzer & Tscharnuter, 1982).

It is important to observe, evaluate, and treat feeding and swallowing within a framework of how these mechanisms are influenced by the whole body and its overall postural tone (Morris & Klein, 1987). As with all motor function, a stable base of support is needed to develop movement and functional skills. To facilitate distal movement (i.e., head, upper and lower extremities), central or proximal control is essential either through good pelvic and trunk control or with the assistance of external support such as adaptive equipment. This concept of mobility developing from a base of stability also affects the re-fined development of oral-pharyngeal function. Oral stability is dependent on the development of neck and shoulder girdle stability which are, in turn, dependent on trunk and pelvic stability. The jaw can be viewed as proximal to the lips, cheeks, and tongue; therefore it is important to have jaw stability in order to develop refined tongue, cheek, and lip movement (Morris & Klein, 1987). Stability of the jaw is influenced by the stability of the hyoid cartilage in the neck area which, in turn, is influenced by the development of head, neck, and shoulder girdle control. There is also a relationship between gross and fine motor development. In normal development gross motor skills develop prior to fine motor skills. Feeding is also considered a fine motor progression (Morris & Klein, 1987) that depends on the gross motor base of controlled stability and mobility.

Influence of Muscle Tone on Oral-Pharyngeal Development

Although differences exist among children with developmental disabilities, many of their problems are commonly associated with abnormal development of muscle tone. Drooling, uncoordinated breathing, and inability to initiate, grade, or sustain oral patterns are often seen (Ottenbacher et al., 1983). Hypotonic children lack the ability to stabilize their head and trunk which may, in turn, degrade control for breathing and swallowing. The child with fluctuating tone may exhibit irregular breathing patterns, impaired coordination of swallow, and coughing or choking. In children with fluctuating tone, strong asymmetries often exist that interfere with lip approximation, chewing, and swallowing. Hypertonic children frequently exhibit extensor patterns of head, trunk, and limbs that limit oral and thoracic movement (Ottenbacher et al., 1983).

Postural Control and Oral-Pharyngeal Function

Postural functions, such as head and trunk control and shoulder girdle stability, have a strong effect on oral-pharyngeal movement patterns. Graded jaw movements require some degree of postural stability of the head, neck, and shoulder girdle. Abnormal distribution of postural tonus (e.g., as seen in a strong asymmetrical tonic neck reflex) may be manifested in the oral and facial area, thereby impeding coordination and dissociation of oral movements (Scherzer & Tscharnuter, 1982).

Optimal feeding patterns seem to be linked to optimal positioning in the child with central nervous system deficit. Head position influences oral posture and function. A reclining or semi-reclining position interferes with manipulation of the food. The food falls by gravity toward the pharynx. Therefore, an upright symmetrical position is recommended with postural support and stability (Scherzer & Tscharnuter, 1982). The development of swallowing is dependent on normal tone, alignment, and coordination of the musculature of the oral structures as well as on intact oral reflexes (Meek, 1991). Children with motoric disorders of postural tone and movement often have co-occurring difficulty with closing the mouth, coordinating tongue movement, and swallowing.

Head and neck stability, as noted, facilitate use of the mouth. Shoulder action is also directly related to the functioning of the mouth through the action of the pectoral musculature of the chest on the forward structures of the neck and throat (Nelson & de Benabib, 1991). Lack of head and neck control often results in compensations in the shoulders. They tend to elevate and move forward in an attempt to do the work of the neck, but in turn interfere with neck elongation. Nelson and de Benabib (1991) suggest that elongation of the neck is achieved by simultaneous capital flexion (cranium on the neck) and cervical extension at vertebral level C7–T1, or flexion forward. They further suggest that poor mobility and limited range of movement in the pelvis limit the opportunity for true elongation of the neck by limiting forward movement of the trunk. Abnormal shortening of the neck tends to be associated with a forward position of the chin, rounding of the back, and backward tilt of the pelvis when the child is seated.

If the scapulae are adducted, the shoulders will pull back into a retracted position causing tension that may hyperextend the neck and cause lip, jaw, and tongue retraction. The child will also have difficulty getting the hands to the mouth. If the shoulders are held in abduction (too much forward rounding or protraction), this also influences the position of the neck and will change oral-pharyngeal patterns. In this instance, the pelvis is tilted in a posterior direction requiring the child to strain to extend the neck to get the face upright to receive food. Shoulder protraction also creates excessive muscle tone which affects chewing, sucking, and swallowing patterns (Morris & Klein, 1987).

The presence or absence of righting responses also contributes to the problem and interferes with mouth function. Postural control against gravity develops with the influence of righting reactions which bring the head into proper position in space (Scherzer & Tscharnuter, 1982). In righting reactions, optical, labyrinthine, or tactile stimuli to receptors in the eyes, inner ears, muscles, or skin orient movements of the head, neck, and body to maintain the eyes and mouth in horizontal, head vertical, and body in proper relationship to the head.

Historical Perspective

The Bobath neurodevelopmental approach to the treatment of oral motor dysfunction has been expanded by Mueller (1972) and by Morris and Klein (1987). Emphasis is on the reduction of tactile defensiveness and the use of body positioning. Excessive sensitivity to sensory stimulation may interfere with bottle or breast feeding requiring special handling (e.g., slow vestibular stimulation) to integrate tactile information and reduce sensitivity. Proper body positioning inhibits abnormal muscle tone and reflexes throughout the body while facilitating normal movement patterns. The sitting posture is preferred for feeding. When head control is poor, support must be provided. Midline orientation with slight ventroflexion is generally preferred (Ottenbacher et al., 1983).

The effects of Bobath's treatment principles were investigated in a study by Banerdt and Bricker in 1978 (cited in Ottenbacher, Bundy, & Short, 1983). Development of finger feeding was facilitated in a 2½-year-old child with spastic cerebral palsy. Initially, spasticity was reduced by rocking. Then the child was placed in an adapted highchair which included a rubber mat on the seat to reduce sliding, a footrest, and a peg mounted on the right side of the tray. The child was encouraged to hold the peg to assist him in maintaining a symmetrical body position. The authors concluded that the use of proper positioning and the aforementioned adapted equipment improved the child's ability to move his hand to his mouth and begin to self-feed. It is felt that with proper positioning a child is freer to use his upper extremities and concentrate on the activity itself.

Case study reports have focused on the issue of therapeutic positioning to improve head control during feeding programs. In a study by Hulme, Gallacher, and Hulme in 1981 (cited in Mac Neela, 1987) a model for use of adaptive equipment for children with developmental disabilities is described. The effectiveness of these interventions included improved head and trunk control, sucking

and swallowing ability, and finger feeding. Hulme, Schulein, and Hulme in 1983 (cited in Mac Neela, 1987) further reported functional benefits for clients receiving adaptive equipment. Significant improvement was noted in eating manner, drinking manner, and ability to reach for and grasp an object.

Mueller (1972) suggests supporting the infant with poor head control on a wedge or pillow in a semi-reclined position. The parent sits in front of a table with a large wedge or pillow on the lap supported on the edge of the table. The infant reclines on his back on the wedge or pillow facing the parent (Figure 8–1). Flexion of the head and hips while in this position counteracts abnormal extensor patterns.

Takagi and Bosma (1960) recommend that an infant with severe sucking and swallowing problems or with functional retrusion of the mandible be placed in the prone position for feeding. Lewis and Pashayan (1980) recommend that infants with Robin anomaly, who present with respiratory and feeding problems in the immediate postnatal and neonatal period, be maintained in the prone position at all times, including feeding, to take maximum advantage of the effect of gravity on the tongue and so as not to upset the delicate airway balance. Congenital micrognathia and secondary glossoptosis, with or without cleft palate, constitute the Robin anomaly; and these infants are at risk for life-threatening respiratory and feeding problems. When feeding older children in the prone position, it is important to remember that lack of sufficient extension against gravity, which is necessary for adequate head control in the prone position, will result in abnormal use of extensor tone. Positioning on the prone board in a more upright position diminishes these problems.

Placement of the food and how the parent approaches the infant also influence head position. For example, food presented

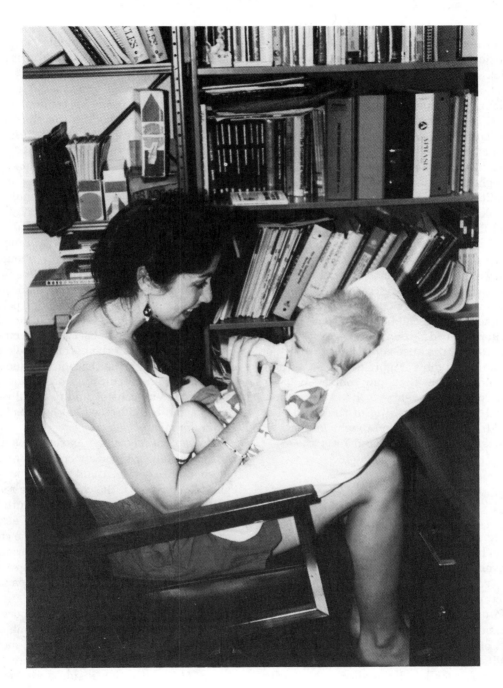

Figure 8–1.
Feeding the infant with poor head control: Support the child on a wedge or pillow in a semi-reclined position. The parent sits in front of a table with a large wedge or pillow on the lap supported on the edge of the table; the child is reclined on his back on the pillow facing the parent. The child's legs are abducted around the parent's waist and flexed at the hips to reduce extensor tone, the head is slightly flexed forward, the arms are facilitated toward midline.

from above results in too much head extension. To correct hyperextension of the neck and reinforce midline orientation, food should be presented from the front in midline and from below the mouth.

By 5 to 6 months of age, the normal baby has sufficient sitting balance to be fed in a highchair. If possible the developmentally impaired infant should also be fed sitting in a highchair or seat insert. It is important to facilitate an upright posture of head and trunk. If fed on the parent's lap, Scherzer and Tscharnuter (1982) recommend that hip flexion be obtained by having the baby's buttocks slide down between the parent's legs. They suggest that placing one foot on a stool helps the caregiver to increase the amount of the infant's hip flexion. The opposite knee can support the child's low and mid-back to influence head flexion. The caregiver's arm can rest on the knee supporting the back or on a nearby table (Figure 8–2). The authors further suggest that "jaw control" helps to correct any tendency to head retraction, head turning, or tilting of the head. The child's arms should be brought forward for proper posture of the shoulder girdle.

Physical Therapy Assessment for Feeding

Feeding difficulties are frequently noted early in life. Children should be assessed for intervention as soon as the problems are observed. The evaluation, for the purpose of therapeutic intervention, should be a team effort including the physical therapist, occupational therapist, speech pathologist, parent or caregiver, teacher, physician, nurse, and social worker, if involved. This allows input from all individuals involved with the child and coordination of treatment and goals.

Prior to the evaluation it is helpful to obtain the child's background history. Knowledge of the child's medications is important because certain medications can influence the child's behavior and response as well as teeth and gum hygiene. The assessment (see Appendix 8A) should include initial impressions and observations without facilitation. What does the child look like? How does the child interact with other people and with the environment?

A physical and gross motor assessment is essential to determine the primary problems. This part of the assessment should address muscle tone, body symmetry, postural reactions, primitive reflexes, spinal and pelvic mobility, abdominal activity, range of motion, head and trunk control, shoulder girdle stability, positions available for function, total patterns of movement, associated reactions, and bony structure (spine, pelvis, and hips as well as oral areas). Much of this can be determined by observing the child's movement, watching the parent handle the child, and through the therapist's handling of the child and facilitation of movement. Body alignment, control, and postural reactions should be addressed as they relate to feeding problems.

Assessment of upper extremity active range of motion is important both in the child old enough to self-feed and in the younger child to determine if the child's active range is sufficient for getting hands to mouth for oral stimulation and investigation. Passive range of motion does not tell you if the child can accomplish these skills. The assessment should determine if the range is greater when the pelvis, trunk, and proximal parts of the body are stabilized.

Sensorimotor assessment is important to determine if and how postural tone and dominant tonic reflexes impact on movement and the reactions of the child to sensation. Oral sensation inside and around the mouth should be observed for the presence or absence of oral reflexes. Auditory sensation, including visual and gross motor responses, should also be noted. The examiner should observe the child's reaction

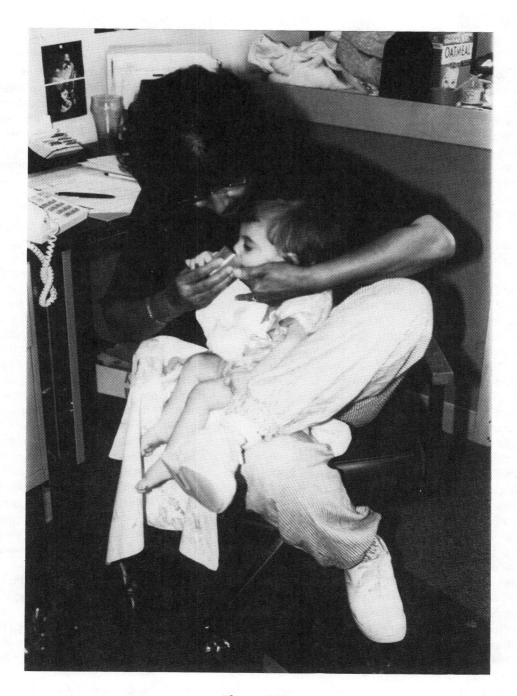

Figure 8–2.
Postural control when feeding the child on the parent's lap: Slide the child's buttocks down between the parent's legs to influence hip flexion, place one foot on a stool to increase hip flexion. The other leg should be used to support the child's back against the knee to facilitate head flexion while resting the parent's arm on the knee for support. This facilitates upright position of the head and trunk, allows for jaw control, and enables the parent to influence the arms forward for proper posture of the shoulder girdle.

to touch in the oral area; to the texture, taste, and temperature of the food; and to the utensil being used. Observe the child's reaction to being held and how the child reacts to being moved in space. Does the infant place his or her hand in the mouth; what is the response? How does the child respond to objects or soft toys around the mouth? It is important to place the stimulus on the body prior to the mouth for desensitization even during the assessment. Look at the teeth and gum area.

The caregiver should be observed feeding the child to assess the impact of the child's position on oral function. Is the infant reclined, upright, aligned and supported sufficiently? Optimally the child should have an upright head and trunk. Support should be given to the low and mid-back to facilitate head flexion. The child's arms should be in the forward position for proper shoulder girdle posture. The child's head position prior, during, and after swallowing of pureed foods, solids, or liquids should be observed. Observe for tongue thrust. How can you position the child better to achieve improved swallow? These observations are important to determine how to position the child to improve swallowing. Position may also affect control of oral secretions. Increased stability can facilitate head control and improved jaw control. Feeding behaviors are further discussed in Chapter 3.

The child's predominant breathing pattern in sitting, standing, supine, and prone positions should be observed because of its influence on swallow. In the older child, observe sound production, initiation of phonation, and prime form of communication. Does the child have to use total extension to produce sound?

Assessment of the facial and oral peripheral area includes observation of facial tone and expression at rest and during activity. Is there a relationship of oral tone to overall postural tone? (Tone in mouth may

be the same as or different from the rest of the body, or may be mixed.) Oral and facial features are observed for asymmetry, structural problems, or dental misalignment due to abnormal movement patterns. Note features of oral anatomy (e.g., cleft lip or palate, facial tremors including jaw clonus and grimacing) that would influence the feeding position decision.

Sensory stimuli within and around the mouth elicit feeding reflexes in the normal baby. The hypersensitive child reacts to stimuli with abnormal tension of lips, cheeks, and tongue. To appreciate subtle tonal changes, the therapist selectively touches the oral and perioral area to stimulate different oral reflexes (Scherzer & Tscharnuter, 1982). Does the position or handling affect oral function? If primitive/abnormal reflexes are present, can they be inhibited by proper handling and positioning? Knowledge of the oral reflexes is important during the assessment.

In assessing the swallow reflex, videofluoroscopy may be recommended. An appropriate seating system should be utilized for this. Special chairs are commercially available (e.g., Hausted's Video-Fluoroscopic Imaging Chair which offers infinite positioning from supine to sitting for full spectrum filming and modular inserts for pediatric patients) (see Figure 8–3). The oral reflexes are discussed in Chapter 3.

Determine the areas of postural development that are limiting or blocking the acquisition of new skills or the improved quality of skills. This provides the therapist with the basis of the treatment plan.

The Seating Positioning Assessment

Children should be assessed for positioning and seating intervention as soon as oral motor problems are recognized. Feeding problems often cause frustration resulting in a stressful family situation in both the

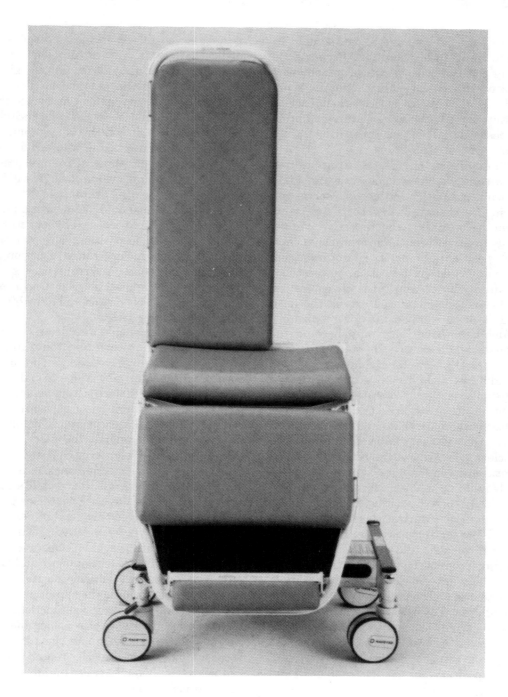

Figure 8–3.
The Hausted Video-Fluoroscopic Imaging Chair with a modular seating system to feed, hold, transport, and position the pediatric patient. Chair has a built-in abductor, safety vest, and positioning belt with contoured interior for posturally correct seating alignment. The chair is illustrated here with a Tumble form feeder seat for use with a small child.

normal and at-risk infant and should be given immediate attention. Proper positioning of the body is critical to achieving positive changes in feeding. Therapy to improve oral skills for eating should not be initiated until a team has addressed proper positioning (Bergen, Presperin, & Tallman, 1990).

To determine the best seating position for a child, we need to observe the child's postural strengths and needs. Morris and Klein (1987) suggest that there are orthopedic, respiratory, and digestive components to all positions. For example, a chin-tuck position may be an appropriate goal for many children, but not appropriate for children with certain types of respiratory problems. Some children extend the head and neck to compensate for respiratory difficulties. Breathing may become too stressed when we provide neck elongation and capital flexion for the ideal chin-tuck. In addition, a child with extreme extensor spasticity may not tolerate the more upright position with knee and hip flexion. A better position for that child may be reclining on the right side, which facilitates more efficient emptying of the stomach. Therapeutic intervention may be needed to gradually build up tolerance for the more physiologically correct position and to facilitate the transition during this skill development. The seating posture must be individualized to each child's needs. In addition, positioning must be altered or modified as new skills develop and to accommodate to growth and body changes.

Children with severe involvement may develop fixed deformities that need to be considered in creating an effective positioning system for feeding. There are different positions for feeding: seated (weight bearing on arms with head forward), on a prone board (weight bearing on arms with chin tuck), or on a propped pillow or wedge (on the lap against a desk or table).

In the seating positioning assessment (see Appendix 8B) the child's medical histo-ry must be considered, including diagnosis, medical prognosis, medical problems that may affect positioning for feeding, surgical intervention past and planned for the future, and adaptive equipment and orthotics in use. Background history should include the environment in which the equipment will be used and caretakers who will be using the equipment. Many of the areas assessed in the feeding evaluation also will be included in the seating evaluation.

The evaluation should begin with an assessment on the mat followed by an assessment in the sitting position. The mat assessment should include range of motion of all extremities, pelvis, and trunk because of the influence of limited lower or upper extremity range or pelvic and spinal mobility on the positioning decision.

The evaluation should include an assessment to determine tone and tonal influences on positioning, as well as the presence or absence of postural and balance reactions which influence sitting balance. A biomechanical evaluation of postural control and skeletal status including deformities is important to analyze the effect of any externally applied load through positioning and the forces generated in bones, muscles, and joints by these loads. If the child's balance is precarious, the body possesses poor ability to resist forces that tend to destroy the balance. This is important in planning an adaptive seating system. Observe the level of gross motor development and the impact of abnormal motor patterns of movement to determine the appropriate influence required for improved function.

The assessment should consider the effect of sensory problems and their impact on positioning. Skin integrity requires special attention. Visual acuity, auditory status, and perceptual ability may need to be addressed in terms of presentation of food and its impact on positioning. Perceptual ability is the ability to organize and interpret the sensations received from internal and external stimuli and the ability to effectively respond motorically. Inaccurate visual or auditory perception or deficient awareness of limb position or body position in space may cause inappropriate movement responses which should be considered in positioning for feeding. Observe fine motor skills and Activities of Daily Living (ADL) skills to determine how the positioning equipment can facilitate or improve these skills. Assess cognitive and behavioral status in terms of ability to utilize technology in an adapted positioning system. It is also important to look at communication status, in terms of receptive and expressive skills, as well as special positioning equipment that may be needed to facilitate the use of augmentative communication. Home, work, and educational environments, and transportation needs must be considered to ensure that the positioning equipment will be appropriate for the life style of the child and his or her caretakers.

During the assessment it is important to observe the reaction of the child's body to each influence provided in a positioning system. A seating simulator, such as the Kiss or Flamingo (see Figure 8–4), is helpful if used during the evaluation to visualize which influences result in the desired effect.

It is important to take into consideration the aesthetics of the positioning equipment being considered. Acceptance of the equipment by the child and caretaker is essential if the equipment is going to be utilized. Involving the family and child in the choice of the equipment, including color and style, is helpful.

Strategies for Providing Competent Body Postural Control

Proper positioning and seating is an important priority in the management and development of the disabled child. It is a prerequisite to learning and to functioning, as well as feeding. Good therapeutic seating is an adjunct and a continuum of ther-

apy that has a role to play in helping the child achieve therapeutic goals of treatment that lead to increased functional ability. For the child with cerebral palsy, these therapeutic goals include reducing or normalizing muscle tone, as well as abnormal patterns of movement, to allow development of more normal patterns of movement. Improvement of proximal control is essential to establish improvement in distal control which includes head, neck, and all extremities. The goals of seating include providing appropriate support to facilitate this needed proximal control.

The ideal position for feeding includes a good base of support, balance of the trunk over the base of support, good alignment between the head and trunk, decreased elevation of shoulders, hands toward midline, chin tucked in, and vertical face position. If additional stabilization is needed, weight bearing on elbows or forearms on an upper extremity support surface will be helpful.

Proper positioning begins with a firm stable base of support. Proper support of the pelvis and hips is the key to functional seating and therefore the place to begin. The goal is to obtain a level or neutral pelvis. The solution should begin with the pelvis and its relationship to spinal alignment which influences the position of the head, shoulders, and upper extremities (see Appendix 8C). Improved stability of the pelvis will facilitate control of trunk, head, respiration, mouth, and self-feeding. Obliquity of the pelvis will cause spinal asymmetry with resulting impact on breathing, swallowing, and digestion. An anterior pelvic tilt may cause a reaction of pulling back the shoulders for balance. This retraction of the scapulae results in tightness of the neck muscles influencing jaw mobility and swallow. A posterior pelvic tilt influences the lower extremities into hip adduction and internal rotation, forward flexion of the trunk and head, compression on the diaphragm, decreased respiration, difficulty in swallow, with a low-

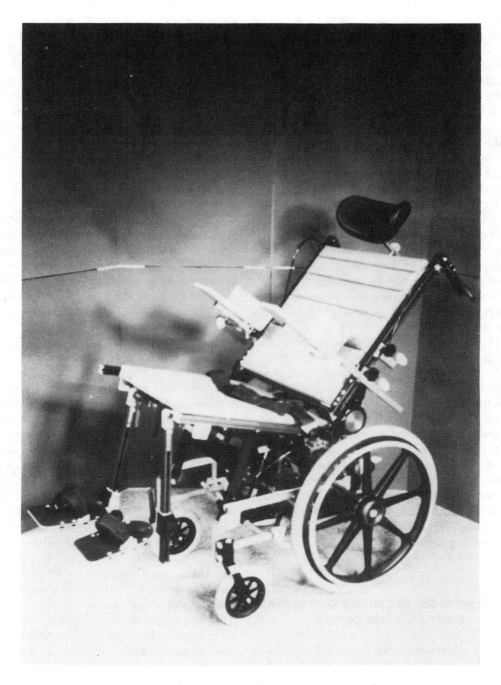

Figure 8–4.
The Flamingo Seating Simulator is a clinical tool for seating evaluation and functional positioning. Problem-solving strategies can be tried. Planar, as shown in the photo, and contour approaches are available and interchangeable on the Flamingo.

ered eye gaze. The aim is to get the pelvis in as close to neutral position as possible, which will facilitate improved spinal alignment and increased spinal mobility to avoid the above-mentioned problems and facilitate improved respiration, oral motor control, and swallow.

In positioning the pelvis, the depth and width of the seat is important. The child's thigh should be fully supported almost to the popliteal space to support the body weight. Full support of the femur facilitates proper pelvic alignment and inhibits extensor posture which may occur as a result of a short seat. If the seat is too deep, the pelvis will tilt posteriorly and the spine will round. A seat that is too narrow may force the legs together, narrowing the base and requiring a greater amount of trunk control for balance; a seat that is too wide may allow for too much movement and lack of symmetry.

The seat-to-back angle is an important consideration. Changes in seat-to-back angle can influence tone and posture (Bergen et al., 1990). Decisions on seat-to-back angle are based on the results of the mat assessment of the child's abilities. Some clinicians recommend using increased hip flexion of more than 90°, by wedging the seat or the back, to control the child's extensor thrusting. Others consider a 90° seat-to-back angle to produce the least amount of extensor tone. Recently, Zacharkow (1988) recommended opening the seat-to-back angle slightly to accommodate for the natural contours of the upper thorax and to ensure balance. A rigid seat-to-back angle is not appropriate for the child who does not have 90 degrees of hip flexion. Children with spasticity may experience reduced hypertonicity in the anterior muscles by opening the angle to 95°. In the hypotonic child, opening the angle may decrease the tone by decreasing the co-contractions occurring between flexor and extensor muscle groups and may result in increased hypoactivity of the trunk, decreased stabili-

ty, and therefore decreased active control for movements of the head, upper torso, and upper extremities. It may even result in increased extensor activity. The proper angle, therefore, is often determined by the amount of hip flexion required to maintain a neutral pelvic position and the amount of hip flexion available.

Tilting the seating system slightly in space may help maintain postural alignment in children who have difficulty fighting the pull of gravity when in a fully upright position. A chair with mechanisms that permit adjustments for changes in orientation in space allows the child to be upright for practice in developing head and trunk control. This type of chair will also allow for tilt backward when the child begins to fatigue. When utilizing a tilt-in-space chair, a headrest is needed to support the head and maintain proper alignment of the face, mouth, and chin.

For a symmetrical seating base, proper positioning of the legs is important. The legs must be positioned to inhibit the influence of abnormal tone and muscle imbalance and to assist in maintaining proper pelvic position for a stable base on which to build trunk, upper extremity, and head stability (Bergen et al., 1990). A medial knee support will inhibit hip extension and adduction as is seen in associated reactions during activities. The medial knee support should be placed between the knees but not have contact with the mid-thigh which may stimulate the adductor reflex. Use of lateral knee supports will limit excessive abduction of one or both legs and help to maintain a symmetrical position.

To achieve good stability, a footrest or foot support is needed. If the child's range allows, the hips, knees, and ankles should be positioned at 90° to inhibit extensor tone. Footrests that are too high will cause the child to sit on a small area of his or her bottom. This provides an unstable sitting base with excess pressure on the buttocks resulting in discomfort or skin breakdown (McEwen & Lloyd, 1990). Securing the feet on the footplate, in a neutral position, enhances stability especially if there are associated reactions during activities or if extensor tone is present.

A positioning belt is needed to maintain the pelvis back in the seat and for safety. It is usually recommended that the belt be placed at a 45° angle to the seat. However, if the child slips forward or the belt limits neutral pelvic position, the belt may be placed at 90°, at the thigh/hip junction. Some belts are fabricated with four attaching points to pull in both the 45° and 90° direction (both back and down) for improved pelvic positioning.

After positioning of the pelvis and lower extremities, attention should then be given to the trunk. It is important to observe the trunk for tone and symmetry. Poor trunk control leads to poor head control (Morris & Klein, 1987) because the neck needs a stable support surface for precise head control. Consider seating systems that provide adequate trunk support when needed.

Children who are mildly impaired may need only a firm back support with perhaps a lumbar pad to increase anterior pelvic tilt. For more involved clients, lateral trunk support may be required as well as hip guides to facilitate symmetry and postural control. Lateral supports can be bilateral or provide three-point control for a curvature. In the three-point system, two of the supports counter each other on each side of the trunk (over the apex of the curve on one side; placed higher on the opposite side which is the side to which the child usually leans), and the third is lateral to the pelvis stabilizing the pelvis so it does not shift in response to the forces applied to the trunk (Bergen et al., 1990).

The type of seat back recommended depends on the amount of trunk support needed. If the child has a spinal deformity or significant skeletal involvement, a more contoured back or custom-molded back might be considered to accommodate the deformity and provide postural control. This type of seat back affords more or maximum contact with the body and covers or surrounds the skeletal deformities fully, lessening the chance of pressure at bony prominences. Increased contact will provide increased stability and increased comfort with decreased pressure over the points of contact. However, the molded back does not allow for movement and should be used only when maximum control and support are needed. A custom carved solid back may provide sufficient support and can be fabricated to allow for accommodation of deformities that would be difficult to position in a straight or flat planar surface.

If shoulder retraction is present, it will affect the child's ability to bring the hands together and impact on neck position resulting in abnormal oral motor function. Upper arm blocks attached to the chair or tray may help to inhibit the arms from going back. They also inhibit shoulder retraction and facilitate a more midline upper extremity position. Increased shoulder protraction will also cause changes in oral motor patterns. An anterior chest support attached to the chair can provide trunk extension and inhibit shoulder protraction. An upper extremity support system (tray) will also be helpful.

The importance of the position of the child's head has been stressed. The position of the head influences the way we swallow, and change of head position affects the swallow. Changes in the hips, pelvis, trunk, and shoulder girdle allow the head to assume a more normal posture. The angle formed by the back and seat of the chair will influence head position. The more upright the position, the more the head and neck need to work. To give the child with poor head control better support, a slightly reclining position will reduce the amount of effort that is involved.

A variety of headrests are available to assist the child in maintaining a more normal head and neck posture. The child may not need a headrest at all times. The headrest can be used for safety when riding a school bus, when being fed, or any other time when more support is needed. It can be removed at other times so that continued development of head control can occur (Morris & Klein, 1987). An occipital contour incorporated into the headrest encourages cervical flexion and discourages hyperextension of the neck. Hyper- and hypotonic individuals may benefit from this type of support. Excessive pressure at the base of the skull where there is no bony protection should be avoided. The neck roll provides occipital support without contacting the occiput. It is placed behind the neck and below the occipital contour. The neck support frees the child to make small head adjustments which are helpful in using eye gaze (Bergen et al., 1990). It is important to understand that the headrest may need to be removed during feeding if "jaw control" is utilized to facilitate oral posture and movement or to inhibit head retraction, turning or tilting.

Although appropriate positioning greatly improves oral function, further control of oral responses may be indicated for the severely involved child. This control can be achieved with a facial grasp or "jaw control" to facilitate proper head flexion and midline orientation. The facial grasp may be applied from the side and from the front. In the side grasp, the caregiver's arm is placed behind the child's head together with the grasp around the chin to prevent the child from pushing the head back (Scherzer & Tscharnuter, 1982). In this case, removal of the headrest is required. In the front approach, the headrest can remain in place.

During the assessment it is important to continually observe the response of the child's body to each influence provided in a positioning system to afford maximum postural control for feeding.

Therapy Treatment for Feeding

The use of positioning and handling is important to facilitation of normal gross motor development. Mastery of fine postural adjustments around the vertebral midline is reflected in improved mouth symmetry and control. There is a close relationship between the state of the mouth and that of the body (Nelson & de Benabib, 1991). Postural difficulties should be addressed by clinicians skilled in dealing with mobility and alignment problems. Positioning of the child must take into account the findings and observations of postural control assessment (Nelson & de Benabib, 1991).

Chin tuck, abdominal control, and balance of flexion and extension for upright head control bring the tongue and lips into more forward position and reduce inappropriate posturing of the mouth and pharynx. Improving the strength of the abdominal muscles promotes stability and mobility of the rib cage for improved respiration. Morris and Klein (1987) have found that promoting upper body and abdominal stability may reduce excessive burping and gastroesophageal reflux. Other positional strategies which may reduce postprandial gastroesophageal reflux (GER) include feeding on the right side and prone positioning at a 30 to 45° angle for 1 hour after meals. The Reflux Wedge (Figure 8–5) is a commercially available piece of equipment specifically designed for postprandial positioning to reduce gastroesophageal reflux in infants. It will hold the child comfortably prone at a 30° angle (see Appendix 8D).

Infants with difficulty in maintaining control of the pharyngeal airway may have

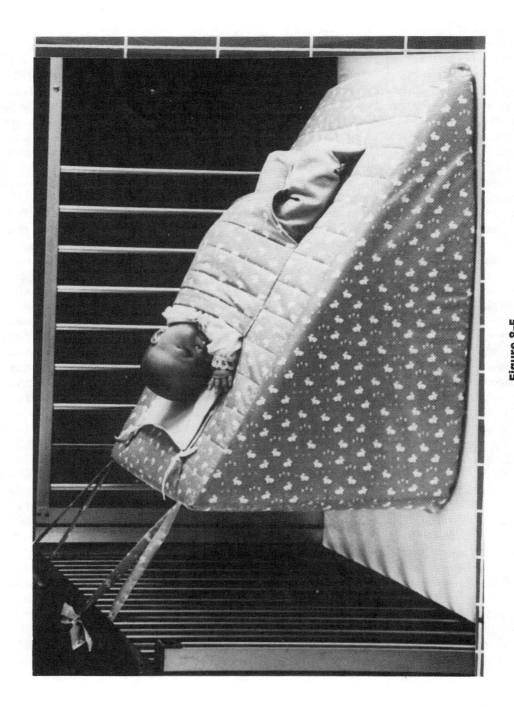

Figure 8–5.

The Reflux Wedge for postprandial positioning to reduce gastroesophageal reflux in infants. It holds the child prone at 30° angle.

the problem of the tongue falling back into the airway when placed in a supine position. These children benefit from prone lying or forward side lying during nippling.

It is important for the therapist who is doing the treatment to identify and analyze abnormal patterns. In the young infant postural control against gravity develops with the influence of righting reactions which bring the head into proper position in space. At approximately 4 months of age, neck extension and flexion begin to be integrated, permitting chin tuck and neck elongation. This brings the face into vertical and the mouth into a horizontal position. Free head movement is then able to occur against a stable shoulder girdle (Scherzer & Tscharnuter, 1982). In the baby with abnormal development, head posture is often affected. Retention of the primitive Asymmetrical Tonic Neck Reflex (ATNR) or a pattern of head and neck hyperextension and shoulder elevation only allows movement of the head and shoulders as one unit. An abnormal flexor pattern may limit the ability of the child to lift the head against gravity. Strong extensor tone may restrict movement and cause asymmetry. This sets the stage for problems in oral motor development and dysphagia. Treating these problems requires the utilization of specific handling techniques for influencing posture as well as the utilization of external support for seating and positioning to inhibit poor postures and facilitate more normal movement for improved feeding and function, as discussed previously (see the case study in Appendix 8E). Because of the intimate relationship between the head, neck, and oral motor structures, problems at this early stage of development can have a serious impact on the development of oral motor skills including feeding and communication.

Treatment and handling techniques should be aimed at having the child learn new motor skills; the focus is mainly on the coordination of movement patterns and their accompanying postures, which are changing and therefore dynamic. The infant with a restricted repertoire of postures is limited in purposeful movement. Normal postures and movements require normal strength and normal distribution of postural tone. Movement, tone, and posture are dependent on one another. Modification of any one of these functions will affect the other two. For example, correcting abnormal postural alignment can change tone and make possible more normal movement patterns. This is applicable to positioning for improved feeding. Proper adaptation of posture and tone, and maintenance of balance are normally regulated by subcortical centers. Postural adaptations are mostly automatic, freeing higher cortical centers for planning intentional motor acts. Patterns of voluntary movements are based on automatic postural reactions, such as righting, equilibrium, and protective reactions. The goal of therapy is to elicit appropriate automatic reactions in response to handling. The fact that motor responses can be elicited on an automatic level makes the treatment approach, of handling to facilitate normal movement and inhibition of abnormal movement, independent of the child's cooperation and level of cognition and is therefore well suited for the infant (Scherzer & Tscharnuter, 1982).

Summary

The concept that any influence on muscle tone, movement, or posture will cause a reaction, and that a desired automatic response can be facilitated through appropriate handling is applicable to the decision-making process in the treatment of dysphagia. Any influence to the child's position through handling or an adapted seating insert system will cause the body to react. Observation of the body's reactions to the seating and positioning help to determine the final positioning decisions. Utilization of a seating simulator has been found to be one effective way to observe how the child's body reacts to each change or influence offered and helps to ensure selection of the most appropriate seating system. Children grow and change rapidly, and positioning must change as the body changes. Therefore, frequent reassessment is required to ensure that the treatment provided is eliciting the desired response for swallowing and the child's other functional needs.

References

Bergen, A. F., Presperin, J., & Tallman, T. (1990). *Positioning for function*. Valhalla, NY: Valhalla Rehabilitation Publications.

Farber, S. D. (1982). *Neurorehabilitation: A Multisensory Approach*. Philadelphia, PA: W. B. Saunders.

Lewis, M. B., & Pashayan, H. M. (1980). Management of infants with Robin anomaly. *Clinical Pediatrics, 19,* 519–528.

Mac Neela, J. C. (1987). An overview of therapeutic positioning for multiply-handicapped persons, including augmentative communication users. *Physical & Occupational Therapy in Pediatrics, 7*(2), 39–60.

McEwen, I. R., & Lloyd, L. L. (1990). Positioning students with cerebral palsy to use augmentative and alternative communication. *Language, Speech and Hearing Services in Schools, 21,* 15–21.

Meek, M. (1991). Alternate feeding methods. In M. B. Langley & L. J. Lombardino (Eds.), *Neurodevelopmental strategies for managing communication disorders in children with severe motor dysfunction* (pp. 81–111). Austin, TX: Pro-Ed.

Morris, S. E., & Klein, M. D. (1987). *Pre-feeding skills*. Tucson, AZ: Therapy Skill Builders.

Mueller, H. A. (1972). Facilitating feeding and pre-speech. In P. H. Pearson & C. E. Williams (Eds.), *Physical therapy services in the developmental disabilities* (pp. 283–310). Springfield, IL: Charles C Thomas.

Nelson, C. A., & de Benabib, R. M. (1991). Sensory preparation of the oral motor area. In M. B. Langley & L. J. Lombardino (Eds.), *Neurodevelopmental strategies for managing communication disorders in children with severe motor dysfunction* (pp. 131–158). Austin, TX: Pro-Ed.

Ottenbacher, K., Bundy, A., & Short, M. A. (1983). The development and treatment of oral-motor function: A review of clinical research. *Physical & Occupational Therapy in Pediatrics, 3*(2), 1–13.

Scherzer, A. L., & Tscharnuter, I. (1982). Early diagnosis and therapy in cerebral palsy. In *Pediatric habilitation* (Vol. 3). New York: B. C. Decker.

Takagi, Y., & Bosma, J. (1960). Disability of oral function in an infant associated with displacement of the tongue. *ACTA Paediatrica, 49*(Suppl. 123), 62–69.

Zacharkow, D. (1988). *Posture: Sitting, standing, chair design and exercise*. Springfield, IL: Charles C Thomas.

APPENDIX 8A

Physical Therapy Assessment for Feeding

Name: _____

Date of Birth: _____ Date of Evaluation: _____

Evaluating Team:_____

Diagnosis: _____

    I. General Observations
       A. Interaction with others
       B. Description of child's looks
       C. Alertness
   II. Background Medical History
       A. Birth history
       B. Medical problems
       C. Medication
       D. Surgical history
  III. Gross Motor Assessment
       A. Muscle tone
       B. Body symmetry and alignment
       C. Postural reactions present
       D. Primitive reflexes present
       E. Spinal mobility
       F. Pelvic mobility
       G. Range of motion: upper and lower extremities
          1. Passive range
          2. Active available range with stability
       H. Head control
       I. Trunk control
       J. Shoulder girdle stability
       K. Patterns of movement
       L. Associated reactions during feeding
       M. Abnormal reflexes and postural responses affecting position and feeding
  IV. Sensory Assessment
       A. Observe presence or absence of oral reflexes
       B. Visual and gross motor responses to auditory sensation
       C. Reaction to touch in the oral area
       D. Reaction to texture, taste, and temperature of food
       E. Reaction to utensils utilized
       F. Reaction to being held and moved in space
       G. Reaction to soft toys around mouth
       H. Child's ability to bring hand to mouth and reaction

   V. Observation of Child Being Fed by Parent
      A. Position held for nursing, bottle drinking, cup, or spoon feeding
      B. Type of swallow, chew, lip closure; and influence of position
      C. Oral posture and tone during feeding
      D. Phase of swallow in which problems exist
      E. Coordination of suck/swallow/breath and impact of position
  VI. Breathing Pattern in All Positions and the Influence of Position on These Patterns
      A. Sitting
      B. Prone
      C. Sidelying
 VII. Facial and Oral Peripheral Status
      A. Oral tone; relationship to overall tone
      B. Symmetry of facial features
      C. Structural deviations (e.g., cleft lip and palate, dental misalignment)
      D. Drooling
      E. Observe for jaw clonus, grimacing
VIII. Conclusion
      A. Effect of posture on existing feeding skills
      B. Effect of posture on improving feeding skills
      C. Effect of posture on airway protection

APPENDIX 8B

Seating Positioning Assessment

Name: _____

Date of Birth: _____ Date of Evaluation: _____

Evaluating Team: _____

   I. Medical History
      A. Diagnosis
      B. Medical problems
      C. Surgical history and future planned surgery
      D. Adaptive equipment and orthotics in use
      E. Present programs and related services (i.e., PT/OT/SpT)
  II. General Impression
      A. Adjustment to handling
      B. Alertness
      C. Social interactions
      D. Present means of parental carrying and equipment utilized
 III. Tone and Postural Reflexes
      A. Determine tone and its influence
      B. Balance reactions present
      C. Note pathological reflexes or reactions
 IV. Biomechanical Issues
      A. Skeletal status including deformities and their affect on positioning and handling
      B. Strength of trunk and extremities
      C. Range of motion; upper and lower extremities
         1. Passive range
         2. Active available range with stability
   V. Sensory Status
      A. Skin integrity should be watched in seating
      B. Visual and auditory status (e.g., influence on placement of food presented)
      C. Perceptual-motor status as it relates to response to position in space and movement
 VI. Functional Gross Motor Status (refer to Appendix 8A)
      A. Gross motor skill level
      B. Head and trunk control
      C. Sitting, pull to stand, standing skills
      D. Contractures and deformities which restrict movement and mobility
      E. Ambulation status and gait pattern
 VII. Fine Motor and ADL Skills
      A. Functional abilities (e.g., dressing, feeding, toileting)
      B. Eye-hand coordination and relation to self-feeding
      C. Grasp patterns
      D. Postural reactions interfering with feeding
      E. Hand dominance
VIII. Cognitive and Behavioral Status and Their Influence on the Use of Adapted Positioning Equipment and Technological Aids
 IX. Receptive and expressive communication status and use of augmentative communication devices
  X. Home, school, transportation, and environmental needs and limitations

APPENDIX 8C

Possible Seating Solutions to Feeding Problems

A careful mat assessment in supine, sidelying, and sitting positions is an essential part of the decision making process to find solutions to feeding positioning problems.

Problem	Impact	Possible Solutions
Pelvis		

Posterior pelvic tilt	Lower extremities adduct, internally rotate
	Rounded spine creating eating, and respiratory problems
	Difficulty reaching forward
	Excessive neck flexion or extension causing visual, eating, and respiratory problems
		Support pelvis in optimal position:
		  Firm seat, good back support, appropriate seat/back angle
		Correct seat depth for optimal support (too deep results in posterior tilt)
		Correct knee flexion angle to eliminate hamstring pull on pelvis
		Lumbosacral pad to block posterior iliac crest and support lumbar curve
		Maintain pelvis at rear of seat using:
		Properly placed lap belt
		  Aggressive seating contours to discourage sliding
		  Anterior knee block (MD must check to confirm hip and knee integrity)
		  Alter tilt of system to change gravitational pull

Excessive anterior pelvic tilt	Shoulders pulled back for balance with secondary tightness in neck muscles influencing jaw mobility and swallow	Support pelvis (same as above) Use of belly binder Second belt across anterior superior iliac spine or 4-point belt

Asymmetrical pelvis	Asymmetry of trunk, head, and lower extremities	Fixed:
		  Support pelvis in optimal position and attempt to maintain level head and shoulder alignment
		  Contoured seating system for increased control and comfort, decreases pressure
		Flexible:
		  Lateral hip supports or positioners
		  Contoured seating system for increased contact and increased control
		  Special placement of positioning belt

Lower Extremities		
Hip abduction, external rotation	Asymmetrical positioning Decreased stability	Correct seat depth for full thigh support Lateral knee blocks

Problem	Impact	Possible Solutions
Lower Extremities (Continued)		
	Posterior or anterior pelvic tilt	Increased contour of seating system
Hip adduction, internal rotation	Narrow, unstable base of support Increased total extension Posterior pelvic tilt	Correct seat depth for full thigh support Medial knee contour or block Foot positioners: heel cups, shoeholders, straps
Trunk		
Trunk instability	Inadequate base for head control Compensatory "fixing" positions for stability Respiratory and feeding problems	Provide adequate trunk support with: Appropriate back height and width Lateral hip support for symmetry Lateral trunk support Anterior chest support Contoured or molded back for increased support and control
Rounded spine (fixed, postural)	Poor head/neck alignment Difficulty sitting upright Difficulty with breathing and swallowing	Decrease influence of gravity by: Tilt in space seating system Anterior chest support Shoulder support Change in seat-to-back angle
Trunk asymmetry	Asymmetry of head and neck resulting in respiratory, oral motor, and feeding problems	Accommodate, support, and/or provide postural control using: Contoured or molded positioning system for maximum control and support 3-point control
Shoulder Girdle		
Shoulder retraction; scapular adduction	Difficulty bringing hands together or to mouth Increased muscular tension may hyperextend neck causing lip, jaw, and tongue retraction Poor neck position causing abnormal oral motor function	Support pelvis and trunk as discussed above Facilitate scapular protraction by using: Upper extremity support system Upper arm blocks attached to back support or tray Facilitate upright position of head by: Opening seat/back angle Tilting system back a few degrees
Shoulder protraction; scapular abduction	Poor position of head, neck and oral structures Upper trunk rounding requiring the child to strain to get face	Support pelvis and trunk as discussed above Upper extremity support at proper height and pitch Alter tilt and/or seat/back angle

(Continued)

Problem	Impact	Possible Solutions
Shoulder Girdle (Continued)		
	upright to receive food Increase flexor tone affecting chewing, sucking, and swallowing pattern	

Head and Neck
Hyperextension
	Swallowing problem
	Poor lip approximation
	Lip, jaw, and tongue retraction
	Compensatory posture: elevation of shoulders and forward movement of shoulders interfere with neck elongation
	Long-term compensation: posterior pelvic tilt, rounded back, forward chin, neck shortening
		Facilitate neck elongation and improved head control by:
		  Properly positioning and supporting pelvis, trunk and shoulder girdle
		  Headrest with occipital contour
		  Open seat/back angle to align shoulders over hips to improve head position
		  Tilt system to allow head to rest on head support
		  Neck support which allows small head movements for adjustment
		  Providing upper extremity support
		  Pressure over anterior chest wall

Neck flexion	Swallowing problem
	Limited respiration
	Visual gaze problem
	Forward position of chin, rounding of back, and posterior pelvic tilt
		Facilitate upright head position by:
		  Upright position of pelvis, trunk and shoulder girdle (including upper extremity support)
		  Headrest with extra surface area, side support, anterior forehead support
		  Tilt-in-space to reduce effect of gravitational pull
		  Open seat/back angle as noted above
		  Anterior neck support
		  Presenting stimuli on easeled surface

Tone
Increased extensor tone
	Posterior pelvic tilt
	High guard position of upper extremities
	Hyperextension of neck with secondary respiratory and feeding problems
	Limited oral movement
	Limited thoracic movement
		Decrease tone by:
		  Adjust seat/back angle to decrease tone
		  Accommodate natural body contours by surface shaping and/or opening of seat/back angle
		  Alter orientation in space to maintain joint position, seating angles, and pelvic stability
		  Inhibit posterior pelvic tilt as noted above

Decreased tone	Inability to sit upright
	Inability to stabilize head and trunk causing compromised respiration
		Provide increased support by:
		  Contoured or molded seating surface
		  Lateral and/or anterior trunk support as needed

(Continued)

Problem	Impact	Possible Solutions
Tone (Continued)		

	and swallow	Counteract hypotonicity by:
		  Adjusting tilt in space and/or seat/back
		    angle to minimize influence of gravity
		  Open seat/back angle and forward
		    slope seat to facilitate active trunk
		    extension

Associated Reactions
  Adduction of
  hips
	Unstable sitting base
	Asymmetrical pelvis
	Poor stability for trunk,
	  head, and upper
	  extremity control
		Provide supportive seated position by:
		  Supportive seat and back with
		    aggressive contour and/or control
		    blocks
		  Proper seat depth and back height
		  Correct seat/back angle and tilt
		  Proper foot support (correct height,
		    sufficient controls)
		  Increase hip abduction beyond neutral
		    but within available range of motion

Reflexes
  Asymmetrical
  tonic neck
  reflex (ATNR)
	Postural asymmetry
	Impedes coordination
	  and dissociation of
	  oral movements
		Reduce influence of reflex by:
		  Appropriate positioning of pelvis
		    and trunk to facilitate midline
		    symmetrical positioning
		  Head support to facilitate neck
		    elongation and midline head position
		  Upper extremity support to facilitate
		    arms forward and in midline
		  Shoulder blocks on back or upper
		    extremity support surface for midline
		    positioning
		  Orientation of stimuli in midline

Absence of
  righting
  responses
	Lack of postural control
	  against gravity
	Unable to bring head into
	  proper position in space
	Unable to maintain head
	  eyes and mouth in
	  horizontal, head neutral,
	  and body in relationship
	  to head
		Influence upright midline posture by:
		  Providing lateral pelvic and trunk
		    positioners for support and symmetry
		  Providing appropriate back height
		    to support shoulders in neutral
		    or slightly protracted
		  Appropriate tilt in space

*Gastroesophageal
reflux (GER)*
		Provide sufficient support to promote
		  upper body and trunk stability to
		  reduce reflux
		Use alternate positioning after meals:
		  30–45° angle in prone for 1 hour
		  after meals
		Reflux wedge for postprandial positioning

APPENDIX 8D

Resources

Video-Fluoroscopic Imaging Chair (VIC)

Hausted
927 Lake Road
P.O. Box 710
Medina, OH 44258-0710
Fax: (216) 725-0505
Phone: (800) 428-7833 / (216) 723-3271

Reflux Wedge

Pedicraft
2014 Perry Place
Jacksonville, FL 32207
Phone: (904) 396-9627

Flamingo Simulator

Tallahassee Therapeutic Equipment
9601 Miccosukee Road #13
Tallahassee, FL 32308
Phone: (904) 877-0488

Kiss Simulator

Pin Dot Products
6001 Gross Point Road
Niles, IL 60648

Head and Neck Supports

Danmar Products Inc.
221 Jackson Industrial Drive
Ann Arbor, MI 48103

Mulholland Positioning Systems Inc.
215 N. 12th Street; P.O. Box 391
Santa Paula, CA 93060

Otto Bock Orthopedic Industry, Inc.
3000 Zenium La., North
Minneapolis, MN 55441

Whitmyer Biomechanix, Inc.
848 Blountstown Hwy. Suite H
Tallahassee, FL 32304

Ortho-Kinetics, Inc.
W220 N507 Springdale Road
Waukesha, WI 53187-1647

Miller's Special Products
284 East Market Street
Akron, OH 44308

Wheelchairs

Invacare Corporation
899 Cleveland Street
Elyria, OH 44036

Sunrise Medical/Quickie Designs
2842 Business Park Ave.
Fresno, CA 93727

Adapted Utensils

Therapy Skill Builders
3830 E. Bellevue/P.O. Box 42050-H92
Tucson, AZ 85733

Contour-U

Pin Dot Products (see above)

Etran (Eye Transfer)

Zygo Industries, Inc.
P.O. Box 1008
Portland, OR 97207

Introtalker

Prentke Romich Co.
1022 Heyl Road
Wooster, OH 44691

Prone Standers

Equipment Shop
P.O. Box 33;
Bedford, MA 01730

Kaye Products, Inc.
535 Dimmocks Mill Road
Hillsborough, NC 27278

Rifton for People with Disabilities
Route 213
Rifton, NY 12471

Medco Adaptive Equipment Ltd
P.O. Box 645
Merrick, NY 11566

Maddak, Inc.
6 Industrial Road
Pequannock, NJ 07440

Mulholland (see above)
Ortho-Kinetics, Inc. (see above)

Theradapt Products, Inc.
17 W. 163 Oak Lane
Bensenville, IL 60106

Tumbleforms
P.O. Box 89
Jackson, MI 49204

Etac USA
2325 Parklawn Drive, Suite P
Waukesha, WI 53186

Snug Seat, Inc.
10810 Independence Pointe Pkwy
Matthews, NC 28105

Supine Standers

Theradapt Products, Inc. (see above)

Consumer Care Products, Inc.
P.O. Box 684
810 N. Water Street
Sheboygan, WI 53082

Rifton (see above)

Ortho-Kinetics, Inc. (see above)

Tumbleforms (see above)

Snug Seat, Inc. (see above)

Sidelyers

Preston, Inc.
P.O. Box 89
Jackson, MI 49204

Rifton (see above)

Tumbleforms (see above)

APPENDIX 8E

Case Study

Name: Lauren

Medical Diagnosis: Chromosomal abnormality; cerebral palsy with spastic quadriparesis; seizure disorder

Age: 10½ years old

Cognitive Status:

Lauren exhibits scattered skills ranging from 3–3½ years. She is distractible; needing verbal prompts to maintain attention. She is sociable; has a sense of humor; directs self-care.

Functional Status:

There is very little volitional movement of upper extremities. Lauren postures and fixes with scapular elevation and shoulder protraction bilaterally. Lauren primarily utilizes a light pointer to access a communication device and for educational activities. She utilizes a wobble switch with her head to access switch toys and a computer. Lauren also uses a head pointer for communication as well as education and leisure activities. Head control is limited, and she fatigues easily. She wears glasses for myopia and astigmatism. She is able to fix and follow objects in all directions. She is dependent in all areas of self-care.

Physical Findings:

There is increased tone in all extremities with decreased tone in trunk and oral facial areas. There is some tightness in the lower extremities. Lauren has had bilateral varus derotational osteotomies. There is a functional and structural kyphosis and mild thoracolumbar scoliosis. The right leg is three quarters of an inch shorter than the left leg. There is pelvic obliquity with the left hip rotated anteriorly. Lauren does not demonstrate any independent mat mobility except limited rolling. She requires maximum assistance to maintain all upright sitting postures. She is on an alternate positioning program which includes sidelyer, prone positioning, and standing on a prone stander. She wears Zimmer splints at night to stretch out existing knee flexion contractures. Lauren sits in a wheelchair with an adapted seating system for functional activities. Out of the wheelchair she exhibits hyperextension of the head and neck area. There is an open mouth posture with tongue retraction influenced by gravity and muscle pull. Lauren exhibits elevation of the shoulder girdle to provide stability to assist in holding her head erect. Scapular protraction is noted, influenced by tight pectoral musculature and poor scapular adduction (Figures 8–6 through 8–9 at age 6).

Communication Status:

Receptive language skills are at the 3-year-old level. Lauren vocalizes sounds on occasion to indicate pleasure or gain attention. Hearing status is within normal limits. Lauren demonstrates a yes/no response using eye gaze which she also uses for pointing. She has several overlays for her Etran eye gaze system. She is training for use of an electronic voice output device, the Scan and Point Introtalker, which she accesses by using an optical indicator mounted on a head mount. She also utilizes a single switch on the left side of her

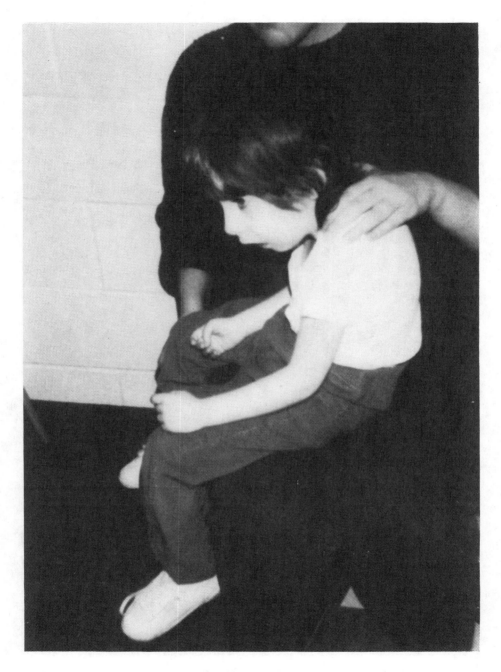

Figure 8–6.
Unsupported sitting posture, age 6 (side view), showing kyphosis, open mouth posture, elevation of shoulder girdle to assist in holding head up, scapular protraction, and tight pectoral musculature.

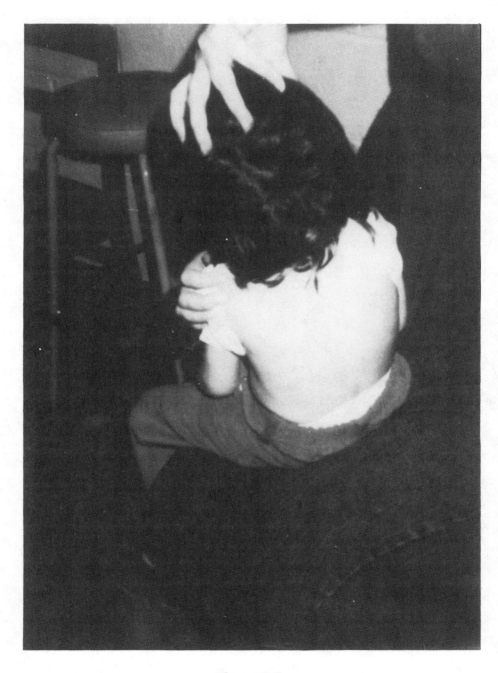

Figure 8–7.
Unsupported sitting posture, age 6 (posterior view), showing kyphosis, posterior pelvic tilt, trunk rotation, and lack of head control.

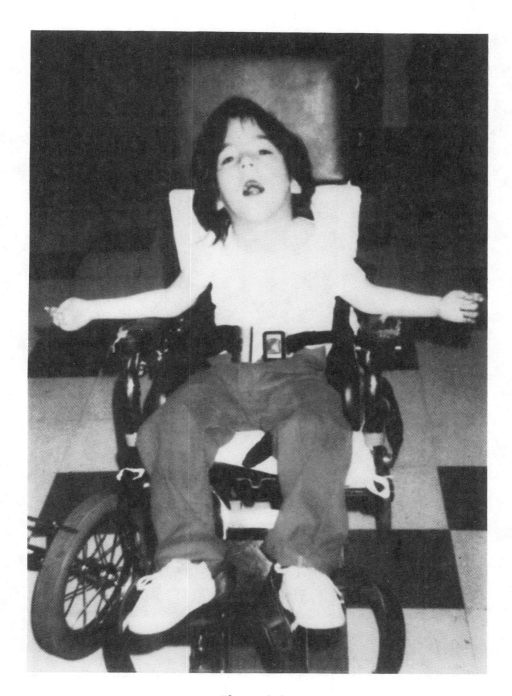

Figure 8–8.
Supported sitting without adapted positioning insert, age 6 (anterior view), showing posterior pelvic tilt, kyphosis, hyperextension of head, open mouth posture, and inability to bring upper extremities to midline.

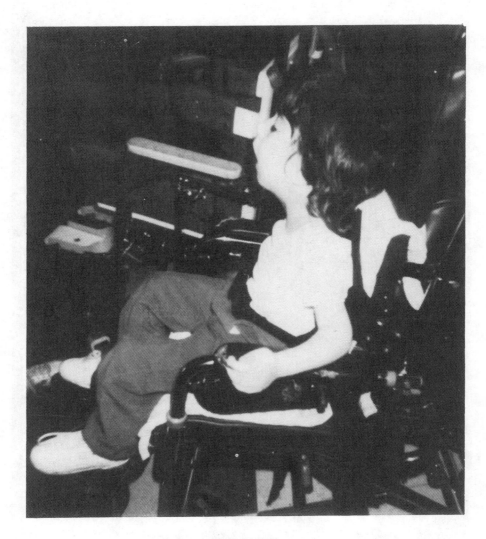

Figure 8–9.
Supported sitting without adapted positioning insert, age 6 (side view), showing posterior pelvic tilt, kyphosis, neck hyperextension, open mouth posture, and inability to bring upper extremities to midline.

head, attached to the wheelchair back, to access the computer, switch toys, or page turner. The goal is to incorporate use of the augmentative communication equipment into all aspects of daily living including mealtime. The rehabilitation team feels that Lauren's optimally fit positioning system has also assisted in providing the required stability to efficiently use a variety of augmentative systems.

Feeding Status:

Lauren presents with severe limitations in oral motor skills for feeding. Open mouth posture is observed with drooling noted. Lauren is not fed out of her wheelchair. She exhibits Stage I oral preparatory dysphagia. She eats soft and pureed foods from a spoon and some finely chopped or soft chewable foods. Finger foods are presented to the right or left molar area. She uses a phasic bite-release pattern with an open mouth posture. She does not exhibit adequate pressure and jaw grading to utilize a sustained bite. Mastication is achieved through an up/down munching pattern. There is limited tongue lateralization to transfer the bolus; however, this skill is emerging. There is need for oral control at the front for some textures, and Lauren requires frequent verbal cuing to maintain her head upright. Support is provided at the crown of the head, as needed. Lauren utilizes a suckle (extension-retraction tongue movement) pattern for spoon feeding. During cup drinking she requires two point oral control from the front. She uses a 4012 (Therapy Skill Builders) cut out flexi cup and takes 2 to 3 consecutive sips of thin liquids. Lauren's swallow appears functional for most textures when provided proper positioning. A modified barium swallow, investigating the pharyngeal stage of the swallow, has not been conducted; however, the procedure is being considered.

Wheelchair and Positioning System:

Lauren's significant motoric and neurological involvement necessitates the need for adaptive seating to maximize her oral motor/feeding function. Lauren is seated in a Quickie Zippy tilt-in-space wheelchair with a Contour U seat and back insert system (Figure 8–10). The positioning system was designed to facilitate the most stable base of support through positioning of her pelvis and trunk. The Contour U seating system was molded with lateral trunk and pelvic support as well as lateral knee influence to provide stability and support while accommodating Lauren's scoliosis, trunk rotation, and pelvic obliquity and allowing maximum hip abduction post bilateral varus derotational osteotomies. A positioning belt is used to maintain the pelvis in an appropriate position as well as for safety during travel. The footrests have sandals with ankle and toe straps to maintain the feet on the footplates for stability and for better positioning/alignment of the feet. An anterior chest support is utilized to facilitate the erect upright posture as well as for safety during travel.

The tilt-in-space feature affords Lauren the opportunity to be tilted back in space, as she tends to fatigue and cannot maintain an upright position against gravity for long periods. The system also allows for relief of pressure on the buttocks.

An Otto Bock neck ring is provided for symmetrical head positioning for all activities. A flat headrest and Danmar Hensinger anterior neck support are used for travel. Lauren has been evaluated with several types of halo anterior head supports to facilitate an upright head position for longer periods of time. The Mulholland (head/neck/shoulder support), the Whitmyer (head support with forehead strap), the Ortho-Kinetics Hans head support, and the Miller forehead support have been under consideration. Lauren utilizes a clear lap tray with protractor blocks to provide upper extremity support and facilitate midline positioning of her upper extremities. Use of the tray also facilitates trunk extension and improved head control. An Etran (clear plexiglass board) is placed at the end of the tray for eye gaze communication.

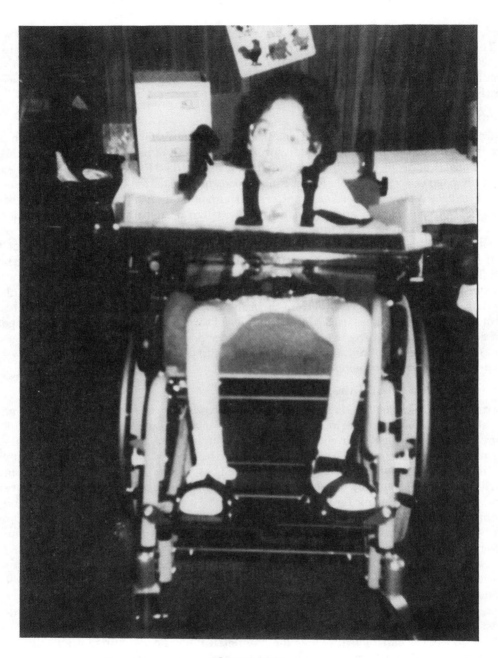

Figure 8–10.
Wheelchair with adapted positioning system, age 10 (anterior view): Tilt-in-space wheelchair, Contour U seat, and back insert. Note improved position of pelvis and trunk; maximum support and accommodation of pelvic obliquity, scoliosis, and kyphosis; and abduction of hips, especially on the left to accommodate limited hip adduction post varus derotational osteotomies. Anterior chest support, and Otto Bock neck support facilitate improved head position and mouth posture for feeding.

Use of the Contour U positioning system helps to establish a stable base through positioning of the pelvis and trunk. This improved stability assists Lauren in establishing control of her head and neck which in turn helps to provide jaw stability distally. The increased jaw stability provides the foundation for use of the intrinsic musculature within the oral mechanism and enables Lauren to eat functionally and as efficiently as possible. The tilt-in-space feature assists with the mealtime process as the chair may be tilted a few degrees when necessary to assist with head control. A pillow is inserted behind the occiput to facilitate a safer position for swallowing through head flexion.

Lauren's positioning system has had a positive influence on her tone, pelvic and trunk alignment, and head control which in turn has improved her position for oral motor and feeding function.

Radiologic Assessment of Pediatric Swallowing

JAMES MARQUIS, M.D., AND HILDA PRESSMAN, M.A.

CONTENTS

Swallowing disorders in children with developmental disabilities present special challenges to the clinician and to the radiologist. Abnormal swallowing can present at any age from newborn to adolescent, and the symptoms can be varied and subtle. Indeed, the cough reflex may be absent, resulting in so-called "silent aspiration." In some instances severe swallowing problems may be ignored or misunderstood by the caregiver. The techniques and type of radiographic study vary with the age of the child and type of disability. Patient cooperation frequently is limited or absent.

Although the radiologist plays the key role in imaging these problems, a combined approach utilizing the expertise of the dysphagia team is an important part of a successful study. It is essential that a clinical examination by the speech pathologist, or other feeding specialist, precede the Modified Barium Swallow. This examination is necessary to devise a plan for the study that includes positioning, bolus viscosities and textures to be used, and the order and method of presentation. The method of conducting the clinical examination is presented in Chapter 3.

The complex mechanism of swallowing is best studied by means of videofluoroscopy. With this technique, precise evaluation of the entire swallowing process can be obtained with the least discomfort to the patient. Swallowing may also be assessed by use of the modified barium swallow which is discussed in this chapter. This is a special study that is different from the usual barium esophogram, and requires unique techniques and positioning. Unless specifically requested by the clinician, it usually is not done, and valuable information may be overlooked.

Radiation Dose

Radiation exposure is inevitable during videotape recording, but it is essential that every effort be made during the procedure to reduce the radiation level. It is beyond the scope of this chapter to discuss this topic completely, and there are numerous references in the literature for those who wish to read more (Beck & Gayler, 1991; Committee on the Biological Effects of Ionizing Radiations of the National Academy of Sciences-National Research Council, 1980; Hall, 1988; Keriakes & Rosenstein, 1980;

National Council on Radiation Protection & Measurements, 1987). Radiation dose should be kept at the lowest level consistent with acceptable diagnostic images.

The primary x-ray beam is the x-ray energy directly emitted from the x-ray tube. It is directed through the area of interest in the patient. Scattered radiation results from x-rays that bounce or scatter in all directions from the patient's tissues. These x-rays do not contribute to the x-ray image, and although of low energy, they are the major cause of acquired radiation exposure during fluoroscopy. The radiation stops when no fluoroscopy is taking place. It does not contaminate the surrounding room or equipment.

Patient radiation occurs over the area of interest, and should be limited only to that area. X-ray beam collimation, careful fluoroscopy, and a constant effort to decrease the total time of fluoroscopy should be basic practice. The use of lead aprons to protect the body and gonads of the patient offers additional protection from any scattered radiation outside the primary beam. The modified barium examination of the child with dysphagia and developmental disability requires approximately 5 minutes of fluoroscopy time. (Beck & Gayler, 1991, Griggs, Jones, & Lee, 1989). If related areas of interest are included, such as distal esophagus, stomach, and duodenum, additional fluoroscopy time will be needed.

The best radiation protection for medical personnel is to remain outside the fluoroscopy suite. Unfortunately, this ideal situation is seldom achieved when very young or neurologically impaired children are studied. Therefore, it is essential to reduce radiation exposure to the fullest extent. The radiologic and dysphagia team personnel should remain outside of the primary beam, and every effort should be made to reduce exposure to any scattered x-rays. No radiation worker should be permitted to be in the primary x-ray beam. If it becomes necessary for some reason, lead gloves should always be used. Lead aprons and shields should always be used, and radiation film badges worn on the collar outside the lead apron. Although the level of permissible dose for radiation workers is never to be exceeded, it is essential to try to keep exposure to the absolute minimum. Periodic review of all film badge readings should be done at regular intervals by the radiation safety officer. Any unexpected exposure warrants immediate investigation into possible errors in technique with appropriate corrective actions initiated.

Every effort should be made to keep the assistant out of the primary beam and as far away from the scattered x-ray as possible. X-rays are subject to the inverse square law which states that increasing the distance from the source by two will reduce the exposure to one fourth. Thus the use of long-handled clamps, or syringes with tubing attached, helps to reduce total radiation dose to the assistant.

We do not allow a pregnant parent or nonradiation worker to be in the fluoroscopy suite during the examination. However, it should be emphasized that with wraparound lead aprons and proper fluoroscopy techniques, the radiation dose to a fetus should be so low as to be almost unreadable.

Purpose of Modified Barium Swallow

The conventional barium swallow study usually only includes a cursory evaluation of the swallowing mechanism, and many subtle interactions of swallowing can be missed. In the modified barium swallow, the oral cavity, pharynx, and cervical esophagus are carefully imaged and closely studied. The distal esophagus, stomach, and duodenum may also be included if it is clinically indicated. The purpose of the modified barium swallow is to evaluate motility disorders of swallowing and to determine

the textures and viscosities that can be safely fed to the patient. The study is geared to prevent aspiration or at least to keep the amount aspirated to the absolute minimum. *Aspiration* as used in this text is defined as passage of material into the trachea during swallowing usually, but not always, resulting in a cough (Dodds Stewart, & Logemann, 1990) (Figure 9–1). The radiologist and speech pathologist watch, discuss, and review the proceedings to determine whether it is safe to continue and if there is a need to modify the plan as the examination proceeds. Portions of the videotape are reviewed with the family to demonstrate any significant findings.

Tracheal aspiration can occur prior to swallowing by leakage from the oral cavity into the unprotected larynx, during swallowing due to abnormal oral pharyngeal coordination, or following swallowing due to retention of material in the pharynx or obstruction at the pharyngoesophageal segment. *Laryngeal penetration* is defined as passage of material into the laryngeal vestibule, usually with rapid expulsion back into the pharynx during swallowing (Figure 9–2). If there is passage below the level of the vocal cords, tracheal aspiration then occurs. Although some transient laryngeal penetration may occur as a normal phenomenon, we consider it to be an ominous sign in the developmentally disabled child with neurological deficit and feel that the patient is at increased risk for aspiration.

Imaging Equipment

The type of x-ray fluoroscopic unit will vary from department to department, but any good unit will be satisfactory if an adequate image can be produced at an acceptably low radiation output. For very small infants, some modification in x-ray output

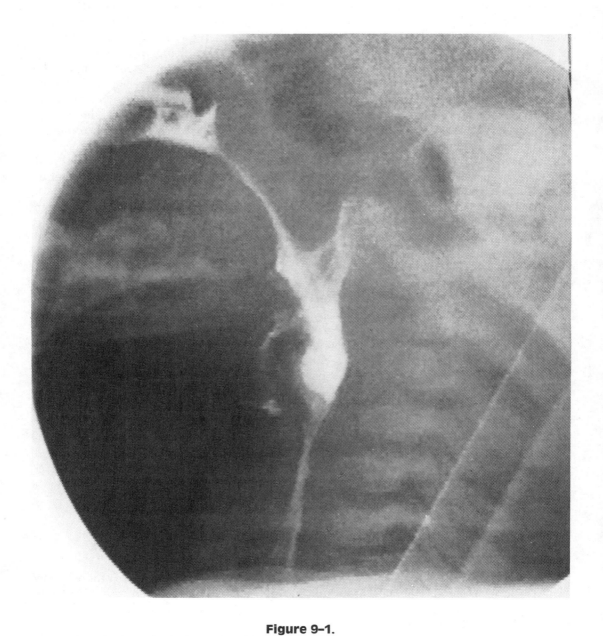

Figure 9–1.
Tracheal aspiration. Single frame image from a videotape recording. Note contrast below the level of true cords in the trachea *(arrow)*.

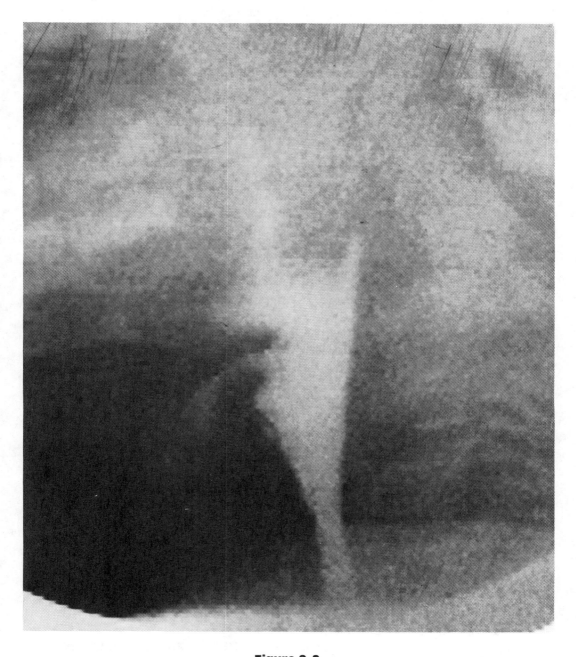

Figure 9–2.
Laryngeal penetration. Single frame image from a videotape recording. Note contrast beneath epiglottis entering larynx but above level of true cords *(arrow)*.

may be required to ensure the minimum radiation exposure. It is necessary for the table to rotate into a 90° erect position. A fluoroscopy timer is mandatory, and total fluoroscopy time should be monitored and kept as part of the patient's record. The maximum distance between the table top and the fluoroscopic carriage is very important, because the patient chair must be able to fit between them.

Videotape recording of the fluoroscopic image permits review of the study in real time as well as slow motion and still images. The radiation dose to the patient is only slightly increased over conventional fluoroscopy. The use of cinefluoroscopy is no longer recommended for this procedure. The slight increase in image detail is outweighed by the marked increase in patient radiation exposure and the complexities involved in developing and viewing the images.

We use a modified digital method to freeze the last fluoroscopic image, and the entire study is recorded on high resolution VHS tape using a Sony videocassette recorder (Model Number SVO9500MD). During review of the videotape, selected images are copied on hard film using a conventional camera printer (Matrix Model Number MP4000, Series III). These selected images are obtained at no additional radiation to the patient.

Other radiographic capabilities, such as digital fluoroscopy, have advantages and disadvantages but are beyond the scope of this chapter. The basic concept is to reduce patient radiation exposure to the minimum while preserving a diagnostic image. Electronic manipulation and digital forms of imaging are used in conjunction with the conventional fluoroscope and image amplification techniques. The resultant images are viewed on a cathode ray tube (CRT) similar to the conventional television screen. The resultant image can be manipulated and enhanced as needed to bring out various areas of interest that would not be demonstrated by conventional x-ray tech-

niques. This is done with a substantial reduction in patient x-ray exposure. The images are then printed using a laser type printer processor.

Other imaging techniques, such as computed tomography and magnetic resonance imaging (MRI), can demonstrate exquisite anatomic detail but generally lack real-time capability. Their use in pediatric swallowing problems tends to be limited at present. Ultrasound is an emerging technique that has some potential advantages. The procedure is noninvasive, requires no radiation, and is relatively nontraumatic to the patient. The image quality however, is generally poorer than with other techniques, and it has not been useful in identifying aspiration. The technique also requires considerable skill and experience by the operator and is therefore quite operator-dependent (Shawker, Sonies, Stone, & Baum, 1983; Weber, Woolridge, & Baum, 1986). Lastly, nuclear medicine or radioisotope studies have a limited but definite role to play in specific situations, particularly gastroesophageal reflux. The milk scan is a very sensitive test for reflux from the stomach to the esophagus. The level of reflux in the esophagus can be assessed, and any aspiration into the lungs can also be documented. The radiation dose is generally quite low. Anatomic detail is poor with this technique, and conventional barium study may be required prior to any surgical intervention.

An emerging radioisotope study for the detection of lung aspiration is the salivagram. A small drop of radioisotope is placed on the tongue, and the patient's lungs are monitored. Any activity that is noted in the lungs is presumptive evidence of aspiration of saliva because of the small amount of isotope originally placed on the tongue.

Radiographic Techniques

The radiographic techniques used vary with the age of the child and the information required. Each examination is tailored to fit the individual patient. In general, an attempt is made to parallel the feeding environment of the patient and, if possible, find the best feeding position, feeding techniques, and/or consistency of food.

For early morning studies, the caregiver is advised that the patient should be NPO from midnight, except in the case of children under 6 months of age who are NPO from 3:00 A.M.. For afternoon studies, the patient is kept NPO for a period of 6 hours, given only a light breakfast. This is done to allow hunger to assist in the child's acceptance of the barium and to provide an empty stomach in case evaluation of reflux is necessary. We do allow medications to be taken, because many of the children are on anti-convulsants. If the patient is taking a drug, such as Reglan®, it is important to determine whether the medication should be given. This will depend on the ultimate goal of the study. One may wish to determine the degree of reflux either with or without medication. Consultation with the physician who has ordered the study and/or the physician who has prescribed the medication may be necessary. This is usually done in advance by the coordinator.

The clinical examination will have determined the position in which the child is fed at home and in school as well as the position judged to be safest. Observation of the parent feeding the child may show that the position is quite different from what the parent describes or that it changes as the feeding progresses. Many children who are fed in their parents' laps may begin in an upright position but they then progress to reclining or supine positions. The study begins with the patient in the position deemed to be safest. If safe swallows are achieved in this position, the study progresses to duplicate the feeding position at home and/or at school. If safe swallowing is seen in the upright position, the child may be examined in supine, if this is typical of the position that is used at home. If this position is found to be safe for feeding, it will influence the recommendations made (Table 9–1)

Motion is a frequent problem with young, as well as neurologically impaired, children. It is essential that the head and neck of the patient remain in the x-ray field during the examination. If cooperation cannot be obtained, some method to ensure no motion of the head must be used. Gentle restraint of the head with a lead glove usually is sufficient. Infants are generally examined in an upright position first and may later be examined in the recumbent right lateral position. This offers the best view of the oral-pharynx. The patient can easily be rotated into a supine position if an antero-posterior (AP) view is required. The young child who may not be able to sit for the examination can also be examined using this technique.

Table 9–1. Positioning options for modified barium swallow examination.

Position	Equipment
Upright 75–90 degrees	MAMA® Chair Tumble Form® insert Hensinger collar Patient's own wheelchair Hausted® Videofluoroscopic Chair
Angled back to customary position	MAMA® Chair Patient's own wheelchair Stretcher X-ray table Hausted® videofluoroscopic chair

Most children, however, are able to be examined in a seat designed for the evaluation. For children under 60 pounds, a MAMA chair (MAMA® Systems Oconomowoc, WI) (Figure 9–3) is used to position them for the study. This chair allows modifications in the depth of the seat as well as the seat-back angle. It has an adjustable foot plate and supports that can be placed in a variety of places along the seat and/or back. A Hensinger collar is added to provide further head support if indicated (Figure 9–4). For very small children, a Tumble Form® (Tumble Forms Feeder Seat Preston Company, Jackson, MI) seat is placed into the MAMA® chair (Figure 9–5). Both seats have seat belts and chest restraints. Larger children are examined in their own adaptive chairs or in the Hausted® videofluoroscopic chair. Patients may subsequently be placed on the table for additional studies.

A familiar parent or guardian plus caring technologist and team members all contribute to a nonhostile environment which is essential in calming an apprehensive child. The parent is invited to be the feeder, if she is not pregnant and seems to feel comfortable with this role. We observe the parent's style in calming the child to help us to determine if he or she will be an asset in the study. Some parents are intimidated by the examination, and this can be conveyed to the child in nonverbal ways. In some cases, the speech pathologist or other professional from the child's program may be the feeder. Guidance is given throughout the procedure regarding size of bolus and timing. If too much difficulty is encountered, the speech pathologist on the dysphagia team may take over.

The contrast agent of choice is barium sulfate. Barium may be mixed with many

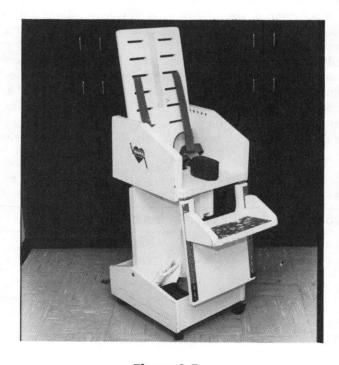

Figure 9–3.
MAMA® chair used for positioning children under 60 pounds (MAMA systems, Oconomowoc, WI).

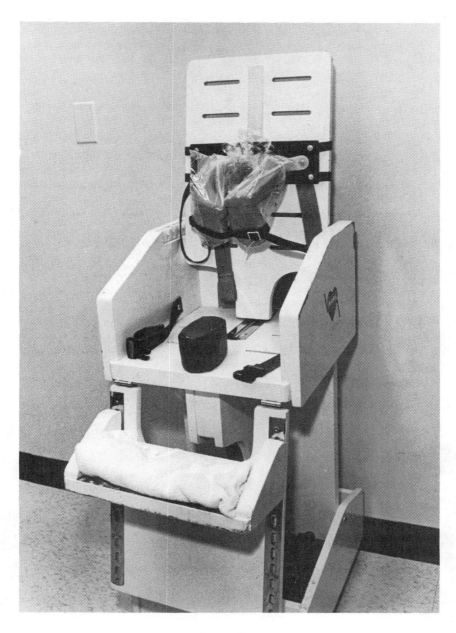

Figure 9–4.
MAMA® chair with Hensinger collar in place to provide added head support.

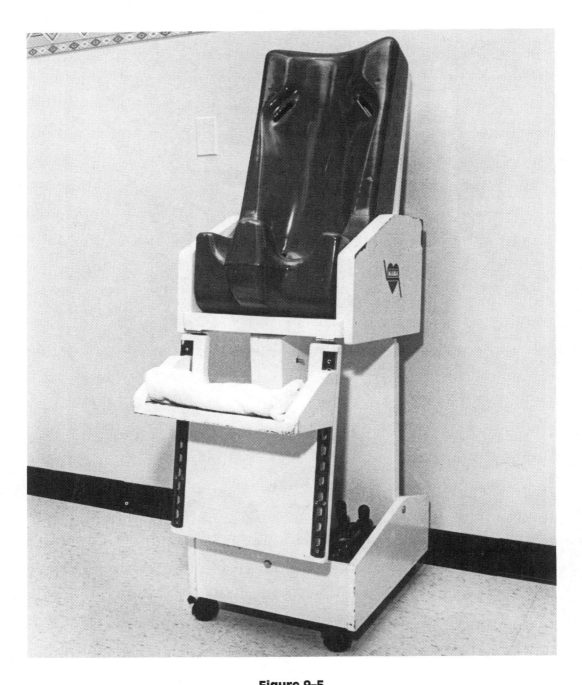

Figure 9–5.
MAMA® chair with Tumble Form® Seat inserted (Preston Company, Jackson, MI). This is used to position small children.

types of food and can be heated or frozen (Table 9–2). Parents are encouraged to bring foods from home, including preferred foods and foods that are causing particular difficulty. Powdered barium is added to thin pureed fruits, such as applesauce or pears. One tablespoon of barium is mixed with 2 oz of fruit. If the barium makes the consistency too thick, small amounts of liquid barium are added as needed. Dehydrated baby cereal with banana flakes is mixed with liquid barium (5 tablespoons cereal to 2 oz of liquid barium) to make a thicker puree, the consistency of hot cereal. The banana flakes have a strong flavor and help to make the taste more palatable. In the same manner, powdered barium is added to puddings, mashed potatoes, chopped meats, and so on. Powdered barium is sprinkled on pieces of graham cracker to evaluate chewables. Alternatively, paste barium may be used. Liquid barium may be presented alone or mixed with cereal as a thickening agent to evaluate the swallow for thick liquids which may be swallowed more safely than thin liquids. Liquids may be thickened to nectar or milkshake consistency. The amount of cereal added is recorded so that the viscosity can be duplicated for feedings, if recommended. It is important to remember that liquid barium is somewhat thicker than milk or water. Flavorings such as chocolate or strawberry powder may be added. One parent brought vanilla extract, as that was her child's preference. Foods may be warmed in a microwave oven if available. Liquid is usually warmed to at least room temperature for infants.

The food judged to be the safest is presented first, working backwards to the food which may be least safe. This determination is made during the clinical examination that precedes the study (Table 9–3). Typically, we offer a thick puree, thin puree, thick liquid, and thin liquid. If there is poor anterior containment for liquids, a slight change in positioning may be necessary to assist with oral transport. Chopped foods and chewables may be used as appropriate for developmental level and goals of the study. Iced foods or liquids may be presented to study their effect on the swallow.

Water soluble contrast agents (Hypaque®, Renografin®) are not routinely used in swallowing studies. They taste bad, many are irritating to the lungs, and they can be more easily aspirated, especially in the very young infant. Nonionic contrast Omnipaque®) is potentially less harmful due to its isotonic osmolarity. Bad taste remains a problem and at present cost is excessive.

The method of feeding the patient is extremely important and varies with the pa-

Table 9–2. Barium mixtures used for modified barium swallows.

Viscosity or Texture	Mixture
Chewables (table foods)	Powdered barium sprinkled on top or paste barium on cookies
Pudding or thick puree	5 tablespoons dehydrated baby cereal (not rice)/2 oz liquid barium
Thin puree	1 tablespoon powdered barium/2 oz pureed fruit (applesauce)
Thick liquid	2 tablespoons rice cereal/2 oz liquid barium
Thin liquid	6 oz powdered barium/6 oz water

Table 9–3. Plan for modified barium swallow study.

Study Options	Indications for Use
Oral feeding	
Chewables (table foods)	Intermittent gagging, choking; limited intake of table foods
Pudding or thick puree (bananas)	Coughing or limited intake of thin puree
Thin puree (applesauce)	Coughing; limited intake; respiratory symptoms
Thick liquid (malted)	Coughing; refusal of thin liquid; respiratory symptoms
Thin liquid (milk)	Coughing; refusal; respiratory symptoms
Tube feeding	
NGT including pullup into esophagus	Refusal; aspiration precludes oral feeding with need to assess esophagus
GT	PO feeding refused; aspiration precludes oral feeding; assess stomach emptying and reflux
GI Series	
Esophagus	Rule out dysmotility, cricopharyngeal achalasia, esophagitis, stricture, hernia, TE fistula
Reflux study	Vomiting; gastrostomy tube being considered
Stomach emptying	Vomiting; Refusal of feedings or limited intake; gastrostomy tube being considered
Chest x-ray	Aspiration occurred during study

tient. Solids are presented by spoon. A Kelly Clamp may be used to keep the feeder's hand out of the x-ray field and a lead glove is always used for protection. Liquids are presented by cup or bottle, as preferred by the child.

For children who cannot or will not take liquid in this manner, a gavage is used. For children who will accept a nipple, a catheter is fed through the hole in the nipple and held in place with a clamp held by the feeder (Figure 9–6). Small amounts of liquid are introduced by syringe. Frequently, this will initiate sucking on the part of the child. If not, liquid can continue to be dis-

pensed by syringe. This catheter and syringe technique allows the patient to be fed with the attendant away from the primary x-ray beam (Poznanski, 1976).

Care must be taken with this strategy to control the size of the bolus presented to prevent inadvertent aspiration. Even a neurologically intact child might aspirate if a large bolus is injected or presented too rapidly. We prefer to observe fluoroscopically the contrast in the plastic straw while slowly injecting to the level of the nipple, thus allowing precise control. Most infants will begin to suck and swallow at the first few drops of barium. For those for whom a nipple is not

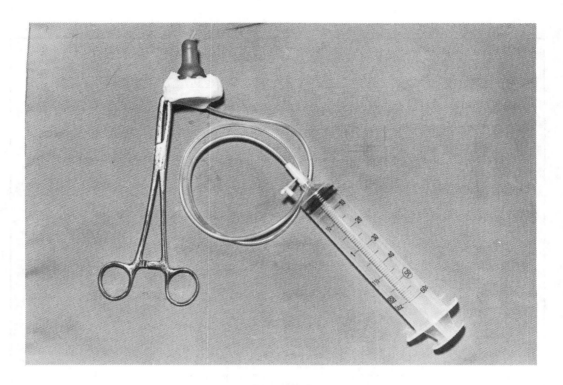

Figure 9–6.
Nipple gavage with clamp. A catheter is fed through the hole in the nipple which is then fixed to the mouth with tape or held in place with a clamp held by the feeder.

appropriate, a catheter is cut to the size of the individual's mouth and attached to a syringe. The catheter is then placed lateral to the tongue and the liquid dispensed slowly. The presentation is monitored on the video screen, and a lead glove is always used to protect the hands of the feeder.

The modified barium swallow usually starts in the erect lateral position centered over the mouth and pharynx. This view allows the best study of the mechanism of swallowing, and in many cases is all that is required. Antero-posterior views of the mouth and pharynx are used occasionally in special instances, particularly to evaluate asymmetrical bolus transit swallowing and tongue movements. The thoracic esophagus, stomach, duodenum, and small bowel also may require study; and recum-

bent prone, oblique, and supine views are used as needed. The sequence of positions and foods offered are recorded on a form (Figure 9–7).

Radiologic Evaluation

The radiologic evaluation of a patient using the modified barium swallow is similar for any age group. The type and consistency of food and the method of administration may vary, but the assessment follows a similar path. The oral phase, pharyngeal phase, and pharyngo-esophageal phase must all be studied carefully. Certain anatomic variations occur in different age groups, and these need to be included in the assessment. The examination may be altered to fit certain

VIDEOFLUOROSCOPY EXAMINATION FORM

Name _____Date_____DOB _____

Reason for referral_____

Check if any of the following apply:

_____Tracheostomy _____Trach value _____GT _____Altered Structure

Comments: _____

Pt. State: _____Alert _____Cooperative _____Crying _____Drowsy

Positions: Upright _____AP   Recumbent _____AP

                _____Lateral   _____Lateral

Procedures:

Modified barium swallow	_____	Fluoro time	_____
Esophageal motility	_____	Stomach emptying	_____
Gastroesophageal function	_____	Chest x-ray	_____

Bolus delivery/order/amt.   Bolus type/order

_____ Spoon 3, 5, 10cc	_____	Thin liquid
_____ Cup	_____	Thickened liquid
_____ Bottle	_____	Puree
_____ Nasopharyngeal gavage	_____	Pudding
_____ Oral gavage 3, 5, 10cc	_____	Cookie 1/8 graham cracker
_____Other	_____	Other

Compensatory strategies   **Response**

Posture: Chin tuck   _____

         Head turn R/L   _____

         Head tipped R/L   _____

         Recline   _____

         Other   _____

Intake: Liquid washdown   _____

         Cold food   _____

         Other   _____

Figure 9–7.
Videofluoroscopic examination form used to record sequence of evaluation and findings.

Bolus Motility disorders	Cookie	Pudding	Puree	Thick Liquid	Thin Liquid
Oral Preparatory Stage					
Anterior containment	_____	_____	_____	_____	____
Bolus formation	_____	_____	_____	_____	____
Posterior containment	_____	_____	_____	_____	____
Oral Stage	_____	_____	_____	_____	____
Delayed initiation of swallow	_____	_____	_____	_____	____
Piecemeal delivery of bolus	_____	_____	_____	_____	____
Piecemeal deglutition	_____	_____	_____	_____	____
Nasopharyngeal reflux	_____	_____	_____	_____	____
Pharyngeal Stage	_____	_____	_____	_____	____
Preswallow filling	_____	_____	_____	_____	____
Postswallow stasis	_____	_____	_____	_____	____
Valleculae	_____	_____	_____	_____	____
Pyriform sinus	_____	_____	_____	_____	____
Laryngeal vestibule	_____	_____	_____	_____	____
Preswallow aspiration	_____	_____	_____	_____	____
Laryngeal penetration during swallow	_____	_____	_____	_____	____
Tracheal aspiration during swallow	_____	_____	_____	_____	____
Postswallow aspiration	_____	_____	_____	_____	____
Asymmetrical transit	_____	_____	_____	_____	____
Esophageal stage: Anatomy _____	_____	_____	_____	_____	____
Peristalsis _____	_____	_____	_____	_____	____

Related Disorder: GE Reflux _____

Gastric stasis_____

Other _____

Comments and Recommendations: _____

_____

_____

Figure 9–7.
(Continued)

clinical circumstances if needed. (Dodds et al., 1990; Griggs et al., 1989; Jones & Donner, 1988, 1991; Kramer, 1989; Poznanski, 1976)

The oral phase is important to assess the child's ability to maintain oral containment. Anterior and posterior leakage of the contrast agent is noted. Tongue blocking frequently alerts the radiologist to a protective effort by the patient to prevent overfilling and potential aspiration. Bolus formation and tongue motion should be carefully noted. Posterior displacement of the bolus is monitored with attention being paid to apposition of soft palate and the superior pharyngeal wall and naso-pharyngeal reflux, if any. If posterior displacement is decreased or absent, the bolus may pass over the tongue by gravity. This results in rapid or ineffectual filling of the pharynx.

The pharyngeal phase can occur rapidly, and videofluoroscopy allows repeated review of this complex process. If the posterior displacement is relatively normal, barium is delivered to the pharynx in one well-contained bolus. This is followed by a rapid pharyngeal swallow. The larynx lifts upward and the epiglottis tilts backward, the glottis closes, peristalsis starts proximally and contracts the pharynx in a smooth cephalocaudal motion. Disturbances in either oral or pharyngeal swallow will result in abnormalities in this process. If small or varying amounts of food pass over the tongue by gravity without the patient's control, the valleculae and the pyriform sinuses fill at a variable rate, and leakage into the unprotected trachea can occur. The completeness of pharyngeal emptying and the progression of peristalsis are assessed. Laryngeal penetration and possible tracheal aspiration are monitored. If tracheal aspiration occurs, the study may need to be terminated. The examination is continued if the aspiration appears to have been an isolated incident or if the exact nature of the problem is not clearly defined. It may also be important to find an alternative mixture or consistency that will be tolerated without as-

piration. Careful planning between the speech pathologist and radiologist allows for initial presentation of textures that are anticipated to be the safest. In most instances, the information needed has been obtained before aspiration occurs. Review of the videotape helps to determine the cause of aspiration. The character and effectiveness of the cough reflex should be noted, because some chronic or neurologically impaired patients may have lost the cough reflex. Following the examination, a posterior-anterior chest x-ray (Figure 9–8) is usually obtained to assess possible lung disease or aspiration. During the modified barium swallow, various techniques and positions can be attempted by the dysphagia team, as mentioned earlier, to try to find the best method to feed the patient.

The pharyngo-esophageal phase is important and should be carefully observed. Failure of relaxation, stasis, strictures, and cricopharyngeal achalasia must be excluded (Mendelsohn & McConnel, 1987). Occult foreign bodies, congenital tracheoesophageal fistulae, and the rare laryngotrachael cleft must all be looked for.

Following the modified barium swallow, the lower esophagus, stomach, and duodenum should be studied in the prone and supine positions, if they have not been previously found to be normal. Peristaltic stripping of the esophagus should proceed normally in a cephalo-caudal motion with satisfactory emptying of the esophagus. Any retention or reverse peristalsis should be noted. Tertiary contractions are unusual in children and indicate abnormal or ineffectual peristaltic activity. Other esophageal abnormalities, such as achalasia or cardiospasm, and acquired or congenital strictures should be excluded. Hiatal hernias and gastroesophageal reflux can have a profound influence on swallowing abnormalities (Tuchman, 1989). If a feeding gastrostomy is contemplated, gastroesophageal reflux should be noted, because a fundoplication may be required. In patients with previous fundoplica-

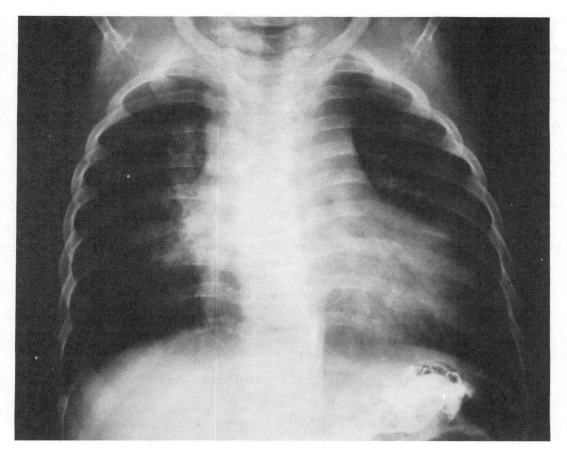

Figure 9–8.
Aspiration pneumonia. Note pneumonia in typical location in right upper lobe and adjacent to the spine on the left lung.

tion, careful assessment of the esophagogastric-junction should be done to ensure that there is no recurrent reflux.

Gastric or duodenal obstructions, ulcer disease, and various anomalies should be excluded because they can all have an adverse affect on the young child's feeding patterns. Occasionally, small bowel disease such as Crohn's disease can affect feeding and swallowing, particularly if the patient is young or neurologically impaired and cannot communicate.

Radiologist Report

The radiologist should provide a written report for each modified barium swallow, and it should be placed in the patient's chart, with copies made available to the dysphagia team as well as the referring agencies and physicians. A combined report from the dysphagia team is separate from the radiology report and typically includes the radiology report as part of the total evaluation.

The radiology report should include a statement about positioning the patient, the various types of contrast used and how they were offered to the patient, and a detailed analysis of the findings during each phase of swallowing. If the rest of the esophagus, stomach, and small bowel were also examined, the report should include a description of these findings as well. A conclusion is necessary to summarize the important findings. If a follow-up study is indicated based on the radiologic findings, this should be included in the report. The modified barium study may be repeated for several reasons. Reassessment of a new feeding technique and reevaluation for potential improvement in the swallowing mechanism are the most common indications. Occasionally, a repeat study will help to convince a reluctant parent that the current feeding method needs further alteration or even complete cessation. Acquired or organic disease distal to the oro-pharynx, such as stricture, peptic ulcer disease, or occult foreign bodies, may require follow-up or additional studies.

Summary

The radiologic imaging of swallowing is frequently the pivotal study in the evaluation of dysphagia in the pediatric patient with developmental delay. The use of videofluoroscopy for modified barium swallow and upper GI series allows careful study of all phases of swallowing, and even minor alterations of normal function can be documented. The radiologist plays an important role in the diagnosis of pediatric swallowing abnormalities; however, for a complete evaluation a combined study using the members of the dysphagia team is essential. The examination can be tailored to fit the individual patient, and specific questions and problems can thus be addressed. The pediatric patient with a swallowing abnormality can present a complex and difficult challenge to the clinician. Many times the exact nature of the problem is not appreciated or is even denied by the parent. A clear demonstration of the dynamics of swallowing can be of immense help in guiding the clinician, and especially the concerned and often confused parent, in managing the disorder.

REFERENCES

Beck, T. J., & Gayler, B. W. (1991). *Radiation in videorecorded fluoroscopy*. In B. Jones & M. W. Donner (Eds.), *Normal and abnormal swallowing—Imaging in diagnosis and therapy* (pp. 1–6). New York: Springer Verlag.

Committee on the Biological Effects of Ionizing Radiations of the National Academy of Sciences-National Research Council. (1980). *The effects on populations of exposure to low levels of ionizing radiation*. Washington, DC: National Academy Press.

Dodds, W. J., Stewart, E. T., & Logemann, J. A. (1990). Physiology and radiology of the normal oral and pharyngeal phases of swallowing. *American Journal of Roentgenology, 154,* 953–963.

Griggs, C. A., Jones, P. M., & Lee, R. E. (1989). Videofluoroscopic investigation of feeding disorders of children with multiple handicap. *Developmental Medicine and Child Neurology, 31,* 303–308

Hall, E. J. (1988). *Radiobiology for the radiologist* (3rd ed.). Philadelphia: Lippincott.

Jones, B., & Donner, M. W. (1988). Examination of the patient with dysphagia. *Radiology, 167,* 319–326.

Jones, B., & Donner, M. W. (Eds.). (1991). *Normal and abnormal swallowing—Imaging in diagnosis and therapy* (pp. 51–75) New York: Springer-Verlag.

Keriakes, J. G., & Rosenstein, M. (1980). *Handbook of radiation doses in nuclear medicine and diagnostic x-ray*. Boca Raton, FL: CRC Press.

Kramer, S. S. (1989). Radiologic examination of the swallowing impaired child. *Dysphagia, 3,* 117–125.

Mendelsohn, M. S., & McConnel, F. M. S. (1987). Function in the pharyngoesophageal segment. *Laryngoscope, 97,* 483–489.

National Council on Radiation Protection and Measurements. (1987). *Recommendations on limits for exposure to ionizing radiation* (Report No. 91). Washington, DC: Author

Poznanski, A. K. (1976). *Practical approaches to pediatric radiology* (pp. 98–100). Chicago: Year Book Medical Publishers

Shawker, T. H., Sonies, B., Stone, M., & Baum, B. J. (1983). Real-time ultrasound visualization of tongue movement during swallowing. *Journal of Clinical Ultrasound, 11,* 485–490.

Tuchman, D. N. (1989). Cough, choke, sputter: The evaluation of the child with dysfunctional swallowing. *Dysphagia, 3,* 111–116.

Weber, F. L., Woolridge, M. W., & Baum, J. D.(1986). An ultrasonographic study of the organization of sucking and swallowing by newborn infants. *Developmental Medicine and Child Neurology, 28,* 19–24.

CHAPTER

10

Otolaryngology Considerations

JOSEPH HADDAD JR., M.D., FAAP, AND
CYNTHIA PRESTIGIACOMO, M.D.

CONTENTS

Children with developmental abnormalities make up a diverse group; and swallowing, feeding, and airway difficulties in these children can result from a number of different problems. Factors that play a role in one child's dysphagia may or may not have bearing on another child's, and there may be as many different combinations of problems as there are children. In this chapter we will discuss various

anatomic, neurological, and acquired causes of dysphagia in the head and neck, and
review otolaryngologic methods of treatment and correction of these problems.

Diagnosis/Evaluation

The evaluation of swallowing problems in
a child requires a detailed history (see
Chapter 12) and physical examination, an
observed feeding session (see Chapter 3),
and other laboratory evaluations when indicated. Table 10–1 summarizes important
aspects of the physical examination.

Dyspnea or stridor at rest which is exacerbated by feeding may be seen in a child
with upper airway obstruction. Typically,
there is a normal arousal mechanism and
feeding is normal for a short time, with
subsequent rapid fatiguability marked by
choking, sputtering, gasping, and development of stridor and cyanosis. Similar findings are seen in patients with congenital

defects of the larynx, trachea, or esophagus
such as tracheoesophageal fistula or cleft
larynx. In patients who tolerate liquids but
have difficulty with solids, stricturing obstruction from foreign bodies or tumors
should be suspected. Voice changes may indicate laryngeal clefts, webs, cysts, or adductor paralysis. Common causes for stridor are listed in Table 10–2.

Laboratory tests which may be useful in
the evaluation of a child with dyspnea are
summarized in Table 10–3. An initial examination should include (1) routine chest
films to aid in the diagnosis of bronchial or
pulmonary infections or to identify the
presence of congenital heart disease or
mass lesions of the mediastinum, which
could lead to esophageal or airway obstruction, and (2) magnification views of the airway to help identify any existing areas of
obstruction. Other tests are reserved for
patients with a high index of suspicion for
a specifc problem based on history, physical examination, and initial tests.

Table 10–1. Physical examination in the child with nutritional disabilities and dysphagia.

Examination	Example of Problem
Facial morphology	Small chin
Head shape	Craniosynostosis
Oropharyngeal anatomy	
Palate configuration	High arch
	Cleft defects
Tongue size and motility	Drooling
	Tongue–tie
Nasal anatomy and patency	Cleft deformities
	Choanal atresia
	Choanal stenosis
Neurologic	
General—Arousal and sensorium	Poor head support
Cranial Nerves VIII, IX, X, and XIII	Facial paralysis
Reflexes and muscle tone	Diminished gag
	Poor tongue thrust

Table 10–2. Common causes of stridor in infants and children.

Supralaryngeal

Nasal obstruction
Lingual thyroid
Adenotonsillar hypertrophy

Laryngeal

Laryngomalacia
Laryngeal web
Cleft larynx
Saccular cysts
Vocal cord paralysis
Allergic edema
Croup
Intubation injury
Stenosis

Tracheal

Stenosis
Granuloma
Tracheaomalacia
Vascular malformation
Foreign body

The initial evaluation is most often combined with a *flexible fiberoptic examination* of the nasopharynx, oropharynx, and larynx. The fiberoptic scope can safely be used in most children in the office. Lubrication and decongestion of the nose will aid in passage of the scope transnally, and it provides a dynamic view of the upper airway, including palate movement, configuration of the epiglottis, and vocal cord mobility. If the child is in respiratory distress, the procedure should be deferred to a more controlled setting (see Figures 10–1 and 10–2).

Videofluoroscopy is a valuable study in a child with dysphagia, because it has the ability to document the entire functional sequence of the swallowing mechanism: the effectiveness of tongue movements and pharyngeal motility; the occurrence and degree of nasopharyngeal reflux; the presence of obstruction in the nasopharynx, at

the upper esophageal sphincter, or in the esophagus itself; and the existence of laryngeal aspiration or a tracheoesophageal fistula (Weiss, 1988).

Laboratory examinations and tests should be selected with the individual child in mind. Often history, physical examination, and observation of a feeding session can provide an experienced clinician with enough information to form a diagnosis with a minimum number of laboratory studies (Cohen, 1990).

Disorders Resulting in Dysphagia

Disorders that result in dysphagia can be anatomic, or they can occur in any of the neuromuscular or sensory components of the various phases of swallowing. They can be congenital or acquired as a result of trauma, infection, neoplasia, or even as a result of treatment procedures for other head and neck disorders. The wide range of abnormalities are characterized according to the phase of swallowing most affected.

Arousal/Response Phase

Alterations in the arousal or stimulation/response phase of feeding in an infant are summarized in Table 10–4. Infants are obligate nose breathers in the first few months of life, and dysphagia due to nasal or nasopharyngeal obstruction may be mistaken for a disorder of the arousal phase of feeding. Both present with an infant who is unable to initiate feeding, as in the case of bilateral choanal atresia. With less severe obstruction, as in choanal stenosis or nasal infection, the infant fatigues rapidly and feeds without appropriate strength and vigor. Unilateral choanal atresia, nasal septal deviation, and allergic rhinitis rarely interfere with feeding (Weiss, 1988). Because anatomic factors such as nasopharyngeal obstruction may mimic problems in the

Table 10–3. Laboratory tests used in evaluating the child with stridor and/or dyspnea.

Test	Example of Problem
All patients	
Chest x-ray	Bronchial or pulmonary infection Heart disease Mediastinal mass
Magnificaiton airway x–ray —posterior–anterior and lateral views	Adenoid hypertrophy Constricting lesion of airway External compression
Selected patients	
Barium swallow	Tracheo–esophageal fistula Vascular anomaly
CT scan MRI	Mass lesions
Angiography	Vascular anomaly
Videofluoroscopy	Functional problems in breathing and swallowing
Endoscopic Procedures Laryngoscopy Bronchoscopy Esophagoscopy	Upper and lower airway problems such as stenosis, foreign body

arousal phase of deglutition, the physical examination of infants with feeding problems should include the attempted passage of a number 8 French catheter bilaterally through each nostril into the pharynx.

Treatment of dysfunctions in this phase of swallowing depends on the specific disorder. For example, a trial of edrophonium chloride is helpful in an infant with suspected myasthenia gravis. In cases of confirmed bilateral choanal atresia, the treatment is surgical and involves computer tomography (CT) scan of the atresia plate to determine the degree of bony and/or membranous blockage. Surgical repair may be done transnasally or transpalatally and usually involves postoperative stenting for a significant period of time. In general, the mainstays of therapy are to protect and support the infant's airway, even to the point of intubation or tracheostomy in severe cases, and to provide the infant with an alternative method of nutritional intake in the form of nasogastric or gastrostomy tube feeding (see Figures 10–3 and 10–4).

Case 1: Choanal Stenois

The patient is a newborn male who was normal at birth, with a good cry. When the baby was quiet, he became cyanotic, with respiratory distress. When he cried, the cyanosis resolved, and his color returned to pink. Passage of 8 French red-rubber catheters was impossible, and CT scan confirmed bilateral choanal atresia. The child had an oral airway placed to ensure mouth-breathing, and was given gavage feedings until surgical repair of the stenosis.

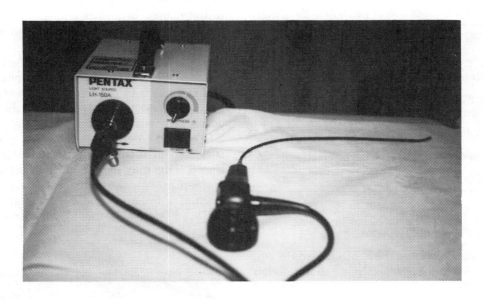

Figure 10–1.
Flexible fiberoptic nasopharyngoscope with light source.

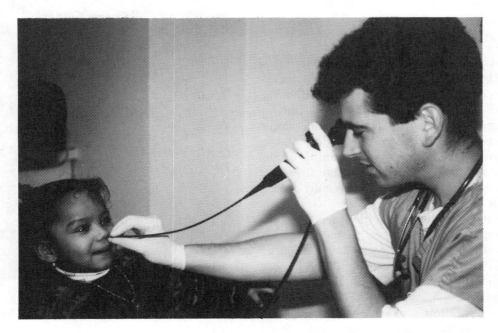

Figure 10–2.
Use of a flexible scope in a small child.

Table 10–4. Disorders in the arousal or stimulus/response phase of feeding in infants.

Failure to awaken for feeding

Failure to latch onto and maintain nipple attachment

Inability to maintain proper nipple position in mouth

Weak tongue motions

Thrusting of tongue

Early tiring during feeding

Case 2: Adenoid Hypertrophy

The patient is an 8-month-old male who was well until 3 weeks prior to admission, when he was noted to have noisy breathing and poor feeding, with weight loss. Examination and magnification x-ray view of the airway revealed adenoid hypertrophy with complete obstruction of the nasal airway. The patient underwent an adenoidectomy with resolution of his symptoms.

Oral Preparatory Phase

In this phase of deglutition, food is mixed with saliva and worked into a bolus of appropriate size and texture for swallowing. This phase is limited in infants but assumes significance as the child adopts more mature patterns of feeding (Logemann, 1988). Proper functioning of the various components of this stage of feeding is necessary to achieve cosmetically acceptable feeding and to prevent aspiration. Deficits in this phase produce different symptoms when different aspects are involved. Lip closure defects such as cleft lip may cause drooling and spillage of food from the mouth during chewing (see Figures 10–5 and 10–6). Feeding deficits similar to those seen with cleft lip may also be found in infants with congenital facial

diplegia (Mobius syndrome), with acquired unilateral or bilateral palsies of cranial nerve (CN) V and/or CN VII, or with weakness of the buccal musculature.

Failure of the soft palate to effect adequate posterior closure of the oropharynx and reduction in the ability of the tongue to control, manipulate, or shape the food bolus are two problems that may allow bits of food to enter the pharynx prematurely, before the laryngeal airway has closed. This may place a child at high risk for aspiration and consequent development of pulmonary disease. Anomalies associated with this form of feeding dys-

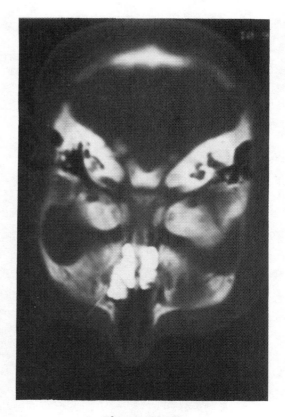

Figure 10–3.
Choanal atresia as demonstrated on a CT scan with barium instilled in the nose.

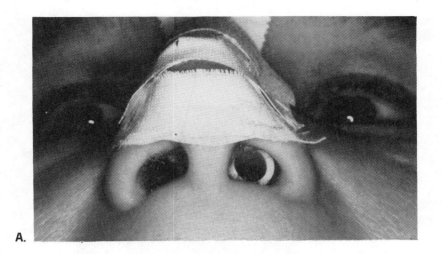

A.

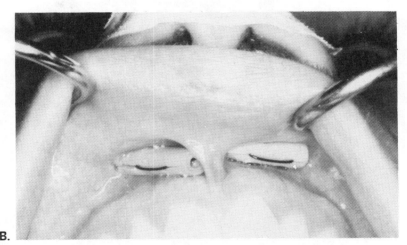

B.

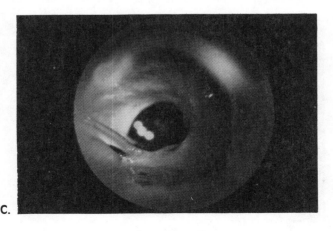

C.

Figure 10–4.
A. Repaired choanal atresia with stents in place **B.** Stabilzation of stents under the lip.
C. Intranasal view of choana after surgery and stent.

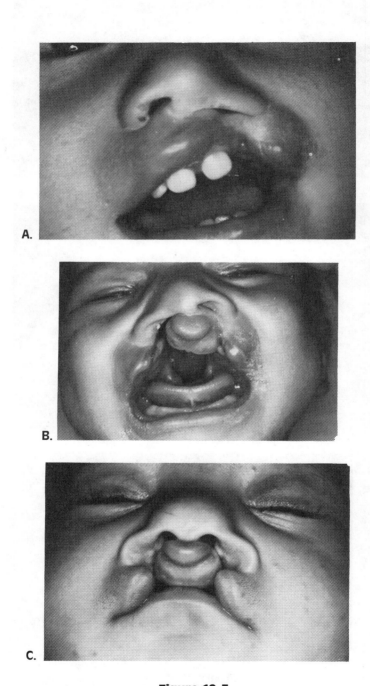

Figure 10–5.
A. Unilateral cleft lip   **B.** Bilateral cleft lip with cleft palate.   **C.** Bilateral cleft lip

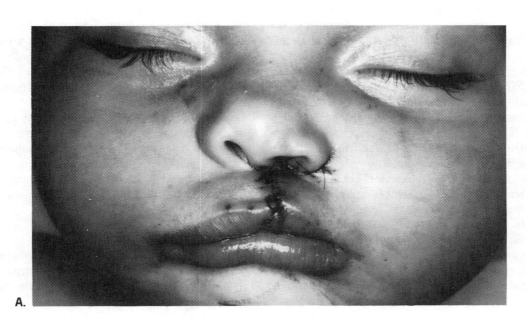

A.

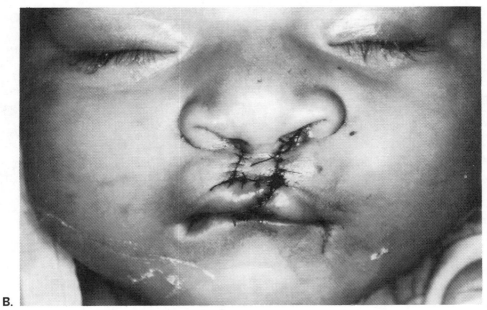

B.

Figure 10–6.
A. Unilateral cleft lip after repair.   **B.** Bilateral cleft lip after repair.

function include congenitally short soft palate, weakness of the palatal musculature, and postadenoidectomy velopharyngeal incompetence. Tongue problems include ankyloglossia, CN XII palsy, or macroglossia due to the presence of a glossal lymphangioma, hemangioma, or lingual thyroid gland. Macroglossia may appear as an isolated congenital anomaly or as part of the syndrome of Trisomy 21 (see Figure 10–7). Tongue weakness and/or incoordination is a recognized problem in many children with cerebral palsy (CP), (Kenny, Casas, & McPherson, 1989), further compromising the ability of these children to feed normally.

Congenital anatomic or neurologic deficits such as cleft lip, macro- or ankyloglossia, or facial muscle weakness or asymmetry may be apparent from early infancy. In such cases, diagnosis is based on physical findings or early symptoms such as dyspnea unrelated to feeding which usually precedes the appearance of symptomatic feeding difficulties.

Other disorders may not appear until later in life and may require more testing to secure a diagnosis or plan treatment.

Other symptoms may be diagnostically useful, such as hypernasal speech in velopharyngeal incompetence or dysphonia and dyspnea from a lingual thyroid gland. Routine tests including chest x-ray and modified barium swallow or videofluoroscopy may be required to document the presence and severity of nasopharyngeal reflux or aspiration into the lungs. In certain cases, more specialized tests may also be necessary. For instance, when the presence of a lingual thyroid gland is suspected, thyroid scanning is done to confirm the diagnosis and to ensure that the patient has additional functioning thyroid tissue.

Surgical Therapy

Therapy for most disorders of the oral preparatory phase of swallowing is surgical in nature. A cleft lip can be surgically ap-

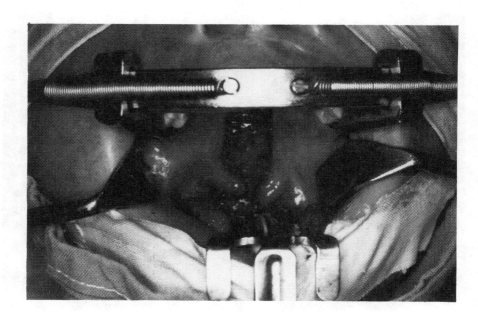

Figure 10–7.
Cleft palate.

posed, tongue size can be reduced by wedge resection of the dorsal midline or trimming laterally, and a tongue tie can be released by clipping the frenulum. In most cases it is possible to achieve both functional and cosmetic results. Neuromuscular deficits including CP are much less amenable to surgical intervention.

Treatment of a lingual thyroid gland can be medical and/or surgical, in the form of either suppressive thyroid hormonal therapy or excision of the ectopic thyroid tissue with or without subsequent need for exogenous thyroid hormone replacement (Parkin, 1990).

Cleft palate is repaired surgically between 12 and 18 months of life. Until surgery is done, breast-feeding is usually not possible, and the child is supported nutritionally with special feeding bottles (see Figure 10–7). The patient should always be examined carefully for other abnormalities, because certain syndrome such as the Pierre-Robin syndrome are associated with cleft palate, and these children are at increased risk for feeding and breathing problems (see Figure 10–8).

When a problem is not amenable to surgical intervention, alternative therapies may be of benefit. For example, maintenance of upright posture during feeding, teaching the child to toss the head back when swallowing, or limiting the patient's food choices to semi-solids may be helpful in some situations. In addition, oral motor therapy with exercises focusing on tongue lateralization have been shown to be useful in children with CP who have oral preparatory phase dysfunctions (Helfrich-Miller, Rector, & Straka, 1986).

Case 3: Macroglossia

The patient is a 1-year-old boy who experienced progressive enlargement of his tongue beginning soon after birth. Complete evaluation including genetic workup revealed no underlying problems. The tongue hypertrophy interfered with feeding and mouth closure, with resultant chronic drooling. The patient underwent wedge resection of the anterior central portion of his tongue with

marked improvement in feeding, speech, and cosmetic appearance.

Case 4: Cleft Palate

The patient is a 1-month-old girl who was noted at birth to have a cleft of the soft palate. There were no associated abnormalities. The patient was discharged home without proper feeding instructions and returned to the pediatrician with failure to gain weight and poor feeding due to rapid fatigue. The mother was instructed in the use of a cleft palate feeding bottle, with a long nipple and squeeze bottle, which puts the milk in the posterior pharynx for easier swallowing. The child's symptoms resolved, and she began to gain weight.

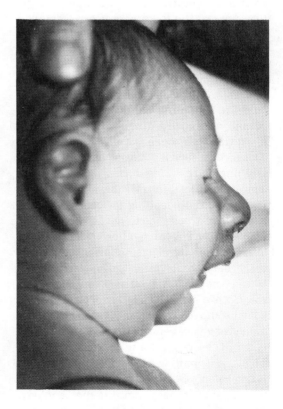

Figure 10–8.
Pierre–Robin sequence with cleft palate and small mandible.

The Oropharyngeal Phase

The exact source of stimulus for the pharyngeal swallow is unclear but probably arises from contact of the tongue with a bolus of food (Logemann, 1988). Sensory receptors in the base of tongue, soft palate, and posterior wall of the pharynx, carry afferent stimuli by the glossopharyngeal nerve, the second division of the trigeminal, and the superior laryngeal nerve to the swallowing center in the medulla oblongata. Efferent impulses then go out to trigger the pharyngeal stripping wave of deglutition.

Congenital sensory impairment or induced anesthesia of any of the afferent tracts of CNS V, IX, or X and destruction of the medullary swallowing center from a central congenital or acquired neurologic disorder are the leading causes of delayed initiation of the pharyngeal swallow. The range of disorders that cause such sensory impairment is beyond the scope of this chapter; however, it is important to recognize that many neurologically impaired children, including children with CP, will exhibit sensory dysfunction leading to delay in the pharyngeal swallow reflex.

Clinically, such a delay is characterized by coughing and choking during feeding and by aspiration of food into the lower respiratory tract, potentially leading to recurrent lower respiratory tract infections. Radiologically, delayed pharyngeal swallow reflex is very difficult to distinguish from premature leakage of bolus material into the pharynx resulting from factors such as poor tongue control. Both disorders are characterized by a delay on modified barium swallow or videofluoroscopy between the time barium is first seen in the pharynx and onset of the pharyngeal stripping wave.

Treatment of delayed swallowing reflex is limited due to its neurogenic etiology. However, Logemann (1986) has advocated thermal stimulation as a useful therapeutic maneuver, and a recent study (Helfrich-Miller et al., 1986) showed that thermal stimulation of the anterior faucial arches of profoundly retarded children with CP and a delayed swallow reflex can produce lasting improvements in pharyngeal phase function. Children receiving this therapy had decreased pharyngeal transit times, reduced number of swallows required to handle a bolus of given size, and decreased level of bolus residue in the pharynx after a swallow.

Pharyngeal Phase

Many anatomic structures and neuromuscular events comprise the pharyngeal phase of deglutition, and it is important that an organized system be used to diagnose and outline the management of patients with dysfunctions of this phase. One convenient system of analysis (Logemann, 1986) involves a determination of whether the risk of aspiration in a given patient occurs *during* the swallow as a result of reduced laryngeal closure or *after* the swallow as a result of diminished pharyngeal peristalsis, cricopharyngeal dysfunction, or anatomic intercommunication between the respiratory and digestive tracts. The treatment implications of such a classification system are great, so this particular system of analysis is especially useful in patient management. It can also help diagnostically because anatomic defects generally result in a postswallow risk of aspiration, whereas neuromuscular pharyngeal phase dysfunction generally produces aspiration during the actual act of swallowing.

The neuromuscular events of the pharyngeal phase of deglutition are complex. Adduction of the true vocal folds, closure of the laryngeal vestibule through posterior movement of the tongue, and downward motion of the epiglottis to cover the laryngeal aditus are all required to seal off the laryngeal opening. Simultaneously, pharyngeal peristalsis requires a strong superior to inferior contraction wave of the pharyngeal constrictor muscles along with pressure contributions from many surrounding structures, including the tongue (Logemann, 1988). Proper and coordinated motor functioning of cranial nerves IX, X, XI, and XII is thus necessary for successful pharyngeal deglutition. This functioning may be disrupted anywhere along the neuromuscular path, so both central disorders (e.g., tumors, kernicterus, hydrocephalus, encephalocele, nucleus ambiguus dysgenesis, or Arnold-Chiari malformation) and peripheral neuromuscular derangements (e.g., myotonic dystrophy, Werdnig-Hoffmann disease, or congenital or neonatal myasthenia gravis) must be considered in neurogenic pharyngeal phase dysphagia.

Vocal Cord Problems

Any of these generalized disorders may cause difficulties in either laryngeal closure and/or pharyngeal peristalsis, yet the heavy dependence of vocal cord closure, the most critical event in laryngeal protection against aspiration, on vagus nerve function places this specific pharyngeal phase event at an even higher risk for neurogenic dysfunction. The vagus nerve has a uniquely long course in the body (see Figure 10–9), and birth trauma to the neck can stretch the nerve and cause transient or permanent vocal cord paralysis. Additionally, the course of the left recurrent laryngeal nerve around the aortic arch subjects it to increased risk of injury. Congenital cardiovascular malformations, such as great vessel abnormalities and patent ductus arteriosus, or cardiomegaly due to anomalies such as ventricular septal defect or Tetralogy of Fallot can stretch or otherwise damage the nerve; and iatrogenic trauma to the nerve can occur during surgical correction of these cardiac abnormalities.

Unilateral or bilateral vocal cord paralysis can result from disorders other than congenital cardiovascular malformations or congenital or acquired neurological disorders. Anatomic anomalies including laryngomalacia, the most common congenital laryngeal malformation, and bifid epiglottis have been associated with vocal cord paralysis and feeding problems in young infants (Cotton & Reilly, 1990). With the advent of antibiotics and routine immunizations, infectious vocal cord paralysis resulting from diseases such as pertussis encephalitis, poliomyelitis, diphtheria, and tetanus is now quite rare (Dedo & Dedo, 1990). Traumatic vocal cord paraly-

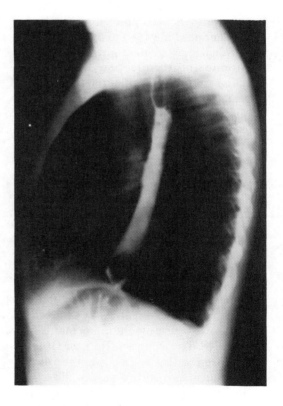

Figure 10–9.
Barium swallow demonstrating a foreign body in the distal esophagus.

sis from blunt neck trauma or postintubation remains a significant problem and should be considered in the evaluation of patients with a suitable history. Unilateral vocal cord paralysis produces a fixed laryngeal opening with frequent aspiration of food. This relatively common form of pharyngeal phase dysfunction must always be ruled out when a disorder of this phase of swallowing is suspected; flexible laryngoscopy as previously described usually allows for a quick diagnosis.

Postswallow Aspiration

Aspiration can also take place *after* the pharyngeal swallow has been completed. This might occur through inhalation of food residue remaining in the pharynx after the passage of a pharyngeal stripping wave rendered ineffectual by a neuromuscular disorder; or it might be due to an anatomic interconnection between the trachea and the esophagus. Esophageal atresia with concomitant tracheoesophageal fistula (TEF) formation is the most common of these anatomic malformations, but posterior laryngeal cleft, an anomaly resulting from aberrant development of the tracheoesophageal septum and cricoid cartilage ring, may also occur. Cricopharyngeal muscle dysfunction, a neuromuscular disturbance resulting in failure of the upper esophageal sphincter to relax when the propelled food bolus reaches the area, is another potential cause of postswallow aspiration. This disorder is rare, but it is known to occur in children with cerebral palsy as well as children with brainstem abnormalities or other CNS disturbances (Painter, 1990).

Children with CP have another disturbance that can result in postswallow aspiration. A study by Kenny et al. (1989) correlating ultrasonic images of swallowing with physiological measurements of ventilation indicated that these children are less able to plan and coordinate swallowing with ventilation than are unaffected children. Children with CP had an increased incidence of failure to close the vocal cords before swallowing and increased inspiration at the end of the swallowing task. It is unclear from this study alone whether the demonstrated incoordination of swallowing and ventilation resulted from sensory or motor dysfunction or some combination of both, but it *is* clear from the study that children with CP are predisposed to pharyngeal phase dysfunctions leading to aspiration both during and after the actual swallowing event.

Signs and Symptoms

Aspiration is the major symptom and aspiration-associated pneumonitis the major complication of dysphagia involving the pharyngeal stripping wave or pharyngeal peristalsis; thus, coughing, choking, and episodes of cyanosis with feeding are all important signs of pharyngeal phase dysfunction. These signs may occur alone, as they often do in cases of unilateral or bilateral pharyngeal muscle paresis, or they may be associated with other signs or symptoms specific to the etiology of the patient's disorder. For example, unilateral vocal cord paralysis usually produces a weak, breathy cry and should thus be suspected in any child with feeding disturbances and such a cry, even in the absence of respiratory dysfunction. Significant respiratory compromise, on the other hand, is often the presenting symptom of bilateral vocal cord paralysis, and dysphagia is often of secondary concern; voice and cry in these children are usually normal.

Excessive salivation or mucus production, with recurrent bouts of abdominal distention and often an absolute inability to accept feeds, are hallmarks of esophageal atresia with TEF and make dysphagia the focus of early attention in affected infants. In contrast, disordered arousal, generalized hypotonia or spasticity, cranial nerve palsies, altered reflexes, and other neurologic manifestations unrelated to feeding, although indicative of neurogenic dysphagia in an infant with a disordered feeding pattern, may serve to divert attention away from dysphagia as a primary concern.

Special aspects of the ENT history include questions regarding neck trauma, infections, and intubation. A thorough physical and neurological examination are very important in any form of dysphagia; however, in contrast to other phases of deglutition where these two elements may be all that is required to render an accurate diagnosis, radiographic studies and sophisticated laboratory tests have a significant place in the evaluation of pharyngeal phase disorders. To begin, modified barium swallow or videofluoroscopy is often useful to distinguish disorders that produce a risk of postdeglutition aspiration from those that lead to aspiration during the swallow (Kramer, 1989), and a routine chest x-ray is always done to document the presence and extent of aspiration pneumonitis. From there, the specific tests chosen depend on the suspected etiology of the pharyngeal dysfunction, and the workup involved can be quite extensive.

For example, when TEF is suspected, physical examination is supplemented by the attempted passage of a number 8 or 10 French catheter through the mouth and into the stomach or by instillation of methylene blue into the esophagus while looking for leakage into the trachea (Adkins, 1990). If these studies are positive, additional contrast studies are then necessary to plan surgical repair. Suspicion of other disorders such as laryngomalacia, laryngeal or pharyngeal edema, or congenital heart disease may be investigated by means of routine chest x-rays or magnification airway x-rays and flexible laryngoscopy; based on these tests, follow-up studies including cardiac angiography and CT or magnetic resonance imaging (MRI) scans may be required. Muscle biopsy and a wide array of laboratory and metabolic tests are important in the evaluation of children for neuromuscular dysphagia. Direct laryngoscopy, rigid or flexible, without anesthesia, is the test of choice in the evaluation of vocal cord mobility. Although esophagography may be useful, bronchoscopy and esophagoscopy are usually the best tests for the evaluation of anatomic respiratory or digestive system abnormalities.

Treatment of pharyngeal phase dysfunction depends on the cause. Certain defects including TEF, posterior laryngeal clefts, and unilateral incompetent laryngeal opening are amenable to surgery. Prior to definitive surgical management, temporizing measures including intubation, gastrostomy feeding, and tracheostomy may be required. The same measures are often necessary in patients with neuromuscular dysfunctions and dysphagia. In the absence of curative treatment, the focus of therapy in the latter group of patients is compensatory, with the goal of therapy being control over the most serious side effect of pharyngeal dysphagia, aspiration.

Making a decision to do a tracheostomy is not easy, because the care of a child with a "trach" is difficult, especially in the home setting. Preoperative discussions with the family are extremely important, and plans for a visiting nurse and home care equipment should be made as soon is surgery is performed. The child should not be sent home until the parents or caretakers have demonstrated facility in tracheostomy care, suctioning, and changing the tube in an emergency situation. Close follow-up after discharge is important to monitor the care and to avoid associated morbidity.

Patients who are at risk for aspiration *during* the swallow may benefit from learning maneuvers such as the supraglottic swallow procedure (holding one's breath at the height of inspiration and swallowing while the larynx is thus voluntarily held closed), from postural assists (turning the head toward the damaged side and tilting it downward during swallowing), or from a program of laryngeal adduction exercises. Children at risk for postswallow aspiration may likewise find postural maneuvers (including lying down in a decubitus position while eating) helpful, or they may find themselves sufficiently protected from laryngeal aspiration simply by coughing after each swallow before taking their next breath (Logemann, 1986).

Case 5: Bilateral Vocal Fold Paralysis

The patient is a 5-month-old boy who presented with intermittent stridor and failure to thrive. At rest there was no audible stridor and his voice was normal; when he cried he showed marked respiratory distress with perioral cyanosis and inspiratory and expiratory stridor. Due to his marked respiratory distress, direct laryngoscopy was done in the operating room, and revealed bilateral vocal cord paralysis. No other abnormalities were noted. A tracheostomy was done with improvement in breathing and feeding and subsequent weight gain. Review of his birth history at another hospital revealed a 7-day intubation for respiratory support after premature birth.

Esophageal Phase

Esophageal phase dysphagia is characterized by symptomatology involving the feeling of food sticking in the throat, partial obstruction with regurgitation and vomiting, and pulmonary symptoms resulting from aspiration of regurgitated gastric contents into the larynx. Constricting lesions causing esophageal phase dysfunction may include congenital esophageal stenosis; vascular rings, webs, or strictures; tumors; irritation resulting from lye or foreign body ingestion, gastric acid reflux, or following the trauma of intubation; and compression of the esophagus by mediastinal masses, tumors, or infections. Also included are neurogenic disorders such as achalasia, denervation injuries, and esophageal spasms which lead to impaired mobility and diminished force of esophageal peristalsis.

Evaluation of these disorders frequently involves barium studies, endoscopy, and manometry, and treatment ranges from medical therapy to surgical repair. The details of these disorders, their evaluation, and their treatment are discussed elsewhere in this book.

Case 6: Esophageal Foreign Body

The patient is a 2-year-old girl who was noted to have a change in feeding, with marked preference for liquids and avoidance of solid foods. This may have been present for as long as 2 months. Barium swallow revealed a foreign body in the distal esophagus; esophagoscopy showed a plastic toy in the distal esophagus, with pieces of food lodged proximally. It was removed and normal feeding resumed.

Aspiration and Aspiration-Associated Pneumonitis

There are three types of aspirated material—orally ingested material, oral and upper-airway secretions, and regurgitated gastric contents (Meyers, 1990). Although at least one study has shown that the degree of pneumonitis resulting from aspiration is inversely related to the pH of the aspirate, aspirate of any pH can produce pulmonary damage (Kirsch & Sanders, 1988). The major causes of aspiration were outlined previously in the discussion of dysphagia. Significant reflux of gastric contents can cause a reflux laryngitis, with associated hoarseness and stridor. Examination on flexible laryngoscopy is notable for erythema and swelling of the arytenoids and posterior larynx.

There are no characteristic roentgenographic findings of aspiration pneumonitis, and findings may range from diffuse bilateral infiltrates in massive aspiration pneumonitis to bibasilar infiltrates in dependent lung segments such as the posterior segments of both upper lung lobes (Kirsch & Sanders, 1988).

Therapy for aspiration pneumonitis consists of tracheal suctioning, oxygen supplementation, and, in extreme cases, even the application of mechanical ventilation and the use of positive pressure. In addition, in patients with rising fevers, increasing leukocytosis, new or enlarging pulmonary infiltrates, and purulent or culture-positive sputum should be provided with appropriate antibiotic therapy (Kirsch & Sanders, 1988). However, where definitive treatments (usually surgical in nature) exist for disorders predisposing a patient to this illness, they should be undertaken.

Temporizing measures may include nutritional support and pulmonary toilet; and often these measures, along with the postural and physical therapy measures previously mentioned, may be all that is available in a given situation. If recurrent aspiration cannot be controlled, surgically closing the glottis and diverting the food stream may be the most viable option (Meyers, 1990).

Summary

Children with developmental disabilities and dysphagia pose many challenges to the health care provider. Understanding the anatomy and physiology of the head and neck as it relates to swallowing provides a good basis for analyzing individual cases. In addition, the study of specific head and neck problems, as presented in the case reports, provides an illustration of the practical difficulties seen in clinical practice.

References

Adkins, J. C. (1990). Congenital malformations of the esophagus. In C. D. Bluestone & S. F. Stool (Eds.), *Pediatric otolaryngology* (2nd ed., pp. 973–984). Philadelphia: W. B. Saunders.

Cohen, S. R. (1990). Difficulty with swallowing. In C. D. Bluestone & S. F. Stool (Eds.), *Pediatric otolaryngology* (2nd ed., pp. 843–849). Philadelphia: W. B. Saunders.

Cotton, R. T., & Reilly, J. S. (1990). Congenital malformations of the larynx. In C. D. Bluestone & S. F. Stool (Eds.), *Pediatric otolaryngology* (2nd ed., pp. 1121–1128). Philadelphia: W. B. Saunders.

Dedo, D. D., & Dedo, H. H. (1990). Neurogenic diseases of the larynx. In C. D. Bluestone & S. F. Stool (Eds.), *Pediatric otolaryngology* (2nd ed., pp. 1172–1177). Philadelphia: W. B. Saunders.

Helfrich-Miller, K. R., Rector, K. L., & Straka, J. A. (1986). Dysphagia: Its treatment in the profoundly retarded patient with cerebral palsy. *Archives of Physical Medicine and Rehabilitation, 67,* 520–525.

Kenny, D. J., Casas, M. J., & McPherson, K. A. (1989). Correlation of ultrasound imaging of oral swallow with ventilatory alterations in cerebral palsied and normal children: Preliminary observations. *Dysphagia, 4,* 112–117.

Kirsch, C. M., & Sanders, A. (1988). Aspiration pneumonia. *Otolaryngology Clinics of North America, 21*(4), 677–689.

Kramer, S. S. (1989). Radiologic examination of the swallowing impaired child. *Dysphagia, 3,* 117–125.

Logemann, J. A. (1986). Treatment for aspiration related to dysphagia: An overview. *Dysphagia, 1,* 34–38.

Logemann, J. A. (1988). Swallowing physiology and pathophysiology. *Otolaryngology Clinics of North America, 21*(4), 613–623.

Meyers, A. D. (1990). Aspiration. In C. D. Bluestone & S. F. Stool (Eds.), *Pediatric otolaryngology* (2nd ed., pp. 1085–1089). Philadelphia: W.B. Saunders.

Painter, M. J. (1990). Neurologic disorders of the mouth, pharynx, and esophagus. In C. D. Bluestone & S. F. Stool (Eds.), *Pediatric otolaryngology* (2nd ed., pp. 1028–1037). Philadelphia: W. B. Saunders,

Parkin, J. L. (1990). Congenital malformations of the mouth and pharynx. In C. D. Bluestone & S. F. Stool (Eds.), *Pediatric otolaryngology* (2nd ed., pp. 850–859). Philadelphia: W. B. Saunders,

Stolovitz, P., & Gisel, E. G. (1991). Circumoral movements in response to three different food textures in children 6 months to 2 years of age. *Dysphagia, 6,* 17–25.

Weiss, M. H. (1988). Dysphagia in infants and children. *Otolaryngology Clinics of North America, 21*(4), 727–735.

CHAPTER

11

Respiratory Conditions and Care

LOURDES LARAYA-CUASAY, M.D., AND SUSHMITA MIKKILINENI, M.D.

CONTENTS

Children with developmental disabilities with dysphagia are prone to respiratory problems that challenge their host defenses and the mechanical aspects of breathing. The usual upper respiratory infection in a normal child can produce irritability, increased nasal and oropharyngeal secretions, and cough. The severely disabled child may not have an effective cough and will rely on external support to clear oropharyngeal and nasal secretions to maintain efficient respiration. This chapter will deal with the various respiratory conditions encountered in children with developmental disabilities and dysphagia and then describe the general principles of pulmonary rehabilitation and respiratory management. The use of tracheostomy and its care will be emphasized because of its relatively common use in these children. Where the discussion is not detailed further use of the references quoted is suggested.

Respiratory Conditions

Associated conditions in children with developmental disabilities and dysphagia that predispose them to respiratory disorders include:

1. swallowing dyscoordination or abnormal neuromotor control;
2. intrinsic and extrinsic congenital abnormalities of the trachea and esophagus;
3. vascular anomalies producing tracheal compression, nervous system disorders, anomalies or defects, or injury; and
4. neuromuscular problems.

Poor neuromuscular function such as that found in congenital muscle disorders as in Werdnig-Hoffman disease or congenital myopathic disorders may be associated with small narrow chest and/or kyphoscoliosis that may develop later due to neuromuscular weakness (Canet & Bureau, 1990). Swallowing dyscoordination or abnormal neuromotor control may coexist in certain conditions with neuromotor dysfunction such as Pierre-Robin syndrome (Bernard, Dupont, & Viala, 1990), and familial dysautonomia (Ganz, Levine, Axelrod, & Kahanovitz, 1983). Aspiration disease may follow. An associated congenital tracheoesophageal abnormality superimposed on a neuromuscular disorder predisposes the child to aspiration pneumonia.

Because of the relative lack of mobility of the disabled child, obesity may occur. Conversely, failure to thrive may result from poor skeletal muscle development, uncontrolled seizures, neurodegenerative disorders, central nervous system abnormalities such as absence of the corpus callosum, or in association with irreparable bilateral cleft palate. Nasogastric or nasojejunal feedings and surgical gastrostomy have improved the nutritional state of most of these children (see Chapter 4).

Behavioral problems complicating the neuromuscular disabilities seen in Lesch-Nyhan syndrome may cause dyscoordination in swallowing function and result in aspiration. Rumination or failure to chew food properly in association with sudden inappropriate laughter in disabled children may sometimes result in fatal aspiration of oral contents.

Figure 11–1 diagrammatically shows the evolution of respiratory problems in the child with developmental disabilities and dysphagia. When there is an associated swallowing problem or oropharyngeal dyscoordination that may or may not also be associated with a seizure disorder or gastroesophageal reflux (GER), aspiration pneumonia may result. This leads to increased mucus production, defective mucociliary clearance, and then atelectasis. Stagnant mucus invites superinfection leading to pneumonia of viral, bacterial, mycoplasmal, or mixed etiology. Failure to resolve the pneumonia causes recurrent obstructive bronchitis (Danos, Casar, Larrain, & Pope, 1976), dilatation of bronchi (bronchiectasis) with subsequent chronic infection or chronic interstitial lung disease resulting in pulmonary fibrosis, restrictive lung disease, hypoxemia, and eventually respiratory failure.

When poor neuromuscular function is complicated by pneumonia, hypoventilation and consequent hypercarbia and hypoxemia will lead to respiratory failure.

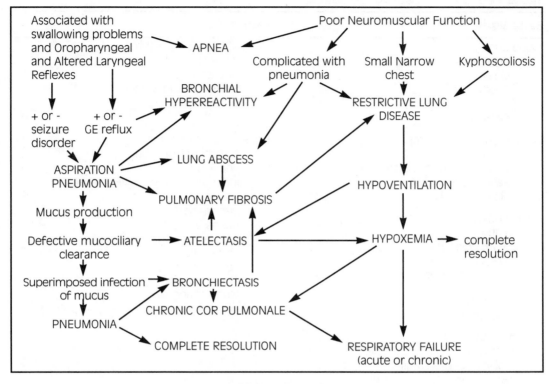

Figure 11–1.
Evolution of respiratory problems in developmentally disabled children with dysphagia.

Patients with kyphoscoliosis may develop restrictive lung disease, leading to chronic cor pulmonale. As soon as pneumonia occurs, the involvement of a pulmonologist will be ideal to assist in preventing the occurrence of the sequelae of unresolved pneumonia. If there is a family history of atopy and asthma, especially when airway irritants such as passive smoke are present, it is more likely that chronic allergic rhinitis and sinusitis will develop which later lead to bronchial hyperreactivity. Obstructive lung disease secondary to bronchospasm, inflammatory edema, and increased mucus production ultimately leads to respiratory failure when unrecognized or improperly treated. For nonverbal patients early recognition of signs and symptoms may not be easy (see Table 11–1).

Upper Respiratory Infection

When there is a strong family history of respiratory allergies and atopy, chronic rhinitis may develop. Enlargement of nasal turbinates increases nasal airway resistance, and in infants who are obligate nose breathers, this increases the work of breathing. At about 6 months of age infants convert to oral breathing so if the nose becomes obstructed, when associated with other craniofacial abnormalities, obstructive sleep apnea may develop (Brouilette, Ferbach, & Hunt, 1982).

TABLE 11–1. Early and late signs of asthma.

Early Signs	Late Signs

Mood Changes
    Aggressive
    Quiet
    Overactive
    Tired
    Easily upset
	Signs of worsening asthma
	    Voice changel
	    Swollen face
	    Shallow fast breathing
	    Quickening pulse
	    Listless

Changes in facial features
    Red face
    Dark circles under eyes
    Pale face
    Flared nostrils
	Signs of severe asthma
	    Breathing from the
	      neck up
	    Indentation at hollow Flared nostrils
	      of neck
	    Perspiration

Verbal complaints
    Fatigue
    Tight chest
    Neck feesl funny
    Don't feel good
    Chest filling up
    Chest hurts
    Mouth dry
	Hands over head
	    Labored breathing
	    Raised shoulders
	    Fearful expression
	    Flared nostrils
	    Blue lips and/or
	      fingernails

Breathing changes
    Coughing
    Taking deep breaths
    Breathing through mouth	

Change in seizure pattern	

Source: Adapted from early warning signs of asthma (1987). In *Living with asthma: Part 2 Manual for teaching children the self-management of asthma* (p. 137). (NIH publication No. 87-236.) U.S. Department. of Health and Human Services, Public Health Services, NIH.

In the acute phase of nasopharyngitis or rhinitis, profuse secretions accumulate in the upper airway which requires frequent gentle nasal and/or oropharyngeal suctioning to keep the airways open. In sinusitis, thick nasal secretions and postnasal drip can make clearing of the upper airway difficult, especially when neuromotor control of upper airway muscles is impaired. This explains the frequent attempts to gag and choke and snorting sounds often observed. Constant and careful observation is needed to determine when antimicrobials are indicated. Maintaining a patent nasal and oropharyngeal airway is crucial as deaths in patients with severe developmental dysfunction have unfortunately occurred from overwhelming amounts of secretions blocking ingress of air and causing asphyxia.

Cough is a common manifestation of respiratory infections. A cough draws attention to a nonverbal and/or otherwise disabled child (Tuchman, 1989). Table 11–2 shows the different causes of chronic cough. Cough that persists over 3 weeks is more commonly due to aspiration pneumonia or infection. Rare causes of persistent cough include congenital abnormalities, tumors, or cardiac failure.

TABLE 11–2. Etiology of chronic cough in developmentally disabled children with dysphagia.

Aspiration	Nonpulmonary
Swallowing incoordination	Stimulation of auricular
Foreign body aspiration	branch of vagus nerve
Gastroesophageal reflex	Irritation of pleura,
	diaphragm or pericardium
Congenital anomalies	Sinusitis with postnasal
Airway malformations	drip
Vascular ring	Esophageal foreign body
Tracheoesophageal fistula	Abdominal distention
Neurological abnormality	Central mechanism
Swallowing dyscoordination	Psychogenic
	Anxiety
Environmental	Habit
Passive smoking exposure	Tic
Air pollution	
Excessive dust inhalation	Vascular
Meteorologic factors	Cardiac failure
Reactive airway disease	
Infections	Inherited disorders associated
Viral: adenovirus	with bronchiectasis
cytomegalovirus	Cystic fibrosis
respiratory syncytial	Immotile cilia syndrome
	Immune deficiency states
Bacterial: pertussis	Reactive airway disease
chlamydia	
tuberculosis	Neoplasm
Mycoplasma	Benign tumors
Protozoal	Malignancies

Apnea

Apnea is defined as cessation of respiration. This may occur in the awake or sleeping state. Apnea may result from a defective control of breathing, structural alterations in the neuromuscular components of the control system, or a combination of various factors that affect the chemoreceptors which respond to blood gas changes. Both upper airway and chest muscles increase inspiratory activity in response to hypercapnia and mild hypoxia. Apnea may also follow acute dynamic airway obstruction as is dramatically illustrated by large mucus plugging of a tra-

cheostomized child that goes unobserved for several minutes. Certain respiratory infections can result in apnea such as bronchiolitis secondary to respiratory syncytial viral (RSV) infection (Abreu, Silva, & Brezinova, 1982).

Several sets of paired muscles act in a coordinated manner to accomplish the functions required of the pharynx: swallowing, protecting the airway, and maintaining airway patency. In Pierre-Robin syndrome, there is strong evidence that simultaneous deficiency of sucking and upper digestive motility, leading to frequent gastroesophageal (GE) reflux, and of cardiorespiratory control (frequent central and obstructive apnea, vagal hyperreactivity) have a common origin which is defective ontogenesis of corresponding neuromotor schemes at the brainstem level (Bernard et al., 1990).

Obstructive apnea is thought to be vagally-mediated by stimulation of laryngeal and nasopharyngeal chemoreceptors. Significant hypoxemia with consequent bradycardia can result when apneic periods are prolonged. No alteration in oxygenation is noted when the apneic event is short.

The developmental status and integrity of the central nervous system are major factors that determine the occurrence of apnea with oral feedings. Infants who are neurologically intact may exhibit dysphagia and apnea when developmental progress is slowed by illness. This is short-lived and improves as developmental catch-up occurs. The coordination of suck and swallow is better with the breast than with the bottle in some infants so that some infants will have nasopharyngeal reflux when bottle feeding even when breast-feeding skills are well-established (Loughlin, 1989).

Central apnea is seen in young infants, usually those born prematurely, who develop apnea and bradycardia during feeding as a manifestation of dysfunctional swallowing with or without aspiration. This apneic event need not follow immediately after a feeding, but can occur several hours later. Gastroesophageal reflux in these infants can be demonstrated by using an extended pH probe monitoring and demonstrating reflux episodes up to several hours postfeeding. Delayed gastric emptying may be present for an extended period of time predisposing to late postprandial reflux and central apnea (Loughlin, 1989).

Aspiration Disease

Aspiration disease in the child with neuromotor retardation is used to denote at least two separate entities: aspiration pneumonitis and aspiration pneumonia.

Aspiration pneumonitis is an inflammatory response to aspirated material not associated with infection and is usually associated with aspiration of sterile gastric contents. *Aspiration pneumonia* denotes the aspiration of infected material leading to infection. Aspiration can be of gastric contents (aspirated from below) which is related to gastroesophageal reflux (Bernard et al., 1990; Danos et al., 1976). This can be a silent, indolent process associated with microaspiration, or it can be a fulminant acute episode associated with massive macroaspiration of gastric contents into the upper or lower airways. Alternatively, aspiration can be from above (i.e., aspiration of oropharyngeal, nasal, and sinus secretions, and food). Detection of pulmonary aspiration in children can be determined noninvasively with radionuclide "salivagram." (Heyman & Respondek, 1989).

Mechanism of Aspiration

The lung is protected from aspiration by three major protective reflexes—cough, laryngeal closure, and swallowing. Laryngeal reflex prevents entry of material into the airway. Cough helps clear the airways of aspirated material. The mechanism of swallowing is a complex one utilizing at least 25 different muscle groups and requiring fine neuromotor coordination. As food is propulsed down from the pharynx into the esophagus, the airway is protected by cessation of respiration, glottic closure, and upward and forward displacement of the larynx. In a child with cerebral palsy and neuromotor retardation, or in a child with neuromuscular disease, all of these reflexes are usually absent or weak and not effective in clearing the lower airways. Approximately 45% of normal healthy people aspirate during sleep, but few develop pulmonary complications because of the presence of normal protective reflexes, mucociliary and cellular defense mechanisms. Children with developmental disabilities and dysphagia not only have impaired protective reflexes, but because of repeated insults to the airway, their mucociliary clearance is slow and cellular defenses are impaired.

Aspiration Pneumonitis

This is associated with instillation of fluid or small amounts of gastric contents into the trachea (Schwartz Wynne, & Gibbs, 1980). It is a chronic process and the incidence is difficult to identify because of varied clinical presentations and an absence of identifiable cause-effect relationship.

CLINICAL PRESENTATION. The child presents with repeated episodes of bronchospasm lasting from a few minutes to hours, associated with arterial desaturations. Increased respiratory congestion with an increase in the amount of secretions may be present although no overt infiltrates may be seen on chest radiographs. If left untreated, long-term sequelae include chronic hyperreactive airway disease, interstitial fibrosis, and bronchiectasis.

GER WITHOUT ACTUAL ASPIRATION. Recent studies have shown that reflux into the lower esophagus can induce a vagally mediated reflex bronchospasm. Presence of mild GER and careful history and improvement of bronchospasm with antireflux and aerosolized medications usually confirm the diagnosis.

Massive aspiration, unlike silent microaspiration, is usually a noticeable event. It may occur during a seizure episode, an emergency intubation, or with vomiting or regurgitation. The resulting respiratory dysfunction is related primarily to the pH of the gastric contents, and the critical pH is believed to be one of less than 2.5 (Mallory et al., 1982), with maximum lung damage seen at a pH of 1.5. The clinical picture may range from a mild condition consisting of a few hours of dyspnea, bronchospasm, and arterial desaturation to a more fulminant condition progressing to an acute respiratory distress syndrome (ARDS) type picture with refractory hypoxemia and diffuse alveolar infiltrate on chest radiographs.

Mild episodes are treated symptomatically with bronchodilator aerosols and oxygen. For the more severe cases, ventilatory support with positive end expiratory pressure (PEEP) is usually required. Antibiotics and steroids have not been shown to be useful in the treatment of aspiration pneumonitis. If particulate matter is aspirated, bronchoscopy is indicated, especially if atelectasis is present.

TREATMENT. Therapy is usually symptomatic with aerosolized bronchodilators; anti-inflammatory agents (cromolyn sodium and occasionally steroids) are usually helpful. Oxygen may be required for acute episodes. Prevention is the hallmark and treatment of GER is essential. If medical management fails, gastrostomy with fundoplication may be needed (see Chapters 12 and 13). If overwhelming oral secretions make suctioning difficult, tracheostomy may be necessary.

Aspiration Pneumonia

This occurs as a result of aspiration of oropharyngeal contents. Human saliva contains 10^6 to 10^8 bacteria per milliliter of saliva (Klastersky, Huysmans, Weerts, Hensgens, & Daneau, 1974). Children with poor oral and dental hygiene have a much greater load of bacteria. The respiratory system is more efficient in eliminating organisms introduced by inhalation than those aspirated. Additionally, when the normal host defense mechanisms are not intact, the incidence of bacterial airway and parenchymal infections increase. Because of the alteration in protective reflexes, especially those involved in swallowing, aspiration of oropharyngeal contents is an ongoing problem in children with neurodevelopmental disabilities.

CLINICAL PRESENTATION. The presence of pneumonia is suggested by the presence of a low-grade fever, irritability, and alteration in the color, consistency, and odor of sputum or tracheal secretions. Chest x-ray shows infiltrates usually in the dependent areas of the lungs, and commonly in the perihilar regions. Necrotizing pneumonia, lung abscesses, and empyema can also be seen. Organisms responsible are usually mouth flora.

TREATMENT. Penicillin is usually the drug of choice. For patients who have been in a hospital setting for prolonged periods, the antibiotic should provide broad spectrum coverage. Once culture results are obtained, the antibiotic coverage can be narrowed to give specific and least toxic coverage (Murray, 1979). Meticulous oral and dental hygiene and frequent suctioning of the mouth are essential (see Chapter 14). The goal is to decrease the bacterial load of the saliva and aspiration into the lower airways. The mouth should be cleaned thoroughly at least twice a day, with special care being taken to clean between the cheek and gums. Frequent teeth cleaning and dental check-ups to avoid gingivitis and pyorrhea are recommended. If secretions are overwhelming, tracheostomy is needed to facilitate tracheobronchial toilet. Cuffed tracheostomy may be a good choice in such cases.

Atelectasis

Atelectasis, or lung collapse, results from extrinsic or intrinsic obstruction of the airways. Extrinsic causes include compression by enlarged lymph nodes or presence of an enlarged blood vessel, mass, or tumor. Mucous plugs or intrabronchial tumors can produce complete or incomplete

obstruction. Other causes of atelectasis are conditions associated with poor neuromuscular function (such as occurs in muscular dystrophy or myotonic disorders) that can lead to hypoventilation. This can be compounded by obesity and decreased mobility. Hypoventilation leads to hypercarbia and arterial hypoxemia which can lead to respiratory failure. Poor mucociliary function can prevent removal of mucus from lower airways. Radiographically, the atelectatic area can be diagnosed and its location and size estimated. The addition of a lateral view to the usual postero-anterior view is most helpful. For children with thoracic deformities and myotonia, specific localization may be difficult.

The most common cause of atelectasis in children who are neurodevelopmentally disabled is obstruction from mucous plug. Due to the oropharyngeal incoordination and/or lack of muscle strength, expulsion of the mucous plug by coughing is not effective. Inability to voluntarily move or change position also prohibits the older child from assuming the posture that will favor expectoration. Severely affected children rely totally on caregivers to change their positions frequently to prevent pooling of secretions, especially when there is a superimposed respiratory infection.

Increased mucous secretion secondary to aspiration pneumonia can increase mucous production and lead to mucous plug formation that can obstruct bronchi and bronchioles. The magnitude of ventilation and perfusion defects will depend on the size of the atelectatic areas. Unless two or more major lobar bronchi are suddenly plugged, the patient may not manifest any rapid respiration or change in respiratory status. Irritability may be present. Decreased breath sounds over the involved area will indicate that a possible volume loss has occurred.

With the advent of pediatric flexible bronchoscopy, large mucous plugs obstructing lobar bronchi can be removed under direct vision with an endoscope. If the plug is very viscous, the use of diluted N-acetylcysteine with saline and a bronchodilator will aid in lyzing the disulfide bonds of the mucus enabling the lavage fluid to be sucked through the bronchoscope. Vigorous chest physiotherapy and postural drainage should follow bronchial lavage to aid in removal of any residual fluid.

Measures to prevent the occurrence of atelectasis are: attention to proper hydration of the patient, proper humidity and environmental temperature especially in tracheostomized patients, endotracheal or oropharyngeal suctioning as often as required, use of anti-inflammatory drugs and bronchodilators as needed in hyperreactive airways, and frequent positional changes.

Bronchial Hyperreactivity

Bronchial hyperreactivity (BH), also known as reactive airway disease or more commonly as asthma, is defined as reversible airway obstruction characterized by bronchospasm, airway inflammation, and mucosal edema. Triggers of airway hyperreactivity may be of allergic or nonallergic nature. The most common nonallergic trigger is passive exposure to an airway irritant such as cigarette smoke. Inflamed airways from aspiration pneumonia may cause airway hyperreactivity and lead to manifestations of bronchospasm. Viral respiratory infections can cause BH (Busse, 1988). Recurrent wheezing was found 2 to 7 years after an initial episode of respiratory syncytial viral bronchiolitis in 56% of 62 children studied by Rooney and Williams (1971). Offspring of parents with atopy were more likely to have persistent wheezing. The severity of these episodes decrease as they grow older.

Table 11–1 shows the early and late signs of asthma in infants and children based on wide clinical experience and as described in the manual for teaching children self-management of asthma (Early warn-

ing 1987). Bronchospasm may manifest only as sudden facial pallor or change in seizure pattern. Wheezing should not be used as the sole parameter to make a diagnosis of BH. BH can present clinically as croup-variant asthma, cough-variant asthma from postnasal drip or sinusitis, or upper airway obstruction variant. The upper airway variant may present with wheezing, stridor, or brassy cough. Facial color change/pallor, or circumoral cyanosis, may be misdiagnosed as seizures. Episodic or recurrent shortness of breath or decreased exercise tolerance may not be recognized as early presentation of bronchospasm. In infants, sudden very rapid respirations and change in volume and quality of laughter or cry may be the earliest sign of BH.

In normal children specific diagnosis can be made by pulmonary function testing before and after bronchodilation. Significant response to bronchodilator is diagnostic of BH. Because children with developmental disabilities are usually unable to perform the proper maneuvers required for accurate pulmonary function testing, the practical approach is to give a therapeutic challenge with a bronchodilator when symptoms suggestive of BH are present. Disappearance of wheezing or of chronic cough or return to usual color instead of pallor after administration of nebulized or oral bronchodilator is considered a positive response.

The major drugs used in the treatment of BH are (a) bronchodilators and (b) anti-inflammatory drugs such as steroids and sodium cromoglycate (see table 11–3). The nebulized method of delivery is the most useful because it relies on the normal tidal volume of the disabled child who may be unable to coordinate breathing maneuvers. At best 10% of the aerosolized drug may deposit in the airway, but this amount is enough to elicit a therapeutic response. Theophylline is safe and effective in therapy of asthma (Hendeles, Weinberger, Szefler, & Ellis, 1992). However, because

Table 11-3. Drugs used as aerosols in the treatment of pulmonary disease.

Drug Category	Form Dispensed	Dosage	Marketed Name	Comments
BRONCHODILATORS				
ALBUTEROL				
Nebulizer Solution	0.5% (5mg/ml) and 0.83%	0.05–0.15 mg/kg every 2–6 hrs. 1–2 puffs every 4–6 hrs. before exercise	PROVENTIL VENTOLIN	More frequent doses of 0.05 mg/kg every 20 min. or continuously have been shown to be more effective in acute asthma attaks than larger doses over longer intervals
Metered Dose Inhaler	90 µg/puff 200 puffs			
METAPROTERENOL				
Nebulizer Solution	5% (50mg/ml), 0.6% unit dose vial, (15 mg in 2.5 ml) 0.4% unit dose vial (10mg in 2.5 ml)	0.25–0.5 mg/kg every 2–4 hr.	ALUPENT	Shorter duration of action than Albuterol or Terbutaline. Not beta-2-selective. Do not use solution if brown or has precipitate.
Metered Dose Inhaler	650 µg/puff 300 puffs	1–2 puffs every 4 hr.	METAPREL	
TERBUTALINE				
Injectable Solution as Sulphate	0.1% (1 mg/ml)	.01–0.3 mg/kg every 2–6 hrs. as needed	BRETHINE	Clinically same effect as Albuterol when given in prescribed doses.
Metered Dose Inhaler	200 µg/puff 300 PUFFS	1–2 puffs every 4–6 hr. and before exercise	BRETHAIRE	
ISOETHARINE				
Nebulizer Solution	1%	0.25–0.5 ml in 2–3 ml NS 4 × a day	BRONKOSOL 1%	May develop bronchospasm from bisulfate preservative.
Metered Dose Inhaler	340 µg/puff	1–2 puff 4 × a day	BRONKOSOL MDI	

Table 11-3. Continued

Drug / Category	Form Dispensed	Dosage	Marketed Name	Comments
ATROPINE SULFATE [+] Ophthalmic Solution	0.5% (5mg/ml)	0.05–0.75 mg/kg every 4–6 hr.	ATROPINE SULFATE	Can be mixed with beta-agonists.
IPRATROPIUM [+] Nebuilzer Solution	500 μg in 2.5 mil unit dose vial	250 μg every 4–6 hr.	ATROVENT	Recently marketed in U.S.
Metered Dose Inhaler	18 μg/ puff	1–2 puffs every 4–6 hr.	ATROVENT	
ANTi-INFLAMMATORY CROMOLYN SODIUM				
Nebulizer Solution	20 mg/2ml ampule	1 ampule in 2–3 ml 0.9% sodium chloride 3–4 × daily	INTAL	During attacks DO NOT discontinue. Switch to nebulizer solution. After control of symptoms, titrate dose to 2–3 daily doses.
Metered Dose Inhaler	800 μg/puff 250 puffs	1–2 puffs 4–6 × daily	INTAL	
Spinhaler	20 mg/capsule	1 cap. 4 × daily	INTAL	
BECLOMETHASONE DIPROPIONATE	42 μg/puff 200 puffs	1–2 puffs 3–4 × daily Max 10 puffs	BECLOVENT VANCERIL	No evidence or superiority of longer action of one product over another.
FLUNISOLIDE Metered Dose Inhaler	250 μg/puff 100 puffs	1–2 puffs BID Max 4 puffs (1 mg)	AEROBID	More frequent administration provides better asthma control using the same daily dose.
Nasal Solution	0.025% or 250 mcg/ml	0.25 ml every 8 hrs. to 1 ml every 6 hrs. as clinically indicated	NASALIDE	Used in asthma and BPD.
Triamcinolone Acetonide	100 μg/puff 240 puffs	1–2 puffs every 8 hrs. Max. 12 puffs	AZMACORT	

Table 11-3. Continued

Drug / Category	Form Dispensed	Dosage	Marketed Name	Comments
<u>ANTICHOLINERGIC</u> Glycopyrrolate	0.2 mg/ml in 1 ml single dose vial	0.02 mg/kg every 4–6 hrs.	ROBINUL Injectable	DO NOT use if solution is discolored. Monitor heart rate and titrate dose accordingly. Occurrence of CNS-related effects are lower.
<u>MUCOLYTICS</u> N-acetylcysteine	10% and 20% solution or 100 and 200 mg/ml	2–3 ml 3–4 × a day with bronchodilator aerosol	MUCOMYST	May cause bronchospasm If administered without bronchodilator.
Sodium Bicarbonate	2% solution	2.5 ml of 2% solution		Bronchodilators break down faster in alkaline solution.
<u>DECONGESTANTS</u> Racemic Epinephrine	25%	1 part vaponephrine to 8 parts diluent: May increase up to 2f: 1 dilution every 30 min.	VAPONEPHRINE	Used for severe croup, not for severe asthma.
Phenylephrine	1/4%	As diluent with bronchodilator or 1:1 ratio with saline	NEOSYNEPHRINE	Vasoconstricts bronchial mucosa. May cause local irritation.
<u>ANTIBIOTICS</u> (Partial List) Tobramycin	80 mg/2ml	80–600 mg with bronchodilator and saline	NEBCIN	Nephrotoxicity and neuro- toxicity have to be moni- tored.
Gentamicin	80 mg/2ml	80–160 mg with bronchodilator and saline	GARAMYCIN	
Polymyxin B	5 mg/ml	10 units/mcg of pure polymyxin base	AEROSPORIN	Concurrent use of amino- glycosides and other nephrotoxic drugs must be avoided.

Table 11-3. Continued

Drug / Category	Form Dispensed	Dosage	Marketed Name	Comments
<u>ANTIPROTOZOAL</u> Pentamidine Isethionate	300 mg dissolved in 6 ml of sterile water administered by the Respirgard II nebulizer	300 mg once a month	NEBUPENT	DO NOT mix with any other drug. DO NOT use saline to reconstitue. Causes local airway irritation. 300 mg dose approved for P. carinii prophylaxis in adults, older children and adolescents with AIDS and high-risk patients.

Source: Adapted from Kelly, W. H. (1987). Pharmacotherapy of pediatric lung disease: Differences between children and adults, *Clinics in Chest Medicine, 8*, 681–694; Alderson, S. H., & Warren, R. H. (1984). Pediatric aerosol therapy, *Clinical Pediatrics, 23*, 555–557; and Tabachnik, E., & Leveson, H. L. (1980). Clinical appication of aerosols in pediatrics. *American Review of Respiratory Diseases, 122* (5, Pt. 2), 97–103.
Note: ⁺Also anticholinergic drugs

    BPD = Bronchopulmonary dysplasia. AIDS = acquired immune deficiency state.

theophylline lowers the esophageal sphincter tone, it is not used for patients with high risk for GER. Infants and children with acquired immune deficiency disease with developmental disability can develop dysphagia consequent to loss of developmental skill and could be compounded by presence of oral thrush or esophagitis. Pneumocystis carinii infection occurs in these patients, and pentamidine aerosol can benefit them.

Bronchopulmonary Dysplasia

Bronchopulmonary dysplasia (BPD) is the chronic lung disease that develops in newborn infants following their treatment with oxygen and positive pressure mechanical ventilation for various neonatal lung disorders.

Very small birth weight and/or premature infants who develop developmental disabilities and dysphagia may have BPD as a complication of their clinical course.

On chronic follow-up, occurrence of aspiration either from oropharyngeal secretion or consequent to associated gastroesophageal reflux can prevent the normalization of radiographic changes and lead to chronic lung disease. In the usual uncomplicated BPD course, very minimal small airway dysfunction may be found by 5 years of age and be detectable only with pulmonary function testing. However, in cases complicated by neurodevelopmental disabilities, findings of new radiographic infiltrates, atelectasis, or pulmonary fibrosis will be present especially in those who had aspiration pneumonia.

Treatment modalities used in BPD are aimed at improving the pathophysiologic abnormalities. Oxygen therapy, mechanical ventilation, fluid restriction, diuretics, caffeine, bronchodilators, steroids, and adequate caloric intake are the mainstay of therapy depending on the severity of the BPD. The exact dosages of the drugs used, the pharmacokinetics, and side effects of these agents have not been well-defined. Commonly used inhaled agents in BPD include isoproterenol, albuterol, metaproterenol, isoetharine, atropine, ipratropium bromide, and cromolyn sodium (see Table 11–3). A diuretic is used when signs of fluid overload are present. Symptomatic apnea is treated with caffeine or theophylline. Methylxanthine may also be needed later in the course of BPD when smooth muscle hypertrophy has developed and bronchospastic manifestations are present. At this point evidence of increased pulmonary resistance or decreased lung compliance are demonstrable by pulmonary function studies. Steroids are used for chronically ventilated infants with significant oxygen and ventilator requirements who have not responded to other more conventional therapies and for those infants with BPD whose reactive airway component and history are more suggestive of bronchial hyperreactivity exacerbation (Konig, Shatley, Levine, & Mawhinney, 1992). Oxygen therapy is chronically used guided by oximetric findings. Supplementation with low-flow oxygen facilitates weight gain in the patients who have adequate caloric intake but fail to thrive. Nutritional requirements may be as high as 150 to 200 Kcal per day, requiring use of nasogastric feeding or gastrostomy tubes to achieve caloric requirement without expending increased energy through sucking. Strict attention to tracheostomy care and prevention of secondary bacterial or viral infection is required. Annual influenza vaccination and proper immunizations will help prevent the occurrence of infection causing further lung injury to a convalescing lung.

Possible outcomes of BPD include:

1. recovery with mild residual small airway dysfunction;
2. development of chronic lung disease characterized by interstitial fibrosis, obliterative bronchiolitis, pulmonary

hypertension, chronic oxygen dependency, reactive airway or recurrent lung infections; or

3. death from acute causes such as sepsis, pneumonia, and apnea or from chronic causes such as respiratory failure, aspiration, and cor pulmonale.

Children who have neurological complications in infancy would develop developmental disabilities (Robertson, Etches, Goldson, & Kyle, 1992) with dysphagia of varying degrees of severity. Fortunately, with the increasing early of surfactant after premature birth, the incidence of BPD has shown a decline.

Bronchiectasis

Bronchiectasis is defined as dilatation of bronchi with distorted architecture. It is usually acquired secondary to recurrent pulmonary infections. In developmentally disabled children, bronchiectasis may follow significant aspiration pneumonia which may or may not be associated with gastroesophageal reflux. Other causes include prolonged retention of a foreign body; complication of viral, bacterial, or mycoplasmal infection; complication of poorly controlled asthma; infections associated with abnormal host defenses as in Down syndrome; and rarely, congenital cartilage deficiency. Pertussis, tuberculosis, measles (Laraya-Cuasay, 1988), and influenza (Laraya-Cuasay, Deforest, Huff, Lischner, & Huang, 1977) have been reported to lead to bronchiectasis.

A plain chest radiograph will show infiltrative changes with suggestive cystic areas. Bronchography used to be helpful in confirming the diagnosis. Computed tomography of the chest, a noninvasive method of diagnosing bronchiectasis, has almost totally replaced bronchography. In kyphoscoliosis the posture and the thoracic configuration could limit interpretation and specific localization of the disease process. Bronchoscopy aids in surgical assessment of presence of proximal suppurative endobronchitis which could complicate pulmonary resection.

Bacteriologic evaluation results in variable organisms including gram-negative and gram-positive bacteria. Enteric bacteria are often isolated when aspiration as in GER is occurring. Antibiotic susceptibility testing of cultured organisms is most helpful for appropriate long-term medical therapy.

Medical management is the usual therapy for diffuse bronchiectasis. Humidification, expectorants, bronchodilators, intensive chest physiotherapy, and postural drainage are very important to successful therapy. Surgical therapy is anticipated in localized bronchiectasis and in cases with massive hemoptysis, provided adequate lung function of remaining lobes is determined. However, with the advent of new and potent antimicrobials and advances in adjunctive respiratory care, surgical therapy is *rarely* indicated. Early diagnosis and prompt, careful removal of the aspirated foreign body will prevent bronchial injury and lung abscess formation.

Bronchiectasis secondary to a pneumonia may resolve after intensive appropriate antibiotic therapy. If secondary to partial obstruction by a foreign body, removal of the object can reverse the bronchiectasis provided proper antibiotic therapy and normal host defenses are present. If due to poorly controlled asthma, maximal and intensive anti-inflammatory and bronchodilator therapy will improve the bronchiectasis.

Lung Abscess

The development of an area of suppuration in the lung can result from aspiration of a foreign body or food with secondary bacterial superinfection. Anaerobic and aerobic organisms may be present. In a severely retarded child the occurrence of fetid odor from the mouth without fever can be a clue that anaerobic infection could be present. The presence of a localized mass in chest radiographs without symptoms of respiratory distress is common. Fortunately, with newer and more potent antibiotics, almost complete resolution of aspiration pneumonia is usually achieved so that progression to abscess formation may not occur.

Restrictive Lung Disorders

The condition of the lung that leads to reduced total lung capacity and small lung is termed *restrictive lung disorder*. Because of the small lung volume and total lung capacity consequent to the scoliosis, pulmonary function is impaired and chronic cor pulmonale may develop. Hence, early orthopedic surgical consultation must be obtained to ascertain proper time for surgical intervention.

Scoliosis can result from *neuropathic*, as in cerebral palsy, *myopathic* as in progressive muscular dystrophy, static myotonias, and Friedrich ataxia, *congenital* as in hemivertebrae, failure of segmentation of vertebra, or both, and *mesenchymal causes* as in Marfan's syndrome (Canet & Bureau, 1990). We had a patient with Duchenne's muscular dystrophy who tolerated scoliosis surgery very well without requiring prolonged mechanical ventilatory assistance.

Certain syndromes associated with developmental disabilities have a small and narrow chest as a component of the disorder. With continuing growth the chest may lag behind so that lung function ultimately is disproportionate to the entire body size. Familial dysautonomia (Riley-Day syndrome) is an example where abnormal autonomic function results in feeding and swallowing difficulties and cyclic vomiting "crises." Pulmonary problems result from repeated aspiration pneumonias and re-

strictive lung disease secondary to spinal curvature abnormalities such as kyphosis and scoliosis (Ganz et al., 1983).

Previous respiratory viral infections which led to significant chronic interstitial pneumonia can produce restrictive lung function because of the pulmonary fibrosis that results (Laraya-Cuasay, 1988). As the pulmonary fibrosis progresses, bronchiectasis, pneumothorax, and oxygen dependency are complications expected to develop.

General Principles in Pulmonary Rehabilitation

The goal in pulmonary rehabilitation is to maximize lung function by breathing retraining, exercise and conditioning, clearing airway of secretions, providing adequate caloric intake to provide energy for the work of breathing and for proper growth, and preventive measures directed to proper environment and infection control.

Chest Physiotherapy and Postural Drainage

Chest physiotherapy and postural drainage (CPTPD) are indicated:

1. When there is excessive bronchial secretion not removed by normal ciliary activity or cough;
2. For atelectasis due to mucus plugging; and
3. To assist removal of fluid by gravity using deep breathing reinforced cough, thoracic "squeeze," cupping, and vibrations on selected patients who can understand the maneuvers needed.

Caution must be exercised when treating children on continuous nasogastric feedings or those with gastrostomy tubes to prevent aspiration of residual gastric contents.

Special Breathing Exercises

Breathing exercises are indicated in bronchial hyperreactivity, kyphoscoliosis, as is seen in familial dysautonomia (Ganz et al., 1983), bronchiectasis, and neuromuscular disorder. The goals are to develop more effective diaphragmatic and lower costal breathing; relax all muscles, especially those of upper part of the chest, shoulder girdle, and neck; and attain good posture. Modification of these techniques are used by physical therapists to achieve the same goals in children who have difficulty in following directions. Music therapists or parents can use certain songs or rhythms that cause the patient to produce an inspiratory hold and then prolong the expiratory flow. This could make these exercises a pleasant task especially for children with short attention spans. Breathing retraining will also help achieve proper postural drainage. The creativity of the therapist is challenged when individualized therapy is planned.

Exercise Training

Swimming is an ideal exercise for children with bronchial hyperreactivity. Involvement in Special Olympic activities for those able to is beneficial. Muscular training and conditioning adds to effective mucociliary clearance and cardiopulmonary function. Whenever possible exercise should be done under the sun to prevent development of rickets and osteomalacia especially in children taking several anticonvulsant medications.

Nutritional Care

Attention to caloric intake to prevent poor weight gain will lead to proper lung growth, prevent immobilization, and enhance exercise capabilities. (Please see Chapter 4 on nutrition for further details.) Certain physical anomalies may require special equipment to maintain proper seating posture during feeding and to adapt to utensils needed to self-feed. Use of numerous anticonvulsants can lead to megaloblastic anemia, vitamin deficiency, and decreased mineral intake. Prevention of anemia (because of its consequent effect on oxygen transport to tissues) is important especially when exercise is prescribed. Early individual or group intervention has been very effective. Utilization of an interdisciplinary approach with inclusion of a nutritionist, an occupational therapist or physical therapist, a behaviorist, and speech therapist is ideal (Pipes & Glass, 1989).

Immunizations

Annual influenza vaccination can prevent morbidity or mortality from influenza which can be very debilitating or life-threatening to children with severe disabilities. For those unable to use influenza vaccine, amantadine can be given orally as soon as the influenza infection is diagnosed. Early detection of pulmonary tuberculosis by Mantoux testing should be performed especially in institutions with a large population of developmentally disabled children.

Respiratory Management

Pharmacologic Approach

Bronchodilators, anti-inflammatory drugs, anticholinergics, mucolytics, decongestants, antibiotics, and antiprotozoal drugs are listed in Table 11–3 with the dosage, various forms dispensed, and the marketed names in the United States (Alderson & Warren, 1984; Kelly, 1987; Tabachnik & Levison, 1980). For the nebulized drugs, the amount of drug deposited in the alveoli is variable and dependent on the mechanical forces necessary to achieve maximal inspiratory flow and maintain the inspiratory hold, as well as the efficiency of the compressor or inhalation device used. At best, about 10% may be deposited in the lower airways by nebulization. Studies of drug deposition have used children with chronic lung disease without developmental disabilities. However, clinical experience shows that even the most ill disabled child with wheezing will respond with clearance of wheeze and better air exchange after high-flow nebulization of appropriately dosed beta-agonist or anticholinergic. In infants, placing the face mask or T-piece near the nose can be effective in delivering the bronchodilator to the lower airways.

For children with excessive secretions, administration (orally, by nasogastric tube, or nebulization) of glycopyrrolate has been very effective. Atropine and atropine-like drugs are also useful. The compatibility with beta-agonists makes it very convenient to use in children with BH who need bronchodilation and reduction of secretions. Overuse of anticholinergic drugs should be avoided because of the danger of drying mucous plugs that could cause atelectasis.

Steroids are very effective anti-inflammatory drugs. The only nebulized form used at present is the liquid beclomethasone intended as a nasal solution, which is dosed from 0.25 ml every 8 hours to 1 ml every 6 hours. When used as clinically indicated, therapeutic response is excellent. The advantage of the nebulized form is the relative lack of systemic effects, which is very important in the growing child. Experience with nebulized flunisolide has been mainly in infants with bronchopulmonary dysplasia with reactive airway disease (Konig et al., 1992). Cromolyn sodium is also a very effective agent used in decreasing secretions by preventing or treating the inflammatory state. It acts by preventing mast cell degranulation, thus inhibiting release of mediators that favor the inflammatory response.

Mechanical Approach

Various respiratory equipment and mechanical devices directed toward pulmonary rehabilitation and chronic respiratory care are briefly discussed in the following sections.

Respiratory Therapy Equipment

COMPRESSORS AND NEBULIZERS. Compressors and nebulizers are used to administer bronchodilators, anti-inflammatory drugs, and/or antibiotics by inhalation. Certain children may be able to learn to execute the inspiratory maneuver necessary to use inhalers or space devices like aerochambers and InspirEase™. Assessment of technique of inhalation for proper drug deposition is crucial for therapeutic success. Usually, the nebulization method is more successful because it does not depend on actuation of spinhalers and utilizes the usual breathing pattern of the patient. For tracheostomized children, nebulized medications are administered through the tracheostomy, thus reducing the dead space.

OXYGEN DELIVERY. Oxygen administration has been successfully administered with nasal cannula, oxygen hood or tent, and face tent or face mask. Oximetric monitoring at home can be done to guide prescribed dose of oxygen flow. Attention to patency of nasal and oropharyngeal airway by removal of secretions is needed for unobstructed oxygen flow. Oxygen concentrators, liquid oxygen, and oxygen in cylinders can be prescribed. For ambulatory use, portable oxygen containers and devices are available. Special nonallergenic tapes are very useful for children with tape hypersensitivity or fine skin. Taping the nasal cannula can be very challenging in some disabled children. Frequent checks on the patency of the nasal cannula must be done to ensure absence of mucous plugs at the tip to maintain efficient oxygen delivery.

VENTILATORS. Ventilator therapy using port-able ventilators can be prescribed either at home or in rehabilitation hospitals. For certain neuromuscular diseases such as Werdnig-Hoffman, and upper motor neuron diseases, only night-time ventilation is needed. A back-up second portable ventilator is also available in the home or institution in case of mechanical breakdown. Home mechanical ventilation has been used since new battery operated equipment have been manufactured. Children with ventilator dependent bronchopulmonary dysplasia, and adolescents with cervical cord injury or severe muscular dystrophy have benefitted from the use of portable ventilators. Nocturnal feedings may be continued as constant drip, but feedings are best given at times when patient is not ventilator-assisted.

SUCTION EQUIPMENT. Suction apparatus is a must for children with developmental disabilities who have excessive oropharyngeal secretions and for the tracheostomized and mechanically ventilated patients. Aseptic catheter technique is required. Portable suction apparatus should be prescribed for mobility and emergency use during transport.

APNEA MONITORS. Apnea monitors are used to document episodes of apnea and bradycardia thus preventing sudden deaths and providing time for intervention.

Bronchial Drainage

Mechanical percussors are available in several models including hand-held types for use in chest physiotherapy. A vest therapy model has been tried in patients with cystic fibrosis over 9 years of age. This has the advantage of simultaneous percussion of several lung lobes in the seated position without postural changes. The vest model could be utilized by children who own special chairs. However, this will require further study.

Flutter valves have been recently used to aid in expiratory flow and mobilization of secretions while maintaining a prolonged expiratory phase.

Special Procedures

BRONCHOSCOPY. Flexible bronchoscopy aids in diagnosing airway problems such as foreign body aspiration or intrinsic obstruction. Its major contribution in the care of the developmentally disabled is in removal of mucous plugs under direct vision, thus opening a collapsed lobe or aiding in removal of secretions. It is also used to obtain bronchial specimens for diagnosis of etiology of pulmonary pathology.

ENDOBRONCHIAL LAVAGE. This invasive procedure can be useful in removal of mucous plugs and as an ancillary procedure after aspirated foreign body has been removed as clinically indicated. Usually, normal saline is instilled through the bronchoscope and lavage fluid is later aspirated. If the mucous plug is very thick, a mixture of mucolytic agent with normal saline is instilled and allowed to stay for a few minutes, then later aspirated. Atelectatic areas may open up after endobronchial lavage.

TRACHEOSTOMY. See discussion below.

GASTROSTOMY AND FUNDOPLICATION. Bul and associates studied whether gastrostomy and fundoplication prevented aspiration pneumonia in mentally retarded individuals (Bul, Dang, Chaney, & Vergara, 1989).

Recurrent aspiration was found least often in subjects without preoperative GER who had both gastrostomy and fundoplication. Feeding gastrostomy alone or with fundoplication does not prevent aspiration (Pearl et. al., 1990). Good weight gain was reported in the malnourished mentally retarded children with GER and recurrent aspiration pneumonia. Further information on these procedures is available in Chapter 12.

NASOGASTRIC FEEDING. See Chapter 12.

ORTHOPEDIC PROCEDURES. The specific procedures directed toward correction of kypho-scoliosis or any correctable thoracic deformity include the use of therapeutic bracing or spinal instrumentation depending on the severity of the curve. In the past two decades, a more aggressive approach in the management of scoliosis has been taken in which restrictive lung disease is prevented and a better quality of life is provided to patients with neuromuscular weakness or any disability that favors development of scoliosis.

Tracheostomy

Tracheostomy is a procedure frequently used in the management of the child with developmental disabilities. It is often viewed as a sign of clinical deterioration, and many emotional and ethical issues need to be discussed with the parents and child before they accept the procedure. In the past tracheostomy was associated with an increased morbidity and was usually used as a life-saving procedure or during end stage disease. With the advent of newer materials and techniques and the availability of skilled home care, tracheostomy is used earlier to *prevent* lung disease and respiratory failure and to improve quality of life.

Indications for Tracheostomy

The main indications for tracheostomy are: (1) to bypass upper airway obstruction, (2) to enhance pulmonary toilet, (3) for long-term mechanical ventilation, and (4) to protect lower airways form aspiration of food particles.

To Bypass Upper Airway Obstruction

During quiet breathing the nasal passages account for about 50% of the total respiratory resistance and approximately 65% of the total airway resistance. Hypotonic pharyngeal muscles, either secondary to the underlying disease or because of loss of motor tone during sleep, can contribute significantly to an increased airway resistance. A floppy tongue that falls backward can also cause significant upper airway obstruction. Normally the genioglossus muscle contracts synchronously with the diaphragm so that during inspiration the tongue is pushed forward and acts as a pharyngeal dilator.

In a child with neurologic impairment, decreased muscle tone may worsen further during sleep and the upper airway resistance consequently may increase several fold. The respiratory muscles in themselves may be weak, as in children with neuromuscular diseases, or the respiratory muscles may be at a mechanical disadvantage, as in the child with severe scoliosis and distorted chest wall. In these cases, the inspiratory muscles cannot generate enough negative pressure to overcome the upper airway resistance. This results in severe hypoxia, increased work of breathing, and increased metabolic demands.

Tracheostomy helps by bypassing the nasal and oral airway. Theoretically, there should be about 50 to 60% drop in airflow resistance; however, in reality, because of the small size of tracheostomy tubes, the difference is not as much but is still significant enough (especially when upper airway obstruction is present) to reduce work of breathing, oxygen consumption, and ultimately improve the child's nutritional status.

Pulmonary Toilet

Children with cerebral palsy, neuromuscular disorders, or any other conditions that alter the swallowing pattern have difficulty handling secretions. These children usually also have a weak cough and laryngeal reflex making them more prone to aspiration of mouth contents. Tracheostomy enhances pulmonary toilet and is an effective way of clearing secretion from above as well as from the tracheo-bronchial tree.

Long-Term Mechanical Ventilation

Improvement in operative techniques of tracheostomy, aftercare, and the availability of newer tracheostomy tubes and home care equipment and home ventilators have made it possible to maintain children on prolonged mechanical ventilation. Children with BPD are now sent home and maintained on mechanical ventilation for a few months up to a few years with ultimately good prognosis. Other children with cerebral palsy or progressive muscular dystrophy may initially need only nighttime ventilation, but as the disease progresses, longer periods on the ventilator will be required.

To Protect Lower Airways From Aspiration of Food Particles

Tracheostomy in itself may increase the incidence of aspiration because of alteration in the cough reflex (Konig et al., 1992) and the protective laryngeal closure reflex (Nash, 1988). However, some patients with severe neuromotor retardation who chronically aspirate gastric contents have severe gastroesophageal reflux in spite of having had a fundoplication and being fed via a gastrostomy tube. In these patients, tracheostomy permits frequent suctioning, thus protecting the tracheobronchial tree from the deleterious effects of gastric contents. A high-volume, low-pressure cuffed tracheostomy tube may be used for this purpose. Pooling of secretions takes place above the cuff, and care should be taken to suction from above the cuff before deflating it to avoid leakage of the secretions into the lower airway. Special tracheostomy tubes with a suction channel above the cuff area are available so that the secretions can be suctioned from the outside. For most cases, cuffed tracheostomy tubes are used primarily for effective ventilation in a ventilator-dependent child.

Complications of Tracheostomy

Complications of tracheostomy can be subdivided into intraoperative, immediate postoperative, and late postoperative complications.

Intraoperative complications include bleeding, tracheoesophageal fistula, pneumothorax, and pneumomediastinum (particularly in children with severe lung disease), recurrent laryngeal nerve injury,and cardiopulmonary arrest, especially in children with chronic carbon dioxide retention who are breathing on a hypoxemic drive. Sudden relief of obstruction may lead to respiratory arrest.

Immediate postoperative complications include bleeding, wound infection, subcutaneous emphysema, difficulty swallowing, and displaced or obstructed tubes.

Late postoperative complications include granuloma formation, tracheoesophageal fistula, tracheocutaneous fistula, scar with keloid formation, laryngotracheal stenosis, and late hemorrhage from rupture of the innominate artery.

Care of the Child with Tracheostomy

Preparation

Although long-term care of the child with tracheostomy is discussed here, preoperative teaching, family counselling, and psychological preparation of the parent and child are important aspects of care (Foster & Hoskins, 1981). Once a tracheostomy is performed, a practical planned approach needs to be developed that will enable parents to understand the function of the tracheostomy tube and the basic physiological aspects of respiratory care and then gradually assume responsibility of all aspects of tracheostomy care—suctioning, changing the tube, and handling accidental decannulation and sudden obstruction of the tracheostomy tube. All parents should be taught CPR (cardiopulmonary resuscitation) before the child is discharged from the hospital. The following issues need to be addressed:

HUMIDIFICATION. Tracheostomy bypasses the nasopharyngeal mucosa which is normally responsible for heating and humidifying the inspired air. Therefore, humidification of the air the patient breathes is necessary to keep the tracheal mucosa moist and to facilitate mucociliary transport, to prevent drying of secretions, and eventual obstruction of the tracheostomy tube. Humidifica-tion is achieved by passing compressed air or oxygen through a reservoir containing sterile heated water and then delivering that air, usually via a mask, to the tracheostomy tube. The mist should be applied continuously at night. During the day, it can be applied intermittently but care should be taken to humidify the air whenever the weather is hot and dry or when driving in a heated car. The temperature of the humidified gas should be checked frequently to avoid overheating. The condensed water vapor in the tubing should be drained frequently, and the tubing changed frequently to avoid bacterial contamination.

SUCTIONING. Tracheal suctioning should be performed as often as necessary. Although a sterile technique is used in the hospital, a clean technique is used at home. Suction equipment is kept at the patient's bedside. The lowest negative pressure needed to remove secretions should be used. The size of the catheter used should be such that there is enough room around the catheter for free flow of air. If the tracheostomy tube is completely obstructed and if the negative pressure used is too high, mucosal trauma or even collapse of the alveoli may occur. Care should be taken to avoid passing the suction catheter beyond the end of the tube. The color, consistency, odor, and amount of the suctioned material should be noted, and any change reported to the physician.

TIE CHANGES AND TUBE CHANGES. The ties used to hold the tracheostomy tube in place need to be changed as often as needed. They should be kept dry, free of secretions. The neck and the stoma should be kept clean and dry, and any signs of infection or inflammation taken care of immediately.

The tracheostomy tube should initially be changed after a tract is formed which is usually within 5 to 7 days of the procedure, and at least once a week thereafter. For long-term care at home the tube should ideally be changed every 7–10 days. The frequency of tube changes may be individualized but it should not be left in place for longer than a month.

EMERGENCY SITUATIONS AND RECOGNIZING SIGNS OF RESPIRATORY DISTRESS. Parents are taught the different emergency situations that may arise and how to respond to each of them. They are taught to recognize the signs of respiratory distress—how to count respiratory rate and to look for nasal flaring and use of accessory muscles of respiration. They should learn to identify breath sounds and change in sound with obstruction due to mucus. Complete obstruction, accidental decannulation, and hemorrhage are some of the emergency situations that parents should be taught to handle.

PREPARATION OF THE HOME. The equipment needed at home should be ordered in advance. This include the suction machine, apnea monitor, humidifier, oxygen, suction catheters, and normal saline solution.

ADDITIONAL CONSIDERATIONS. In addition to problems with swallowing, the patient with a tracheostomy tube may not be able to generate enough intra-abdominal pressure to have effective emptying of bowels. The child's diet should include plenty of fluids and fiber to prevent constipation.

Because cough may be ineffective, chest physiotherapy and suctioning may be needed more frequently than prior to the procedure. The parent should report to the physician if there is a change in the color, consistency, amount, or odor of the tracheobronchial secretions. There is an increased incidence of bacterial colonization of the trachea (especially with Pseudomonas species in the tracheostomized patient (Niederman, Ferranti, Zeigler, Merrill, & Reynolds, 1984). Antibiotics should not be administered in an attempt to prevent colonization or pneumonia because recolonization occurs as soon as antibiotics are stopped. The incidence of pneumonia in patients receiving prophylactic antibiotics is similar to those not receiving any prophylaxis. Infection with resistant organisms and superinfection are other reasons for avoiding prophylactic oral or aerosolized antibiotics (Foster & Hoskins, 1981; Klastersky et al., 1974). However, if there are clinical signs of pneumonia or tracheitis

with increase in the polymorphonuclear cells in the tracheal aspirate, antibiotic treatment should be initiated. Bronchoscopy may be useful in visualizing the appearance of the endobronchial mucosa.

Decannulation

Decannulation is dependent on the underlying pathologic process and the initial indications for tracheostomy. Before decannulation can be considered, both primary and secondary reasons for the tracheostomy must no longer exist.

Evaluating Readiness for Decannulation

Physical examination will help evaluate the patient's readiness for independent respirations. The ability to cough or breathe with the tracheostomy tube occluded either with a finger or with the neck flexed is a favorable sign. The smaller the size of the tube, the closer is the patient to decannulation. Auscultation of the chest should be free of wheezing, rhonchi, or rales. The tracheobronchial secretions should be minimal, and the patient should not require frequent suctioning.

Laboratory studies as aids in decision to decannulation include:

1. *Radiographs*—Antero-posterior and lateral radiographs of the neck and chest should be done to show the size of the air column above and below the tracheostomy. Granulation tissue, stricture or papilloma can often be identified on this film.
2. *Arterial blood gases* (ABG)—The underlying pulmonary disorder must be partially or completely resolved, and normal gas exchange as indicated by a normal ABG should exist before decannulation is considered.
3. *Peak inspiratory pressures* are used to measure respiratory muscle weakness.

Peak inspiratory pressures are measured with a hand-held monitor attached to the tracheostomy site. A negative pressure of greater than 40 cm H_2O is indicative of good muscle strength.

4. *Infant pulmonary function testing*—Flow volume loops are done with the child breathing through the tracheostomy and after temporary decannulation (with stoma closed off) breathing through the mouth. If inspiratory flows via the face mask exceed the flow from the tracheostomy there is a likelihood of successful decannulation (Mallory, G. B., et al).

5. *Endoscopy*—All patients should have an endoscopic evaluation of the trachea prior to decannulation. Laryngo-scopy and bronchoscopy are performed to evaluate anatomy, assess the function of the vocal cords, inspect the subglottic area and evaluate its size by "sounding" (passing different sized bronchoscope to estimate the size). Granulomas if present may be dissected out at that time.

Decannulation Procedure

Once it is determined that the child is no longer physically dependent on the tracheostomy, the patient and the family should be prepared for the decannulation. The actual planned decannulation should always be done in the hospital setting. The child should be weaned to the smallest sized tube. If there are no respiratory problems over the next 24 hours, the tube is occluded with tape. The tape is left in place for the next 24 hours except when the child is asleep. If all goes well, the child can be decannulated. The child should be observed for another 24 hours following decannulation for signs of respiratory distress before discharge. In certain cases the stoma may not close completely so that a residual epithelialized sinus may persist for months or years requiring revisits to the otolaryngologist. In children with excessive drooling this sinus may be a site of infection.

Decannulation Failure

If the child develops signs of respiratory distress the tube should be reinserted. In some children the stoma may close within 6 hours. No attempts to force the tracheostomy tube should be made. If the patient needs reintubation, he should be taken to the operating room for reinsertion of the tracheostomy tube. The size of the tube should be gradually increased to the predecannulation level. No attempts at decannulation should be made for another 6 months.

Comprehensive Care of the Developmentally Disabled Child with Dysphagia and Chronic Lung Disease

When chronic lung disease is diagnosed in a child with developmental disabilities and dysphagia, no curative therapy is available. Caring for children with chronic lung disease can be very satisfying, but is also frustrating, complicated, and emotionally and physically tiring. It becomes much more so when there is an underlying neurodevelopmental disability. Parents of chronically ill children are burdened psychologically, emotionally, and financially, so that their coping mechanisms, which may have been adequate in the first few years, gradually become inappropriate or unbalanced. The pediatrician acts as the medical "director," but he or she has to be assisted by a team of professionals attuned to the needs of the chronically ill. The parents know that they have a defective, disabled or abnormal child who is retarded, but acceptance of the retarded state is most difficult. Subsequent development of secondary psychological and emotional problems in the direct caregivers may complicate the ongoing care the children who are chronically disabled and may progress to such magnitude later, making its management more difficult than the chronic disorder in the patient.

Therefore, *prevention* of the occurrence of these psychosocial disabilities or complications in the direct caregivers is more beneficial for the child (Fisman & Wolf, 1991). Anticipatory guidance and counseling is necessary. Knowledge of the most sophisticated pharmacologic and technological advances in therapy is a great boost to the patient and parents. Very often, the physician becomes "everything" to the families as they travel the long journey of progressive deterioration of lung function, as well as progression of the neuromuscular disorder.

Coordinated long-term medical care is needed by all children with chronic conditions. The advent of home medical care companies that specialize in providing home intravenous antibiotics; parenteral alimentation and enteral feedings; ventilator care, oxygen, respiratory therapy equipment and supplies; tracheostomy care; and physical, occupational, and speech therapy has facilitated the home care of children with chronic lung disease and developmental disabilities. The added emotional and economical benefits of being able to care for a loved one in a familiar environment has to be carefully balanced with the physical, emotional, and mental fatigue that some families experience, especially toward the terminal period. In the case of bronchopulmonary dysplasia, almost complete improvement of lung function is usually anticipated unless complicated by aspiration pneumonia or other causes of lung injury. For children with terminal illnesses such as advanced degrees of severe aspiration pneumonia, severe kyphoscoliosis with cor pulmonale and chronic respiratory insufficiency, and other conditions associated with congestive heart and chronic respiratory failure, pediatric hospice care can be most helpful. Advance directives from the parents or legal guardians must be discussed. When all therapeutic modalities fail, the continuing emotional support of the physician and his or her comforting presence

whenever possible, combined with pastoral care, and the presence of family support and love can provide the ideal atmosphere for the child or adolescent.

References

Abreu, F. A., Silva, E., & Brezinova, V. (1982). Sleep apnea in acute bronchiolitis. *Archives of Diseases of Childhood, 57,* 467–472.

Alderson, S. H., & Warren, R. H. (1984). Pediatric aersol therapy. *Clinical Pediatrics, 23,* 555–557.

Bernard, F., Dupont, C., & Viala, P. (1990). Gastroesophageal reflux and upper airway disease. *Clinical Reviews in Allergy, 81,* 403–425.

Brouilette, R. T., Ferbach, S. K., & Hunt, C. E. (1982). Obstructive sleep apnea in infants and children. *The Journal of Pediatrics, 100,* 31–40.

Bul, H. D., Dang, C. V., Chaney, R. R., & Vergara, L. M. (1989). Does gastrostomy and fundoplication prevent aspiration pneumonia in mentally retarded persons? *American Journal of Mental Retardation, 94,* 16–19.

Busse, W. W. (1988). Respiratory infection and bronchial hyperreactivity. *Journal of Allergy and Clinical Immunology, 81,* 770–775.

Canet, E. & Bureau, M. A. (1990). Chest wall diseases and dysfunction in children. In V. Chernick & E. L. Kendig (Eds), *Kendig's disorders of the respiratory tract in children* (pp. 648–669). Philadelphia: W. B. Saunders.

Danos, O., Casar, C., Larrain, A., & Pope, C. E. (1976). Esophageal reflux—an unrecognized cause of recurrent obstructive bronchitis in children. *The Journal of Pediatrics, 89,* 220–224.

Early warning signs of asthma. (1987). In *Living with Asthma: Part 2 Manual for teaching children the self-management of asthma* (p. 137). (NIH publication No. 87-236.) U.S. Department of Health and Human Services, Public Health Service, NIH.

Fisman, S., & Wolf, L. (1991). The handicapped child: Psychological effects of parental, marital and sibling relationships. *Psychiatric Clinics of North America, 14,* 199–215.

Foster S. & Hoskins, D. (1981). Home care of the child with a tracheostomy tube. *Pediatric Clinics of North America, 28,* 855–857.

Ganz, S. B., Levine, D. B., Axelrod, F. A., & Kahanovitz, N. (1983). Physical therapy management of familial dysautonomia. *Physical Therapy, 63,* 1121–1124.

Hendeles, L., Weinberger, M., Szefler, S. & Ellis, E. (1992). Safety and efficacy of theophylline in children with asthma. *The Journal of Pediatrics, 120,* 177–183.

Heyman, S., & Respondek, M. (1989). Detection of pulmonary aspiration in children by radionuclide "salivagram." *Journal of Nuclear Medicine, 30,* 697–699.

Kelly, W. H. (1987). Pharmacotherapy of pediatric lung disease: Differences between children and adults. *Clinics in Chest Medicine, 8,* 681–694.

Klastersky, J., Huysmans, E., Weerts, D., Hensgens, C., & Daneau, D. (1974). Endotracheally administered gentamicin for the prevention of infections of the respiratory tract in patients with tracheostomy: double blind study. *Chest, 65,* 650–654.

Konig, P., Shatley, M., Levine, C., & Mawhinney, T. P. (1992). Clinical observations of nebulized flunisolide in infants and young children with asthma and bronchopulmonary dysplasia. *Pediatric Pulmonology, 13,* 209–214.

Laraya-Cuasay, L. R. (1988). Interstitial pneumonias. In L. R. Laraya Cuasay & W. T. Hughes (Eds.), *Interstitial lung diseases in children* (pp. 140–144). Boca Raton, FL: CRC Press.

Laraya-Cuasay, L. R., Deforest, A., Huff, D., Lischner, H., & Huang, N. (1977). Chronic pulmonary complications of early influenza virus infection in children. *American Review of Respiratory Disease, 116,* 617–625.

Loughlin, G. M. (1989). Respiratory consequences of dysfunctional swallowing and aspiration. *Dysphagia, 3,* 126–130.

Mallory, G. B., Motoyama, E. K., Gibson, L. E., Reilly, J. S., Stool S. ., & Weng, F. T. (1982). Physiological approach to decannulation of tracheostomy in infants and young children. Abstract No. 1658. *Pediatric Research, 16,* 355.

Murray, H. W. (1979). Antimicrobial therapy in pulmonary aspiration. *American Journal of Medicine, 66,* 188–190.

Nash, M. (1988). Swallowing problems in the tracheotomized patient. *Otolaryngology Clinics of North America, 21,* 701–709.

Niederman, M. S., Ferranti, R. D., Zeigler, A., Merrill, W. W., & Reynolds, H. Y. (1984). Respiratory infection complicating long-term tracheostomy: the implication of persistent gram-negative tracheobronchial colonization. *Chest, 85,* 39–44.

Pearl, R. H., Robie, D. K., Ein, S. H., Shandling, B., Wesson, D. E., Superina, R., McTaggart, K., Garcia, V. F., O'Conner, J. A., & Filler, R. M. (1990). Complication of gastroesophageal antireflux surgery in neurologically impaired versus neurologically normal children. *Journal of Pediatric Surgery, 25,* 1169–1173.

Pipes, P. L., & Glass, R. P. (1989). Nutrition and feeding of children with developmental delay and related problems. In I. Krieger (Ed.), *Nutrition in infancy and childhood* (pp. 361–386). St. Louis, MI: Times Mirror/Mosby.

Robertson, C. M. T., Etches, P. C., Goldson, E., & Kyle, J. M. (1992). Eight-year school performance, neurodevelopmental, and growth outcome of neonates with bronchopulmonary dysplasia: A comparative study. *Pediatrics, 89,* 365–378.

Rooney, J. C. & Williams, H. E. (1971). The relationship between proven viral bronchiolitis and subsequent wheezing. *The Journal of Pediatrics, 79,* 744–747.

Schwartz, D. J., Wynne, J. W., Gibbs, C. P., Hood, I. C., & Kuck, E. J. (1980). The pulmonary consequences of aspiration of gastric contents at pH values greater than 2.5. *American Review of Respiratory Diseases, 121,* 119–126.

Tabachnik, E., & Levison, H. L. (1980). Clinical application of aerosols in pediatrics. *American Review of Respiratory Diseases, 122* (5, Pt. 2), 97–103.

Tuchman, D. N. (1989). Cough, choke, sputter: The evaluation of the child with dysfunctional swallowing. *Dysphagia, 3,* 111–116.

CHAPTER

12

Gastrointestinal Problems

MARIA R. MASCARENHAS, M.B.B.S., AND JAY DADHANIA, M.B.B.S.

───────────── **CONTENTS** ─────────────

Gastrointestinal (GI) problems are frequent in children with developmental disabilities. They include motility disorders, gastroesophageal reflux (GER) and its complications, peptic ulcer disease, and constipation. These conditions present clinically as difficulty swallowing, rumination, vomiting, hematemesis, anemia, failure to thrive, gastric distention, abdominal pain, irritability, and constipation. In this chapter we will discuss briefly these common GI symptoms and then review in depth gastroesophageal reflux, motility disorders, peptic ulcer disease, constipa-

253

tion, and the placement and care of percutaneous gastrostomy tubes. Because dysphagia is reviewed elsewhere in the book it will not be discussed here. The surgical aspects of fundoplication are covered in Chapter 13 so only the indications for a fundoplication will be mentioned.

Common GI Symptoms

Rumination, also called merycism, is a syndrome in which previously ingested food is voluntarily regurgitated, rechewed, and partially swallowed. The exact relationship between rumination and gastroesophageal reflux (GER) is unclear. It usually starts between 3 and 12 months of age and can lead to significant loss of food and malnutrition with associated developmental and growth delays. It is seen in association with moderate and severe mental retardation. Emotional and sensory deprivation coupled with anatomic and physiologic disturbances are contributory factors. Treatment consists of treatment of GER and behavior modification. Surgery, sedatives, and antispasmodics also have been tried with varying success.

Dysphagia or difficulty sucking and swallowing is a frequent symptom in children with developmental disabilities. Because swallowing includes the integration of sucking, swallowing, and breathing, any structural impairment in the mouth and pharynx as well as in its neural and motor control both centrally and peripherally will produce dysphagia. These problems can be manifested by poor suck, coughing, and choking during the feeding of foods of different textures. Nasal regurgitation without vomiting is also indicative of a problem. Observation during feeding is invaluable for both the diagnosis and management of these patients, and observation combined with videofluoroscopy is helpful. If the disability results in significant morbidity (i.e., aspiration pnueumonia), the patient should not be fed orally.

Regurgitation or GER is otherwise effortless spitting up of food or ingested material. It is noted first in infancy and is present to varying degrees in most infants. It will be discussed in detail later in the chapter.

Vomiting is the forceful ejection of stomach contents and needs to be differentiated from GER, especially in infancy. It may be related to GI and non-GI conditions. Careful history and physical examination are usually sufficient to make this differentiation. The amount, nature, color, frequency, presence of digested food, blood, or bile in the vomitus and precipitating and relieving factors need to be determined. The pattern of vomiting is also important (i.e., time of day, relationship to meals, and associated symptoms). Early morning vomiting may be a sign of increased intracranial pressure. The presence of associated symptoms of headache, abdominal pain, irritability, diarrhea, fever, constipation, and poor weight gain also need to be determined. Any child with weight loss has significant ongoing pathology, is at nutritional risk, and needs to be investigated immediately. In the child with developmental delay, the usual causes of vomiting include ventriculo-peritoneal shunt malfunction; GER; motility disorders of the oropharynx, esophagus, and stomach; esophagitis; gastritis; urinary tract infections; gastric outlet obstruction (i.e., related to migration of an improperly secured gastrostomy tube); severe constipation; and acute gastroenteritis. Prompt diagnosis and appropriate therapeutic measures should be instituted because of the risk of weight loss in these children, a significant number of whom are already at nutritional risk and for ease of care.

Abdominal pain is a difficult symptom to assess in the child with developmental delay. The child's usual caretaker may sometimes be able to recognize that the cause of the child's discomfort is the abdomen. If possible one must ascertain the chronicity, type, location, frequency, relationship to meals, and other symptoms and relieving and precipitating factors. Whenever possible acute surgical causes should be ruled out first. In a child with developmental disabilities, these will include intestinal obstruction, perforation, ventriculo-peritoneal shunt-related complications, peritonitis, volvulus, renal stones, and so on. A child with GER and abdominal pain is at risk for esophagitis and peptic ulcer disease. Chronic constipation and urinary tract infections also can cause abdominal pain. Appropriate investigations should be done to diagnose the above-mentioned conditions.

Constipation is characterized by a decrease in frequency or change in the consistency of stool. This is a very common problem in the developmentally disabled child and will be covered in some detail later in the chapter.

Irritability is usually a sign that the child is in some discomfort. Knowledge of the child's usual behavior is invaluable. A careful search for any gastrointestinal condition that gives pain should be done. Non-GI conditions should also be considered (i.e., infections, metabolic disturbances, drug-related, etc.). Irritability could also be behavioral in etiology, but organic disease needs to be ruled out first.

Failure to thrive is usually secondary to an inability to meet the caloric needs of the child. This may be due to inadequate intake (i.e., feeding disorders), excessive losses (i.e., vomiting, GER, and diarrhea), or gastrointestinal disease causing malabsorption. Some patients may have an increased caloric requirements related to an underlying condition or intercurrent illnesses.

Gastric distention is frequently seen in children with developmental disabilities. This may be secondary to delayed gastric emptying which seems to be a frequent finding in the patients with scoliosis and GER. Gastric distention may be secondary to swallowing of excessive amounts of air. In patients who have a tight Nissen fundoplication, the ability to burp may be lost,

and they may be in considerable distress because of the bloating sensation they experience. If the patient has a gastrostomy tube, venting of the tube periodically can be helpful.

Hematemesis, anemia, and *GI blood loss* can be seen in patients with esophagitis, gastritis, or peptic ulcers. Vomiting of bright red blood usually means a very recent onset of bleeding or ongoing bleeding. Esophagitis, stress gastritis, gastric and duodenal ulcers, and gastritis secondary to local tube irritation are common causes. Darker or "coffee-ground" material usually indicates old blood or very slow oozing of blood and can also be due to the above-listed conditions. However, the most important first step is to make sure that the material is indeed blood and not food material and that the patient is not having nose bleeds. The clinical condition of the patient will determine the acuity of care required. An unstable patient has to be hospitalized immediately and have an upper endoscopy after initial stabilization. A blood count is invaluable, especially if one has previous values to refer to. Appropriate management can be instituted once the correct diagnosis has been made. Patients with occult GI blood loss may present with anemia and be found on physical examination to have blood in their stools. These patients may also have the same conditions that cause hematemesis. The usual management consists of antacids, prokinetic agents for GER, and anti-acid therapy (i.e., H2 blockers).

Children who ingest *foreign bodies* are commonly asymptomatic. The foreign bodies often are discovered on x-rays obtained for other reasons. Sometimes they can cause intestinal obstruction or constitute the nidus for bezoar formation. In children with developmental disabilities they are usually multiple. Ninety percent reach the stomach uneventfully after being swallowed. Usual regions of hang up are at the tracheal bifurcation, gastroesophageal junction, pylorus, ligament of Treitz, and ileocecal valve. Most foreign bodies pass through the GI tract uneventfully carried along by normal intestinal peristalsis. If there is abnormal motility, erosion, perforation, migration, and diverticular formation occur. Any esophageal foreign body has to be removed. Removal is also indicated if the patient has symptoms suggestive of any GI obstruction. If an object stays in the stomach for more than 21 to 28 days, it is unlikely to pass. Objects that do not pass become embedded in the mucosa and are bound by fibrous adhesions. There is a risk of perforation with sharp objects, although even some of these will pass uneventfully. Sometimes esophageal obstruction with foreign bodies is the first sign of a motility disorder or stricture.

Gastroesophageal Reflux

GER is a frequent and often troublesome problem seen in children with developmental disabilities (Allen, Durie, Hamilton, Walker-Smith & Watkins, 1991; Orenstein, 1991; Roy, & Silverman, 1975). Various clinical studies have reported the overall incidence of vomiting to be 10 to 15% in mentally retarded children (Halpern, Jolley, & Johnson, 1991; Orenstein, 1991; Sondheimer & Morris, 1979). The number could be even higher in institutionalized populations of these children. Often vomiting is considered a symptom of psychogenic origin and is dealt with by a variety of behavioral methods. Many patients are referred for surgical interventions without prior work-up. Using appropriate diagnostic methods in these patients, many studies have concluded that GER accounts for 75 to 80% of causes of recurrent vomiting (Sondheimer & Morris 1979). Furthermore, the incidence of GER is found to be different among institutionalized versus ambulatory patients (Sondheimer & Morris 1979). Diseases of the central nervous system have a well recognized association with GER in children and therefore need to be considered in any diagnostic work-up.

Early intervention and therapeutic management of GER will help in reducing morbidity and prevent future complications, thus improving overall care of these children.

Pathophysiology

With the advent of intraesophageal pH monitoring and various manometric techniques, much attention has been paid to the high frequency of GER-associated disease in neurologically impaired children (Bryne, Campbell, Ashcraft, Seibert, & Euler, 1983; Ross, Haase, Reiley, & Meagher, 1988; Werlin, Dodds, & Hogan 1980). These children often suffer from severe cognitive and motor deficits including seizures and spasticity. Many are nonambulatory and have scoliosis. The factors that contribute to the increased frequency of GER are supine position; increased intra-abdominal pressure from scoliosis, spasticity, or seizures; a co-existing hiatal hernia; decreased lower esophageal sphincter (LES) tone and pressure; increased frequency of transient relaxations of the LES; and motility abnormalities (i.e., delayed gastric emptying and abnormal esophageal motility) (see Table 12–1).

To understand the basic pathophysiologic mechanisms of GER, one needs to understand the dysfunctions that allow

Table 12–1. Factors contributing to increased frequency of GER in children with developmental delay.

1. Supine position

2. Increased intra-abdominal pressure from scoliosis, spasticity, and seizures

3. Hiatal hernia

4. Decreased LES tone and pressure

5. Increased transient relaxations of the LES

6. Motility abnormalities

pathologic GER to occur and eventually cause disease. These events include those that allow reflux events to occur with increased frequency, those that impair the clearance of refluxed material from the esophagus, render the refluxate more noxious to the esophageal mucosa, and permit caloric loss or allow access of the refluxate into the airway. The discussion below will elaborate these events as they relate to children with neurologic impairment (Orenstein, 1991).

In the recent past chronically low LES pressure was believed to be the main factor allowing increased frequency of GER to occur in these patients. However, a recent report of the reflux mechanisms causing GER in six neurologically impaired children (Williams, Tsukada, & Boyle, 1989) showed that 58% were due to transient relaxations of the lower esophageal sphincter (TLESR), 37% were due to increased intra-abdominal pressure, and 10% were due to tonically low LES pressure. Supine positioning is certainly a provocative factor for increased GER as is increased intra-abdominal pressure due to spasticity, scoliosis, and seizures. For some reason many of these patients have a co-existing hiatal hernia which impairs the transmission of intrabdominal pressure to the LES further contributing to GER.

Abnormal esophageal motility and disordered swallowing mechanisms also impair the clearance of refluxed gastric contents from distal esophagus and thus allow complications of GER to occur. The role of delayed gastric emptying in GER remains controversial. Although some authors feel that it contributes to GER, others disagree. Supine positioning and hiatal hernias also impair esophageal acid clearance, thereby contributing to GER disease.

The exact role of gastric acid, bile, and pepsin in making the refluxate material more noxious and its relation to GER and esophagitis in these patients has not been well documented. Whether stress caused by various co-existing medical conditions plays any role in the increased noxiousness

of the refluxate by increasing gastric acid output is also not well understood. Clearly, there appears to be a local tissue resistance to the occurence of esophagitis. Lastly, dysfunctional swallowing mechanisms, poor gag reflexes, and impaired upper airway ciliary function allow easy access of the refluxate into the lungs causing aspiration pneumonia and chronic lung disease.

Clinical Features

The most obvious symptom of GER is regurgitation that is effortless. Often the regurgitation is underreported by caretakers as it is considered "normal" for neurologically impaired children to "vomit" frequently. The regurgitation can be projectile, or forceful, in some cases. Because some children may regurgitate on the basis of rumination, attention must be directed toward behavior that suggests primary rumination such as apparent enjoyment and rhythmicity of movements prior to regurgitation. Most commonly GER tends to occur during feeds or within a few hours of meals. Choking, gagging, and coughing during feeding suggest a swallowing disorder and possible aspiration and need an appropriate evaluation by a feeding therapist.

Accompanying symptoms of hematemesis, occult blood in the stool, anemia, and unexplained irritability suggest esophagitis. Abnormal neck movements and arching of the back may also be a sign of underlying esophagitis. Sandifer's syndrome in which characteristic twisting and arching movements of the head, neck, and upper trunk occur (Nanayakkara & Paton, 1985) exemplifies the neurobehavioral manifestations of GER. Occasionally, head tilting and dystonic neck movements are described in association with severe GER.

Respiratory complications of GER may manifest as recurrent aspiration, pneumonias, recurrent wheezing, apnea, and cyanosis. This may be due to either microaspiration of the refluxed contents into the airway or stimulation of J receptors in the bronchi by the presence of acid in the distal esophagus.

Diagnosis

GER is a frequently considered diagnosis in children with developmental delay. It needs to be considered in patients with chronic vomiting, recurrent pneumonias, irritabiity, anorexia, peptic strictures, rumination, anemia, failure to thrive, wheezing, obstructive apnea, unexplained stridor, occult blood loss, and abdominal pain. In the preoperative evaluation of patients requiring a gastrostomy with or without a fundoplication, GER needs to be ruled out. The various diagnostic methods used to diagnose GER are listed in Table 12–2.

The upper GI barium study is done mainly to evaluate the anatomy and to look for the presence of strictures, diverticuli, or hiatal hernias. It may also provide some idea about grossly obvious reflux, esophageal peristalsis, and the rate of gastric emptying. Other causes of vomiting like intestinal malrotation, duodenal web,

Table 12–2. Diagnostic tests for gastroesophageal reflux.

1. Upper GI barium study

2. Gastroesophageal scintigraphy—milk scan and gastric emptying for solids and liquids

3. 24-hour esophageal pH monitoring

4. Upper endoscopy and esophageal biopsies

5. Barium cine swallowing study

6. Salivagram

7. Esophageal motility

8. Combined esophageal pH probe and pneumogram

duodenal stenosis, or bands can also be easily ruled out.

Currently the most accurate way of diagnosing GER is 24-hour intra-esophageal pH recording. It not only quantifies the amount of GER but also helps in establishing the temporal relationship of GER to the symptom complex in question. With recent technically advanced monitoring systems it has become easier to perform this test even in an outpatient ambulatory set-up. All anti-reflux as well as anti-acid therapies must be stopped at least 24 hours prior to the study. Careful attention should be paid to the position of the patient, time of feedings, and any untoward event occurring during the study which should be accurately recorded so that the study can be better interpreted.

Because there is a higher incidence of delayed gastric empying and some abnormal GI motility in children with developmental delay (Fonkalsrud, Foglia, Ament, Berquist, & Vargus, 1989; Molitt, Golladay, & Seibert, 1985), the work-up should also include radionuclide studies such as a milkscan and gastric emptying scan both for liquids and solids (Figures 12–1 and 12–2). A milkscan helps in demonstrating GER and the aspiraton of the refluxate into the lungs. To differentiate pulmonary aspiration from disordered swallowing and GER, a salivagram (Figure 12–3) can be done in which a small amount of radioactive tracer is placed on the tongue and the lungs are scanned to look for aspiration (Heyman & Respondek, 1989). If positive, this indicates pulmonary aspiration from abnormal swallowing (see Figure 12–4).

When symptoms of esophagitis, such as occult blood loss, anemia, irritability or abnormal posturing, are present, an upper endoscopy with multiple esophageal biopsies should be done to look for esophagitis and Barrett's esophagus.

Rarely other studies like esophageal motility study may be needed to evaluate abnormal esophageal motility. In cases

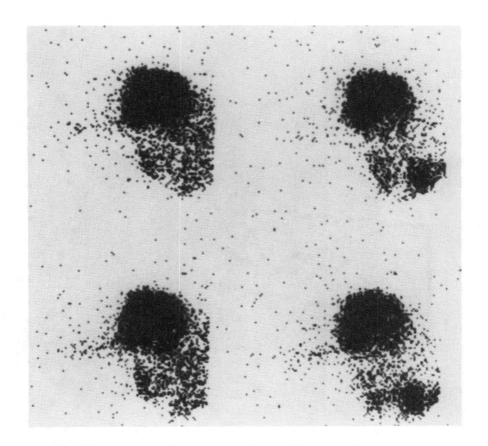

Figure 12–1. This picture shows four sequential nuclear images of distal esophagus and stomach after ingestion of a radio-labeled sulphur colloid tagged liquid meal. The presence of persistent radioactivity in distal esophagus is positive indication of gastroesophageal reflux. Also note that, even minutes after ingestion, the activity in the stomach is significantly higher which suggests the gastric emptying delay often seen in patients with GER.

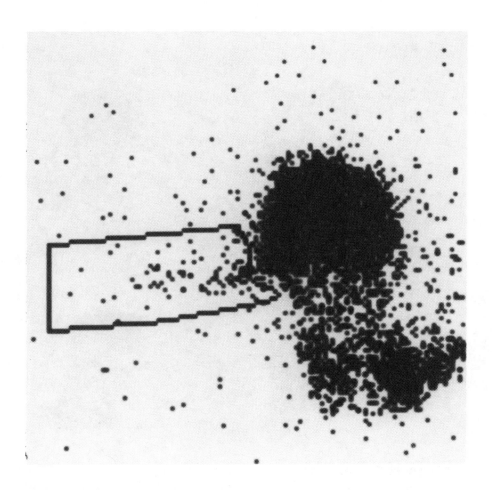

Figure 12–2. Single image view of the stomach and esophagus demonstrating gastroesophageal reflux of radio-labeled liquid meal.

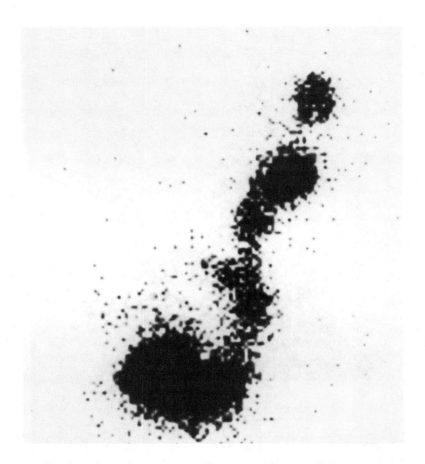

Figure 12–3. Nuclear medicine imaging study using radio-labeled Tc 99 tagged with salivary secretions. The image demonstrates presence of radioactivity in tracheobronchial tree. This study is called a "salivagram."

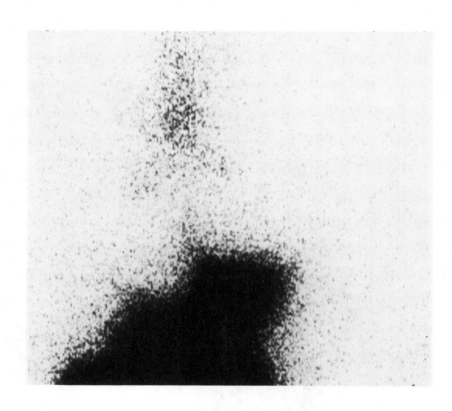

Figure 12–4. Evidence of radioactivity in the airways during the imaging of this nuclear study is suggestive of pulmonary aspiration caused by underlying GER.

where apnea or wheezing is thought to be secondary to GER, a simultaneous pH probe study with pneumogram may be helpful in evaluating these patients to look for any temporal relationship between reflux and pulmonary symptoms.

Complications

Esophagitis, failure to thrive, and various pulmonary symptoms like wheezing, apnea, chronic cough, and recurrent pneumonia are frequently seen complications of GER (see Table 12–3). The most common complication is reflux esophagitis and its sequelae—peptic esophageal strictures and Barrett's esophagus. Unlike in normal children, esophagitis is often asymptomatic in mentally retarded patients and may remain so until the severity of the esophagitis increases resulting in hematemesis and esophageal ulcerations and strictures. Behavioral changes like irritability or refusal to eat may be subtle signs of possible esophagitis and warrant a diagnostic work-up. Most of the children have evidence of chronic esophagitis on esophageal biopsies. Recurrent esophagitis is also a common problem, and some children have to be placed on prophylactic therapy. Difficulty swallowing may be suggestive of a peptic esophageal stricture. Recent data suggest that strictures may develop as early as a few weeks after the onset of severe untreated esophagitis (Orenstein, 1991; Rode, Millar, Brown, & Cywes, 1992). A peptic stricture is diagnosed most clearly by radiography (upper GI series and upper endoscopy). These strictures are usually located in the distal third of the esophagus and often are associated with hiatal hernias. The treatment of reflux esophagitis and strictures consists of the adequate control of reflux and dilataton of the stricture using endoscopic balloon dilators or rubber bougies. These procedures are usually done under general anesthesia, especially in younger children, and may need to be done repeatedly depending on the recurrence of symptoms. The complications of dilatation include perforation, hemorrhage, and infection (mediastinitis). Another significant complication of long-standing GER is Barrett's esophagus, a condition in which the usual squamous epithelium of the esophagus is replaced by columnar epithelium. This complication is believed to arise in areas of chronic reflux esophagitis and appears to be seen fairly frequently in children with developmental disabilities. Overall, the prevalence of Barrett's esophagus varies from 2 to 20% and could be as high as 44% in cases with peptic strictures (Orenstein, 1991). Apart from the usual complications of Barrett's esophagus like ulcerations and stricture, the most important and worrisome complication is the possibility of a malignant transformation of the columnar epithelium to adenocarcinoma. Aggressive medical therapy and regular surveillance upper endoscopies are strongly recommended.

Respiratory complications of GER include aspiration pneumonia, reflex bronchospasm, obstructive apnea, and stridor. These may result either from actual macro- or microaspiration of gastric contents into the lungs or by reflex neurostimulation of the tracheobronchial tree. Often, if untreated, this results in significant chronic

Table 12–3. Complications of gastroesophageal reflux.

Esophagitis

Acute, chronic, and recurrent esophageal strictures, Barrett's esophagus, adenocarcinoma of the esophagus

Failure to thrive

Respiratory

Wheezing, recurrent pneumonias, apnea, and stridor

---

lung disease. Disordered swallowing, poor gag reflex, as well as poor cough reflex also predispose children to chronic lung disease even without obvious aspiration.

Failure to thrive is another very important complication of GER. It generally is the result of insufficient caloric intake due to persistent emesis or poor intake secondary to esophagitis and disordered swallowing commonly seen in these children.

Occult GI blood loss secondary to chronic esophagitis can be seen. This can present with unexplained anemia and on investigation heme positive stools. Rarely, other neurobehavioral manifestations like Sandifer's syndrome, hiccups, belching, eructations, and hoarseness of voice are also seen.

Treatment

Medical Treatment

Although children with neurologic impairment are more likely to have intractable reflux and eventually require some surgical procedure, medical therapy should be tried first. This includes the initiation of some simple measures in feeding and sleeping and medications to control reflux as well as nutritional rehabilitation because these children often have borderline nutritional status. It has been shown that the head-elevated prone position for sleeping results in fewer and less frequent episodes of GER. Smaller more frequent feedings reduce the amount of GER by virtue of the fact that there is less material to reflux. Even though thickening the formula with rice cereal is frequently advocated, it has not been shown in controlled studies to reduce GER.

The medications commonly used in GER (see Table 12–4) consist of prokinetic agents which augment LES pressure and improve gastric emptying and acid reducing agents which decrease acid production in the stomach in an effort to counteract the injurious effects of gastric contents on the esophageal mucosa. Also used are acid neutralizing agents (i.e., antacids and mucosal protective agents such as sucralfate). The most commonly used prokinetic agents are bethanecol and metoclopramide. Less commonly used drugs are domperidone and cisapride. Bethanecol is a cholinergic agonist that acts at the peripheral neuromuscular level to augment LES pressure and the amplitude and duration of esophageal peristalsis. The usual dose is 0.1 to 0.2 mg/kg/dose every 8 hours given 15 to 30 minutes before feeds. Its potential for excacerbating bronchospasm limits its use in children with chronic lung disease. Other less common side effects include irritability, nausea, vomiting, diarrhea, headache, abdominal camps, and urinary retention. Its use is contraindicated in asthma, cardiac arrythmias, hypotension, epilepsy, and intestinal obstruction. The other more commonly used agent is metoclopramide,

Table 12–4. Treatment of gastroesophageal reflux.

Medical	Surgical
Prokinetic agents	Gastrostomy
Acid reducing agents	Jejunostomy
Acid neutralizing agents	Fundoplication
Mucosal protective agents	
Nutrition	

a dopamine antagonist that raises LES pressure and improves gastric emptying and esophageal acid clearance. The usual dose is 0.1 mg/kg/dose every 6 to 8 hours (maximum 0.2 mg/kg/dose) given 15 to 20 minutes before meals. The commonly seen side effects are restlessness, drowsiness, diarrhea, and extrapyramidal dystonic reactions (antidote is diphenhydramine). Its relative contraindications include GI obstruction, perforation, and CNS disease. Although commonly used by many pediatric gastroenterologists, its narrow margin of safety and lack of data about its long-term side effects mandate caution in its use. Domperidone and cisapride are two other prokinetic agents. The former is not approved for use in the United States, and the latter has recently been made available for clinical use.

Acid reducing agents are used to decrease the production of gastric acid to decrease the effects of gastric acid on esophageal mucosa. They include histamine receptor antagonists such as Cimetidine®, Ranitidine® and Famotidine®. Cimetidine® is given at a dose of 5 to 10 mg/kg/dose four times a day, and some of its side effects include headache, pancytopenia, cholestasis, irritability, and gynecomastia. Ranitidine® and famotidine® offer the advantage of less frequent dosing and fewer side effects. Ranitidine® has less liver toxicity and gynecomastia. The usual dose is 2 to 4 mg/kg/day divided two to three times a day. Omeprazole® is a new agent that blocks the proton pump in the parietal cell and so blocks acid production. It is a very potent drug, but its long-term safety record has yet to be established. Because it causes marked elevations of serum gastrin levels in some patients, it is recommended that these levels be followed during therapy which should usually not exceed 3 months. The duration of therapy for esophagitis varies depending on the severity of esophagitis noted on esophageal biopsies. Mild esophagitis is usually treated with 6 weeks of therapy and moderate

to severe esophagitis is treated over 2 to 6 months.

The role of antacids in treating esophagitis is less clear however. They are used mainly for symptomatic relief of pain or irritability and act primarily by neutralizing gastric acid. Traditionally, they are used half an hour before and 2 hours after a meal. In practice this works out to administration between meals. We usually recomend a double dose at bedtime, especially in patients who appear to be more symptomatic at night.

Lastly, mucosal protective agents such as sucralfate may prove to be useful agents in treating severe esophagitis and ulcerations, but data about their efficacy in this context are still limited. An important clinical point to remember is that sucralfate adsorbs any other drugs given at the same time, thus altering drug levels and their efficacy. This is very relevant in children with developmental delay because they are usually on other medications.

Nutritional therapy is an important component of treatment of GER especially in children with weight loss and failure to thrive. It not only improves the response to medical therapy but also makes surgery less hazardous if it is required (Allen, et al., 1991; Orenstein, 1991; Roy & Silverman, 1975). It is always used in conjunction with the above described medications. Initially, the oral route to deliver a higher caloric intake is tried by increasing the caloric density of the formula or food eaten. If this fails, intragastric feeds using high caloric formulas are required to maximize nutrition in these nutritionally deficient children. If bolus feeds produce an increase in GER, continuous intragastric feeds are used. These can be tailored to the individual needs of the patient and for ease of care. We will often try small bolus feeds during the day and continuous feeds at night. For patients who do not tolerate the above, jejunostomy feeds may need to be considered using a nasojejunal tube. These tubes however are difficult to maintain in an adequate position, and this constitutes their biggest disadvantage. Patients who demonstrate a long-term need for tube feeds (more than 3 months) may need to have a more permanent feeding route established (i.e., percutaneous gastrostomy tube [PEG] or surgical jejunostomy tube).

Surgical Therapy

Anti-reflux surgery is required for patients who are refractory to aggressive management of their esophagitis, develop chronic lung disease or complications such as Barrett's esophagus, strictures, and chronic malnutrition unresponsive to therapy. A detailed discussion about the indications, actual surgical procedures, and their complications is presented in Chapter 13. The most commonly performed anti-reflux surgical procedure is the Nissen fundoplication to increase LES pressure. In neurologically impaired children, this procedure is not without significant risks. Major postoperative complications include breakdown of the wrap, delayed gastric emptying, inability to burp causing a gas-bloat syndrome, pneumonias, wound infections, and small bowel obstruction. Recurrence of GER occurs in about 12 to 30% (Vanderhoof, Rappaport, & Paxson, 1978; Wilkinson, Dudgeon, & Sondheimer, 1991). Severe kyphoscoliosis (which is often present), spasticity, and seizures contribute to breakdown of the surgery. Prolonged anesthesia may impose additional risks in these patients and further complicate their postoperative course. Due to improvements in medical therapy for GER and the realization of the limitations of surgery and its risks, the frequency of surgical interventions has been reduced in the last decade. However, when compared to neurologically normal children with reflux, children with developmental delay are more likely to require a fundoplication with gastrostomy

(Fonkalsrud, Foglia, Ament, Berquist, & Vargus, 1989; Wesley, Coran, Sarahan, Klein & White, 1981; Wilkinson, et al., 1991). Most pediatric surgical series report an overall success rate of 90% in terms of reduction or elimination of reflux following surgery (Grunow, Al-Hafidh, & Tunell, 1989; Hillemeier, Grill, McCallum, & Gryboski, 1983; Molitt, Golladay, & Seibert, 1985; Spitz, & Kirtane, 1985; Werlin, Dodds & Hogan, 1980; Wesley, et al., 1981; Wilkinson, et al., 1991). Feeding gastrostomies are commonly required in developmentally disabled children because of failure to maintain optimal nutritional status due to either disordered swallowing or GER. They may also be required in children who suffer from chronic pulmonary aspiration secondary to GER. Percutaneous endoscopic gastrostomy (PEG) placement techniques have become more popular than the conventional Stamm surgical gastrostomy. The advantages of a PEG are shorter anesthesia time, early institution of feeding, shorter hospital stays, and fewer intra-abdominal complications like adhesions, obstruction, and so on. Potential complications include hemorrhage, wound infection, bowel perforation, fistula formation, and recurrence of reflux. A common clinical dilemma is whether a patient requires a simple PEG or a fundoplication with gastrostomy tube. Many surgeons reccomend prophylactic fundoplication in all neurologically impaired children requiring a gastrostomy because thay are at a greater risk for GER, and gastrostomy feeds may provoke reflux in about 30 to 44% of patients (Campbell, Gilchrist, & Harrison, 1989; Grunow, et al., 1989; Langer et al., 1988; Spitz, & Kirtane 1985). However, this approach will subject about 20% of children without reflux to an unnecessary surgical procedure with its concomitant risks (Langer et al., 1988). Therefore, it has become our standard practice to evaluate all patients who need a feeding gastrostomy for GER. This should include a 24-hour pH probe, upper GI barium study, and gastric emptying radionuclear studies. In one study, 35% of neurologically impaired children referred for feeding gastrostomy did not have GER by standard preoperative evaluation which included a 24-hour pH probe study and upper GI barium study. However, 25% of children required a fundoplication at a later date for symptomatic reflux (Byrne, Campbell, Ashcraft, Sebert, & Euler, 1983; Langer et al., 1988). Children in whom a surgical anti-reflux procedure is contraindicated may also be managed with a PEG and then jejunostomy feeds through the PEG if they develop symptomatic reflux. For cases with an initial negative work-up for GER or asymptomatic GER, one must first try a PEG, and if the patient then develops clinically significant GER consider fundoplication. Considerable controversy exists about the need for gastric emptying procedures (i.e., pyloroplasty at the time of fundoplication), and this is not routinely performed at this time. For patients who are not candidates for an anti-reflux procedure and who fail intragastric feeds, a trial of nasojejunal feeds, if successful, can be followed by a surgical jejunostomy.

Motility Disorders

Motility disorders are frequently seen in children with developmental disabilities. As our knowledge of normal GI motility and our investigative tools advance, we are now recognizing that motility disturbances occur far more frequently than previously described. In this chapter we will not deal with oropharyngeal motility disturbances because they are covered in Chapter 10. We will discuss some common motility disturbances by organ system.

Esophageal Motility Disorders

Etiology

Esophageal motility disorders are seen in muscular dystrophies (i.e., myotonic muscular dystrophy, bulbar palsy, brainstem tumors and surgery, myasthenia gravis, poliomyelitis and botulism). Achalasia or incomplete relaxation of the gastroesophageal junction occurs infrequently in children. Children who have had repair of esophageal atresia and a tracheoesophageal fistula also have abnormal esophageal motility. Some infants with chronic GER and esophagitis have been shown to have esophageal dysmotility (Warren & Marshall, 1983). Collagen vascular disorders (i.e., scleroderma and intestinal pseudo-obstruction) can also present with esophageal dysmotility. However, esophageal motility disorders are for the most part idiopathic, as are most motility disorders elsewhere in the GI tract.

Clinical Features

These disorders usually present with dysphagia—a word of Greek derivation (*dys* = with difficulty and *phagein* = to eat). Dysphagia can be divided into oropharyngeal and esophageal types. In oropharyngeal dysphagia the problem lies in the initiation of swallowing or the transfer of food into the esophagus (i.e., the oral, pharyngeal, and cricopharyngeal phases of swallowing). With esophageal dysphagia, patients will complain of food getting stuck in the retrosternal area. Food, either solids or liquids, will leave the mouth without any problem. The severity of the dysphagia may be variable and may be different with solids, liquids, and foods of different temperatures. The onset may be insidious with a variable progression. Regurgitation or GER may also be a common presenting feature and if it occurs high in the esophagus may result in aspiration pneumonias, wheezing, or chronic cough. A resulting esophagitis may produce chest pain, odynophagia, anorexia, and failure to thrive. Chest pain can also be produced by esophageal muscle spasm. Patients with achalasia are often described as slow eaters as they will chew the food as fine as possible so that it will not obstruct at the gastro-esophical (GE) junction. Characteristically, on chest x-ray an esophageal air-fluid level or widened mediastinum may be seen. A barium swallow may show a dilated esophagus with tapering at the GE junction. Esophageal manometry may show elevated LES pressure, absence of esophageal peristalsis, and incomplete LES relaxation.

Disorders of the cricopharyngeal muscle usually present in early infancy with aspiration, choking, and pooling of saliva in the back of the pharynx. They can be diagnosed on barium swallow by a hold-up of barium at the upper esophageal sphincter and a shelf-like impression at the cricopharyngeal level. Various abnormalities have been described and include cricopharyngeal hypertension or spasm, hypotension, incomplete relaxation, premature closure, and delayed relaxation.

Diagnosis

The four available tests are a barium swallow, cine-swallow, radionuclide esophageal clearance scan, and esophageal manometry. The barium swallow is a quick and easy test that usually gives an idea about the anatomy. In uncooperative children the radiologist will put a nasogastric tube into the upper esophagus to facilitate the study.

A cine-swallow is the best way to study all the components of the swallowing apparatus both anatomically and functionally. Because of the rapidity with which radiographs can be taken, a cine-swallow is the most accurate way of identifing swallowing abnormalities currently available. The disadvantages are the subjectivity of the observer, amount of radiation exposure, and the inability to quantify sphincter function.

The radionuclide esophageal clearance scan is used to provide objective evidence of esophageal emptying. The patient is given food tagged with technitium and then scanned under a gamma camera. The advantage of this study is the decreased amount of radiation exposure which permits a longer examination. However, the test does not give any information about the swallowing mechanism or sphincteric function.

Esophageal manometry is the best way to study esophageal motility disorders in children. It uses a pressure-sensing catheter to record pressures at various points in the esophagus. Children can be sedated with chloral hydrate prior to the procedure since this has been shown not to interfere with motility (Ament & Christie, 1977). The catheter is passed into the stomach and then slowly pulled back. Lower and upper esophageal sphincter pressure and relaxation in response to peristalsis and swallowing are assessed. Propagation of peristalsis in the body of the esophagus is also noted. The main disadvantages are the intubation of the GI tract and the noncooperation of infants and some children which can make interpretation of the recording difficult.

Treatment

Treatment of esophageal motility disorders consists mainly of maintaining nutrition and preventing complications related to the underlying disorder (i.e., aspiration pneumonia). Patients who tend to have spasm may benefit from smooth muscle relaxants (i.e., nitrates and calcium channel blockers such as nifedipine). Placement of gastrostomy or jejunostomy tubes and parenteral nutrition may be required. Treatment of achalasia consists of dilatation of the LES using muscle relaxants like nitrates and nifedipine and finally in patients who do not respond to other treatments, a Heller myotomy. Treatment of cricopharyngeal dysphagia is instituted primarily to control the underlying problem and improve the patient's nutritional status. Cricopharyngeal dilatation in cases of cricopharyngeal achalasia may be successful in children and sometimes is followed by spontaneous resolution. Cricopharyngeal myotomy has also been tried with some success.

Disorders of Gastric Motility

Etiology

These disorders occur more frequently than previously recognized, and our knowledge of them is increasing with improving diagnostic methods. Idiopathic delay in gastric emptying forms the largest single etiology accounting for delays in gastric motility (33%). A significant number of the patients are women, who also have associated small bowel motor abnormalities. Primary antral dysrhythmias (i.e., sustained bradygastrias and tachyarhythmias) are seen in these patients. Myopathic disorders affecting the stomach consist of hollow visceral myopathy, collagen vascular disorders, and neuropathic disorders of hollow visceral neuropathy, diabetes mellitus, and so on. Hypothyroidism and diabetes mellitus have been associated with delayed gastric emptying. Clearly, some patients develop vomiting and delayed gastric emptying after a viral illness. The exact pathogenetic mechanisms of this are unclear. Commonly used medications like anticholinergics, narcotic analgesics, phenothiazines, potassium salts, and tricyclic antidepressants can also cause gastric motor abnormalities. Inflammation in the stomach (Helicobacter gastritis) and duodenum (peptic ulcers and inflammatory bowel disease) can also cause gastric motor abnormalities. Delayed gastric emptying is also seen in patients with GER. See Table 12–5 for a list of disorders that cause abnormal gastric emptying. Rapid gastric emptying occurs in some patients with peptic ulcer disease and following surgical procedures.

Table 12–5. Conditions associated with abnormal gastric emptying.

Idiopathic
Myopathic disorders
Neuropathic disorders
Metabolic
Post-viral
Medications
Surgery

Clinical Features

Clinical features are variable depending on whether there is rapid or delayed gastric emptying. The symptoms of delayed gastric empying are nonspecific and include nausea, vomiting, early satiety, abdominal pain, abdominal distention, and bloating. In severe cases food ingested the previous day may be vomited. Rapid gastric emptying may also present with abdominal cramps and diarrhea.

Diagnosis

Two tests are available to detect motor abnormalities of the stomach and duodenum: gastric emptying studies using radionuclide material and antroduodenal manometry. The former test is more widely available; the latter test is available only in a few pediatric centers in the country. Gastric emptying can be assessed for both solids and liquids using 99mTc labeled to a liquid (formula, milk, water) or solid (egg). The stomach is scanned for a 60- to 90-minute period and an emptying rate calculated. Antroduodenal manometry consists of placement of a pressure sensitive catheter in the duodenum and stomach. Motor activity is recorded in the fasting and fed states and in response to certain drugs (i.e., erythromycin). The duration of the study is variable, and patients can be studied for periods up to 24 hours.

Treatment

Treatment for gastric motility disorders consists of maintaining nutrition, pharmacotherapy with prokinetics (metoclopramide, cisapride, and erythromycin), prostaglandin synthetase inhibitors, and supportive therapy (i.e., treatment of bacterial overgrowth). Jejunal feeding tubes may be needed for nutrition. In severe cases, total parental nutrition may be required. Children with significant delays in gastric emptying may benefit from prokinetic therapy as well as pyloroplasty.

Intestinal Motor Disorders

Etiology

Disorders of intestinal motility usually occur in conjunction with motor disorders of other parts of the GI tract, reproductive tract, or biliary tract as well as the urinary tract. These can consist of a variety of abnormalities of the nerves and muscles of the GI tract. Examples of nerve-related disorders are Hirschsprung's disease, neurofibromatosis, drugs (i.e., isoniazid), familial visceral neuropathies, diabetes mellitus, and spinal cord injury. Among the muscle diseases are visceral myopathies, connective tissue disorders, and muscular dystrophies. In chronic intestinal pseudo-obstruction, patients have symptoms suggestive of obstruction without any intestinal obstruction. Patients with hollow visceral disease have abnormalities of either muscle of nerve affecting the GI, gastro-urinary, biliary, and reproductive tracts.

Clinical Features

These diseases are more frequent in women. Common symptoms include nausea, intermitttent vomiting, recurrent abdominal pain, anorexia, early satiety, intermittent diarrhea or constipation, weight loss, excessive flatus, bloating, and abdominal distention. X-ray studies of the abdomen may show dilated stomach, small intestine, or colon. Abnormal intravenous pyelography, barium enemas, upper GI series of the small intestine as well as biliary manometry may be found.

Diagnosis

Diagnosis of intestinal motility disorders can be based on motility testing or biopsy evidence, if available. Formal motility testing at present is restricted to certain centers. Gastroduodenojeujunal recordings using solid state recording techniques are available. The patterns of abnormal motility may be either absent, decreased, or poorly organized and ineffective. Pathologically, degeneration of the enteric neurons and longitudinal muscle or fibrosis of the circular muscle may be seen depending on the disorder.

Treatment

Therapy is primarily supportive in an effort to make the patient's life as normal as possible. In order to maintain nutrition, some patients may require no enteral feeds and receive only intravenous nutrition. Some may be able to tolerate an elemental diet, whereas others require intestinal decompression. Certain prokinetic agents have been tried recently with some success (i.e., metoclopramide, cisapride, erythromycin, and somatostatin). Complications such as bacterial overgrowth and GER may need to be treated as well.

Disorders of Colonic Motility

Because the main function of the colon is to complete water and electrolyte absorption and store stool until elimination, disorders of colonic motility usually present as constipation, diarrhea, and abdominal pain. In this section we will discuss the etiology, clinical features, diagnosis, and treatment of these disorders. A more complete account of constipation is presented later in this chapter.

Etiology

Abnormal colonic motility may be caused by gastrointestinal, systemic, neurological, and drug-related causes. Examples include Hirschsprung's disease, hypothyroidism, intestinal pseudo-obstruction, irritable bowel syndrome, chronic nonspecific diarrhea of infancy, and so on. Studies of colonic motility have shown increased, decreased, or normal activity in a segmental or pancolonic distribution. Reflexes (i.e., gastrocolic and defecatory), hormone levels, and neural elements in the colon can also be abnormal. Different motor abnormalities have been found in patients with irritable bowel disease.

Clinical Symptoms

Disorders of colonic motility usually present with constipation, diarrhea, abdominal distention, and so on. Because diagnosis of a motility disorder is made only after excluding other disease, a work-up to look for colitis, metabolic diseases, and so on is often done first.

Diagnosis

The tests currently performed to evaluate colonic motility include anorectal manometry, the Sitzmark's test, colonic manometry (a technique similar to esophageal manometry), and colonic transit scintigraphy. The former is commonly used specifically for diagnosing Hirschsprung's disease, and the latter two tests are still research tools. Anorectal manometry consists of passing a catheter with three balloons into the rectum and anus. Rectal distention caused by inflating the proximal balloon is used to elicit reflexes of the internal and external anal sphincters. The Sitzmark's test con-

sists of following the progression of colonic markers given orally. Abdominal x-rays are taken at specific intervals over 5 days.

Treatment

In patients in whom symptoms of constipation predominate, regular physical exercise and toilet sitting, a high fiber diet, and laxatives may be used. Drug treatment includes lubricants, stimulant cathartics, hyperosmolar agents, and prokinetics. The safest agents for long-term use are fiber, lubricants, and hyperosmolar agents (i.e., lactulose which acts by increasing the water content of stool). Fiber acts by increasing the bulk of stool, distending the colon, and thereby stimulating motility. Domperidone and cisapride are examples of prokinetic drugs which are under investigation and show promise in being extremely effective drugs in certain groups of patients. Surgery for severe constipation is not commonly performed in children. For patients with symptoms of irritable bowel disease, anticholinergics, fiber containing agents, and stress reduction techniques are used.

Peptic Ulcer Disease

Peptic ulcer diseases include esophagitis, gastritis, duodenitis and ulcers—both gastric and duodenal. Because esophagitis has already been dealt with in detail under gastroesophageal reflux it will not be discussed here.

Gastritis

Gastritis is the term used to describe inflammation of the stomach. It can be primary (due to infection or bile acid reflux) or secondary (due to stress, drugs, etc.) (see Table 12–6).

Etiology

The most common infection causing gastritis is that caused by Helicobacter pylori.

Table 12–6. Etiology of gastritis.

Primary
Helicobacter infection, duodenogastric reflux
Secondary
Drugs, stress, trauma, other

Initially described in 1983 (Eastham, 1990), it has since been documented by microscopy or culture in the antrum of 80% of patients with primary gastritis. A strong association also exists between duodenal ulcers and helicobacter gastritis. Duodenogastric reflux has been proposed as a cause of gastritis in patients who have had prior gastric surgery, with bile felt to be a gastric irritant. Any drug is capable of causing a GI upset, but the drugs causing gastritis commonly are corticosteroids, non-steroidal anti-inflammatory agents (NSAID), theophylline, potassium and calcium salts, and some antibiotics (e.g., cephalosporins). Corticosteroids are thought to cause gastritis, ulcers, and GI hemorrhage by inhibiting local production of prostaglandins and gastric mucus. Inhibition of mucosal bicarbonate secretion and focal loss of gastric mucus are said to result from NSAID use. Stress is a common cause of single and multiple gastroduodenal erosions or ulcers. Sepsis, trauma, respiratory failure, head injury, major surgery, and burns are common stressful situations associated with ulcer formation. Local impairment of gastric blood flow, increased acid and pepsin synthesis, decreased production of mucus, and prostaglandins are some of the causes postulated. Local irritation of the stomach from feeding tubes is another frequent cause of gastritis. Viral gastritis, allergic gastritis, and so on can also occur.

Clinical Features

Patients will usually present with upper abdominal pain, vomiting, excessive heartburn, hematemesis, anorexia, and weight loss. Local epigastric tenderness as well as evidence of GI blood loss (in stools, vomitus, or gastric secretions) may be present.

Diagnosis

Diagnosis is usually made on endoscopy or an upper GI series. Although the latter is noninvasive, the gastritis has to be severe to be detected. An air contrast study may be more sensitive in diagnosing less severe cases. An upper endoscopy (Figures 12–5 and 12–6), although invasive, is the best way of detecting gastritis, which may be seen as erythema, friability, or nodularity. It also allows biopsies and cultures to be obtained. Multiple antral biopsies and cultures are required to make the diagnosis of helicobacter gastritis. The seagull-shaped bacteria are seen within and under the surface layer of mucus both with routine hemotoxylin and eosin stains as well as special stains (i.e., silver stain). The bacteria can also be cultured from antral biopsies and by rapid bedside identification from antral biopsies within 30 minutes using urea broth. Recently, a test for the detection of H. pylori-specific antibodies in blood also became available.

Treatment

The management of gastritis depends on the clinical situation and presentation. Sick patients have to be stabilized and emperic therapy started. Antacids, H2-receptor blocking agents, and sucralfate are commonly used. Duration of therapy (6 weeks–3 months) depends on the severity of clinical symptoms and inflammation observed endoscopically and histologically. For helicobacter infection, a combination of amoxicillin or flagyl and bismuth preparations may be used.

Peptic Ulcers

Peptic ulcers are more common in children than previously thought, and their incidence is believed to be increasing. They oc-

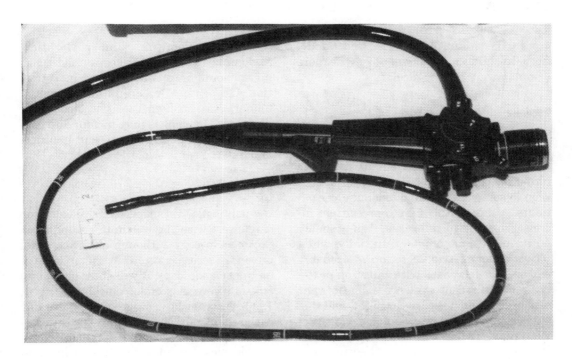

Figure 12–5. This photograph shows a pediatric flexible endoscope (Olympus XP-10) commonly used in patients for evaluation of upper GI diseases such as reflux esophagitis. Also note that the outer diameter of this endoscope is 7.5 mm.

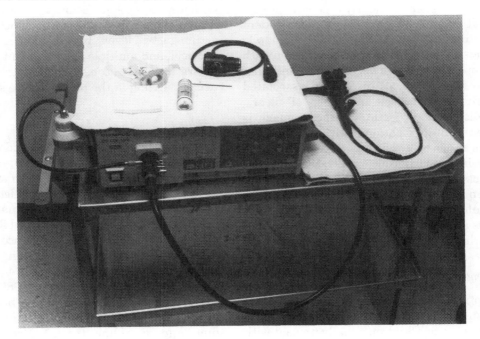

Figure 12–6. This picture shows a typical endoscopy cart containing a flexible pediatric endoscope attached to a light source along with topical anesthetic spray, teaching head for side view by another person, and oral bite lock.

cur in the stomach (gastric) and duodenum. In children, duodenal ulcers are more common than gastric ulcers.

Etiology

The exact etiology of peptic ulcer disease is unknown. Duodeno-gastric reflux of bile and antral stasis may contribute to gastric ulcer formation. Hypersecretion of acid is seen in some but not all duodenal ulcer patients. Although this may represent an increase in parietal cell mass, it is probably an acquired phenomenon. Initially, when ulcers develop, acid secretion is probably normal but increases with duration of the ulcer. Some recent evidence suggests that acid production increases at night, and this may form the basis for timing medication in patients with ulcers and for prophylaxis. Increased levels of pepsin and serum pepsinogen, defective gastric mucous composition, and deficiency of mucosal prostaglandins have been found in some ulcer patients. There is clearly a genetic predisposition to ulcers, and this is more evident in children than in adults. Blood group O tends to be more common in children with ulcers. Diets low in vegetable oil and fiber and high in spices have been associated with an increased incidence of ulcers. Helicobacter infection in the stomach is seen in 50% of patients with duodenal ulcers and is believed to be responsible for relapsing duodenal ulcers. Stress is also felt to cause peptic ulcers. They are usually seen in the same clinical situation that would cause stress gastritis. Cushing's ulcers are seen with intracranial lesions and Curling's ulcers with burns.

Clinical Features

Peptic ulcers can occur at any ages. More than half of all patients are older than 10 years of age. Children usually present with epigastric or periumbilical pain, vomiting, hematemesis, and melena. In the very young the usual presentation is with hematemesis, vomiting, and perforation. Abdominal pain that wakes a child up at night should always warrant an investigation. On physical examination epigastric tenderness and heme positive stools may be found. Duodenitis may be found in conjunction with peptic ulcers and gastritis and has the same etiologic factors.

Diagnosis

If a peptic ulcer is suspected, clinically, the single test with the maximum value is an upper endoscopy. Although an air contrast upper GI series is useful in the absence of an upper endoscopy, it will show only 50 to 80% of ulcers seen endoscopically (Murphy, 1990). Another advantage of an endoscopy is the ability to look for helicobacter infection in the stomach and to obtain appropriate biopsies. In children with multiple and refractory ulcers, it is useful to obtain a fasting serum gastrin level (after all antiacid therapy has been stopped for at least 48 hours) to exclude Zollinger-Ellison syndrome. This is a condition in which high serum gastrin levels, hypersecretion of gastric acid, and multiple and recurrent peptic ulcers in association with a gastrinoma, usually arising in the pancreas, are seen.

Treatment

Treatment is primarily medical and usually consists of 6 to 8 weeks of H2-receptor blocker therapy. Most drugs have similar healing rates, and the choice of which drug to use in an individual patient is made depending on any underlying medical illness, history of drug allergies, and comcommittant medications used. The healing rates for most ulcers are 70 to 80% at 4 weeks and 85 to 95% at 8 weeks (Tam, 1986). The most commonly used H2-receptor blocking drugs in children are cimetidine, famotidine, and ranitidine. Gastric ulcers tend not to be chronic and do not need long-term therapy. Patients (with duodenal ulcers) who relapse after an initial 8 to 12 week course are re-treated and then put on night-time prophylactic doses for up to 1 to 2 years depending on the clinical situation. Antacids can also be used 1 and 3 hours after meals and at bedtime. This usually involves the administration of large doses sometimes with the onset of diarrhea. They tend to be prescribed for symptomatic relief of pain on an as required basis. Sucral-fate, a mucosal protectant agent, is extremely useful for the treatment of active ulcers as well as for maintenance and prophylaxis. It has been shown to be as effective as H2-receptor blocker therapy in children even when used as sole therapy. Peptic ulcer disease frequently persists into adulthood if not treated with H2-receptor blocking agents or sucralfate. Bismuth compounds are useful not only as antacids in anti-acid therapy but also in treating helicobacter infection which predisposes to duodenal ulcer formation.

Surgery is not the mainstay of ulcer treatment and is used only when complications occur (i.e., hemorrhage, perforation, and obstruction). The usual surgeries performed are ligation of a bleeding vessel, closure of a perforation, vagotomy, and pyloroplasty. Patients who have recurrent and refractory ulcers despite intensive medical therapy or who experience complications from medical therapy may also benefit from having a surgical procedure done after the risks and benefits have been assessed.

Constipation

Constipation is the passage of infrequent or hard bowel movements. While the frequency of bowel movements is very variable, it is generally accepted that difficulty passing bowel movements or straining, hard stools, and large caliber stools all qualify as constipation. It is a problem seen very frequently in children with developmental disabilities and one that is often ig-

nored. Its importance must be underscored because it is responsible for significant morbidity in this group of children. Anorexia, frequent urinary tract infections, irritability, abdominal pain, vomiting, soiling, and even intestinal obstruction can be seen as a result of constipation. Various studies have shown that 94 to 99% of adults and preschool children have a stool frequency that varies between three times daily to three times weekly (Rappaport & Levine, 1986).

Etiology

The etiology of constipation is varied. Although the majority of cases fall into the idiopathic category, some systemic as well as neuromuscular conditions can cause constipation (see Table 12–7). Some evidence is available that there may be a genetic predisposition for constipation in some families. Constipation is known to be more frequent in societies where a low fiber diet is consumed. The three primary mechanisms that may lead to constipation are increased absorption of water from the colon, slow colonic transit, and abnormal defecation mechanisms. In an effort to understand the pathophysiology of constipation, numerous manometric and electrophysiolocic studies have been performed in children. Most children with idiopathic constipation have an increased threshold of sensation for rectal distention, with a preserved threshold for reflex inhibition of

Table 12–7. Etiology of constipation.

1. Idiopathic constipation
2. Anatomical disorders of the lower GI tract
3. Myopathies
4. Neuropathies
5. Chronic intestinal pseudo-obstruction
6. Systemic disorders causing constipation

the internal anal sphincter predisposing them to fecal soiling (Rappaport & Levine, 1986). Some children however have evidence of anal outlet obstruction with difficulty expelling rectal contents and failure to relax or actively contract the external anal sphincter during attempted defecation. Constipation is associated with congenital structural conditions of the bowel (i.e., anal stenosis, anterior ectopic anus, congenital and postnecrotizing enterocolitis colonic strictures). Presacral masses can also cause constipation by causing compression on the rectum (i.e., sacrococcygeal teratoma).

Conditions affecting the spinal cord intefere with the sacral reflex causing loss of rectal tone and sensation with preservation of the rectoanal inhibitory reflex. These patients have rectal impaction with soiling. Myelomeningocoele, spina bifida, diastematomyelia, tethered cord, spinal cord tumors, trauma, transverse myelitis, and so on are a few such conditions. Rare familial and nonfamilial visceral myopathies can present with constipation. They are characterized histologically by the presence of degenerating muscle cells and fibrosis. Constipation secondary to diseases of the enteric nervous system can also occur. Aganglionosis, both congenital (Hirschsprung's disease) and acquired, leads to constipation. In Hirschsprung's disease there is a congenital absence of ganglion cells in the myenteric and submucosal plexus in a variable amount of the colon extending proximally from the internal anal sphincter. In 80% of cases the affected segment extends up to the sigmoid colon. In very severe cases, variable amounts of the small intestine are affected. The disease is believed to be secondary to the failure of neural cells to complete their normal pathway of migration from the neural crest. An alternative theory is the failure of differentiation of neuronal survival cells in the affected regions (Tam, 1986). It has been seen in association with numerous congenital anomalies and syndromes (i.e., Down

syndrome). Acquired aganglionosis has been reported in a few infants who experienced necrotizing enterocolitis, sepsis, and shock. Other conditions affecting the enteric nervous system, although rare, can occur (i.e., intestinal neuronal dysplasia which has also been associated with neurofibromatosis).

Chronic intestinal pseudo-obstruction is a disturbance of GI motility in which patients present with a clinical picture of intestinal obstruction but do not have any identifiable obstruction. Systemic conditions like hypothyroidism, diabetes mellitus, chronic lead poisoning, vitamin D excess, uremia, hypercalcemia, and progressive systemic sclerosis can be associated with constipation. Concommitant administration of certain drugs causing constipation (i.e., antacids, anticholinergics, anticonvulsives, phenothiazines, barium sulfate, diuretics, iron) also need to be considered as potential causes of constipation. Local perianal conditions causing pain also cause constipation (i.e., fissures, proctitis, abscesses, sexual abuse). In children with developmental delay, malnutrition, inadequate fluid intake, inactivity, constipating drugs, and low fiber diet are the most frequent causes of constipation.

Clinical Features

Children usually will present with a history of infrequent or hard bowel movements, chronic intermittent abdominal pain, anorexia, abdominal distention, excessive flatulence, and rectal bleeding suggestive of fissures or soiling secondary to fecal impaction. Most children experience transient periods of constipation, which may be related to intercurrent events (i.e., postviral gastroenteritis, psychosocial changes, overzealous toilet training, difficulties of access to toilet facilities, etc.). Often a persistent decrease in stool frequency leads to fecal retention, rectal dilatation, and eventually fecal impaction with soiling (encopresis). By this point the child loses the urge to defecate, is unaware of the episodes of soiling, and will intermittently pass large caliber stools. Stools that have been retained for a long time tend to get hard because of fluid absorption. Passage of such stools causes pain, fissure formation, and fear of defecation leading to further worsening of the constipation. Usually encopresis resolves in adolescence.

Children with hyperactivity and attention deficit disorders tend to have constipation and at times may be resistant to therapy (Rappaport & Levine, 1986). Constipation can also form part of irritable bowel syndrome in which patients have abdominal pain and bouts of diarrhea alternating with constipation. This usually occurs in older children with stress and a low fiber diet as precipitating factors. Children with Hirschsprung's disease usually have delayed passage of meconium after the first 48 hours of life. They will have infrequent stools, which over time occur only after rectal stimulation. These patients tend not to have soiling and large caliber stools and on rectal exam have a small rectum devoid of stool. The exception is in ultra short segment Hirschsprung's disease, where the affected area is very short; these children behave as though they have idiopathic or functional constipation.

In any child with constipation the above discussed conditions need to be considered. Any organic disease especially those that can be corrected surgically (i.e., Hirschsprung's disease) should be ruled out. The most useful test to diagnose Hirschsprung's disease is a suction rectal biopsy showing the absence of ganglia and hypertrophic neural elements in an adequate sized biopsy. Anorectal manometry showing failure of relaxation of the rectosphincteric relaxation reflex can be a useful adjunct diagnostic tool, although it is not always necessary. An unprepared barium enema should always be done to rule out Hirschsprung's disease. This will delineate clearly the transition zone between the normal dilated colon and the undistended aganglionic portion. Films taken 24 and 48 hours later showing significant retained barium in the colon warrant a work-up for Hirschsprung's disease.

Management

Therapy needs to be tailored to the individual patient. The broad principles will be discussed briefly. They consist of dietary modifications, medications, disimpaction if necessary, toilet training if applicable, and behavior modification when applicable (see Table 12–8). Education of the patient and the family as to the etiology of constipation and management plan are vital to the success of the program especially for children with developmental disabilities and encopresis.

Nutrition

For most patients with acute or recent onset constipation a high fiber diet and plenty of fluids will usually be sufficient to alleviate the episode. Limiting the amount of milk to no more than 16 oz per day and also restricting the amount of caffeine in the diet (i.e., in the form of chocolate and iced tea) are also sometimes necessary. It is always preferable to use dietary fiber as opposed to fiber supplements (i.e., Metamucil®, Fiberall®, etc), but the use of these agents may sometimes be necessary in children who refuse to eat fruits and vegetables. Although fiber supplements may be added to food, in an effort to disguise them, care must be taken to ensure that enough fluids are given as well.

Table 12–8. Management of constipation.

1. Dietary modifications

2. Medications

3. Disimpaction

4. Toilet training

5. Behavior modification

Medications

Mineral oil, lactulose, milk of magnesia, and stimulant laxatives (i.e., senna) have been used in patients with constipation once any fecal impaction has been cleared. We prefer not to use stimulant laxatives because of the habituation that can occur. Also there have been reports of nerve damage in the colon with long-term use (Rappaport, & Levine, 1986). Large doses of lubricating laxatives or osmotic agents are more commonly used. Mineral oil, although tasteless and odorless, has the disadvantage of its potential for causing oil pneumonias if aspirated into the lungs. In children with developmental delay, we prefer to use lactulose, an osmotic laxative which works just as well. The dose needed is titrated according to the number and consistency of bowel movements that occur. Once a good stooling pattern has been achieved, the dose of the medication used is maintained for a variable period of time and then tapered off slowly according to the patient's needs. A significant number of children with developmental delay need to be on chronic doses of laxatives in addition to fiber supplements.

Disimpaction

In patients with fecal impaction and encopresis, disimpaction is always necessary. This is best accomplished by a series of enemas, suppositories, or massive doses of oral nonstimulant laxatives. We prefer to use one phosphate enema twice a day for 3 days as an initial regimen. This is usually adequate in most cases. However, in some severe cases enemas may need to be given for a longer period. It is preferable to use enemas only for disimpaction and not on a regular basis as this will encourage habituation. Children under 2 years of age are given pediatric sized enemas, while older children receive the adult sized enemas. Enemas should be used with caution in patients with chronic renal or heart failure

and very young children. It is sometimes useful to use mineral oil enemas in patients with very hard impactions. A polyethylene glycol electrolyte solution may be used for disimpaction. The disadvantage, however, is that children will often refuse to drink the large quantities that are required, and it may then need to be administered via a nasogastric tube. When attempting disimpaction using oral agents, intestinal obstruction should always be ruled out and the agent being used should be stopped immediately should any vomiting occur.

Toilet Training

Any patient with chronic constipation should be encouraged to establish a regular pattern of bowel movements. Complete and regular evacuation of the rectum will result in normalization of rectal size in patients with megarectum, resolution of encopresis, and return of rectal sensation. Regular evacuation results in softer and smaller bowel movements. Stool diameter usually reflects rectal size and may be a parameter to follow in patients. We encourage patients to sit on the toilet for 5 to 10 minutes twice a day usually after a meal to utilize the gastrocolic reflex. Smaller children should have proper foot support so that they can bear down and defecate effectively. Toilet sitting should also be done at the same time every day to establish a routine.

Behavior Modification

All patients are asked to keep a calendar of their stooling pattern. This is very helpful in assessing success of the program. Psychological intervention may be needed in children who do not respond to the above program. These children usually undergo a psychological assessment, and their caretakers are interviewed as well. Ongoing counseling in conjunction with medical therapy is particularly helpful in patients with severe encopresis, behavioral problems, attention deficit disorders, and abnormal family dynamics. We find it useful to explain to the psychologist involved the medical aspects of the case as well the treatment plan.

However, none of the above five parts of this program alone is successful. They all have to be done together. It takes a committed family and physician to achieve success. Regular follow-up is also important to the implementation and success of the program.

Percutaneous Gastrostomy Tubes

Percutaneous gastrostomy tube placement or PEG placement is becoming an increasingly frequent procedure for most pediatric gastroenterologists. It is the placement of a gastrostomy tube using the upper endoscope and usually takes approximately 10 to 20 minutes to do. Its advantages over a conventional gastrostomy are multiple and include avoidance of a laparotomy incision, shorter time under general anesthesia, quicker recovery time, earlier institution of feedings postoperatively, and a shorter hospital stay.

Indications

The indications for PEG are similar to those for a surgical gastrostomy. In the child with developmental disabilities this will include any child who is unable to orally take in sufficient calories to grow or maintain body weight, has significant oropharyngeal and esophageal dysmotility, recurrent episodes of aspiration pneumonia, or progressive neurological disease.

Evaluation

Any child who meets the above criteria is a candidate for a PEG. A complete blood count, chemistry panel, and urine analysis are obtained preoperatively. Patients also have a detailed nutritional assessment so that an appropriate nutritional regimen can be chosen. An upper gastrointestinal series is also necessary to determine any abnormalities in the anatomy of the esophagus, stomach, and duodenum (i.e., exclude malrotation). If there is a history of GER, a 24-hour pH probe recording is performed to estimate the amount of GER. The presence of GER is not an absolute contraindication to a PEG, but because the amount of GER can increase after a PEG, the risks versus the benefits should be weighed to determine whether the patient may be better served by having a fundoplication. Every patient is different, so the decision must be made on an individual basis. The increased GER seems to occur because the PEG "points" directly at the gastroesophageal junction and exaggerates the pathophysiologic events that occur at the LES causing GER. Some patients may also have a gastric emptying scan done preoperatively if they have symptoms suggestive of delayed gastric emptying. Depending on the clinical situation and previous response to prokinetic agents, some of these patients may need a surgical gastrostomy and pyloroplasty. A usual *contraindication* to PEG placement is any previous abdominal surgery because the presence of adhesions puts the patient at risk for intestinal perforation, peritonitis, and subsequent fistula formation. Previous laparotomies may result in complications during a PEG. However, in carefully selected patients in whom surgery is contraindicated, a PEG may be done after the risks have been explained to the family. The presence of a ventriculoperitoneal shunt is not a contraindication, but these patients need to be given appropriate prophylactic antibiotics. In patients on peritoneal dialysis, the presence of peritoneal fluid may make the PEG a little harder to do.

Procedure

Preoperatively patients are admitted the morning of the procedure. We prefer to do the PEGs under general anesthesia because this is a more controlled situation and avoids the agitation commonly seen when patients have their stomachs insufflated. Also in the "pull" technique when the gastrostomy tube and crossbar are pulled through the oropharynx, the intubated airway is less compromised (especially in patients with a tracheostomy tube). However, in a controlled situation, PEGs can be placed under good intravenous conscious sedation. Prophylactic antibiotics (1 dose before surgery and 2 doses after) cover oral flora and staphylococcus.

After induction of general anesthesia and intubation, the patient is maintained in the supine position. The upper endoscope is passed through the mouth down the esophagus and into the stomach. The stomach is then insufflated with air and the tip of the endoscope advanced to the position on the anterior abdominal wall where the light of the endoscope shines brightly. The surgeon, coendoscopist, or assistant usually palpates the area so that the endoscopist can recognize the finger's imprint in an area on the anterior wall of the stomach. This is usually in the body of the stomach adjacent to the antrum. A mark is then made with indelible ink on the anterior wall of the stomach. The skin is then prepared aseptically and a 1 to 2 cm stab wound is made at the site using a surgical blade. A Venocath (14–16 gauge) is introduced through the incision. Two techniques are commonly used—the "pull" or "introducer." Using the "pull" technique, the endoscopist passes a snare through the endoscope and positions the snare around the venocath. The snare is then used to grab the thread that has been threaded through the venocath. The endoscope (along with the snare and thread) is withdrawn from the patient. The gastrostomy tube is then tied to the thread with the tapered end proximal and pulled into the stomach and through the abdominal wall. The endoscope is again passed into the stomach and the site inspected. The esophagus is

also checked for lacerations. In the "introducer" technique, after the venocath is introduced, dilators of various sizes are used over a guide wire until the desired size is reached. The gastrostomy tube is then introduced. In both techniques an external crossbar is placed on the gastrostomy tube. We do not find it necessary to use sutures to anchor the gastrostomy tube and have found a greater incidence of local irritation and infection in patients whose PEGs were anchored to the anterior abdominal wall with sutures.

Patients can usually start feeding within 12 hours of PEG placement. Their feeds can be advanced over 48 hours to the desired nutritional program and when achieved they can be discharged from the hospital. We also advocate rotating the crossbar every 12 hours and cleaning the area initially with half-strength peroxide and keeping it dry. Later, the site may be cleaned with soap and water daily. We have found fewer local complications as well as less pain at the site by making sure the gastrostomy tube enters the abdomen at a right angle. The initial gastrostomy tube usually lasts a few months and can be replaced once a tract has formed. We usually wait 2 to 3 months before replacing the tubes. The tube may be removed endoscopically or by cutting it at skin level and allowing the tube to be passed in the stool.

Complications are usually few. Site infections tend to be the most common and can be avoided by the use of aseptic technique, prophylactic antibiotics, and good local care at the site. If there is a lot of tension and friction at the site, granulomas tend to form which can be cauterized in the office using silver nitrate sticks. Peritonitis, colonic fistulas, and puncture of adjacent organs have been known to occur. Late onset complications are related to improper feeding techniques, formula intolerance, and tube migration of an improperly secured tube.

A gastrostomy tube can be replaced by a *"button"* once the tract has matured. A "button" is a very short gastrostomy tube that is just a little raised over the skin surface. The indication for its use is primarily cosmetic, and it offers no other advantage over a gastrostomy tube. Its care is similar to that of a gastrostomy tube. A variety of buttons are now available, and their advantages vary from manufacturer to manufacturer.

Summary

In summary, a variety of gastrointestinal problems that occur in children with developmental disabilities. Quick, appropriate diagnosis and treatment of these conditions should improve the quality of life for these children. As our understanding of the relationship of the central nervous system to autonomic innervation of the gastrointestinal tract increases, newer therapies may become available.

References

Allen, W. W., Durie, P. R., Hamilton, R. J., Walker-Smith, J. A., & Watkins, J. B. (Eds). (1991). Pediatric gastrointestinal disease: Pathophysiology, diagnosis and management (pp. 417–422). B.C. Decker, Inc.

Ament, M. E., & Christie, D. L. (1977). Upper gastrointestinal endoscopy in pediatric patients. *Gastroenterology 72*, 1244–1248.

Byrne, W. J., Campbell, M., Ashcraft, E., Seibert, J. J., & Euler, A. R. (1983). A diagnostic approach to vomiting in severely retarded patients. *American Journal of Diseases in Children, 137*, 259–262.

Byrne, W. J., Euler, A. R., Ashcraft, E., Nash, D. G., Seibert, J. J., & Golladay, E. S. (1992). Gastroesophageal reflux in the severely retarded who vomit: Criteria for and results of surgical intervention in twenty-two patients. *Surgery 91*(1), 95–99.

Campbell, J. R., Gilchrist, B. F., & Harrison, M. W. (1989). Pyloroplasty in association with Nissen fundoplication in children with eurologic disorders. *Journal of Pediatric Surgery 24*(4), 375–377.

Eastham, E. J.(1990). Peptic ulcer. In W. A. Walker, P. R. Durie, J. R. Hamilton, J. A. Walker-Smith, & J. B. Watkins (Eds.), *Pediatric gastrointestinal disease*. Edinburgh: Blackwell Scientific Publications.

Fonkalsrud, E. W., Foglia, R. P., Ament, M. E., Berquist, W., & Vargus, J. (1989). Operative treatment for the gastroesophageal reflux syndrome in children. *Journal of Pediatric Surgery 24*(6), 525–529.

Grunow, J. E., Al-Hafidh, A. S., & Tunell, W. P. (1989). Gastroesophageal reflux following percutaneous endoscopic gastrostomy in children. *Journal of Pediatric Surgery 24*(1), 42–45.

Halpern, L. M., Jolley, S. G., & Johnson, D. G. (1991). Gastroesophageal reflux: A significant association with central nervous system disease in children. *Journal of Pediatric Surgery 26*(2), 171–173.

Heyman, S., & Respondek, M. (1989). Detection of pulmonary aspiration in children by radionuclide "salivagram." *Journal of Nuclear Medicine 30*(5), 697–699.

Hillemeier, C.A., Grill, B. B., McCallum, R., & Gryboski, J. (1983). Esophageal and gastric motor abnormalities in gastro- esophageal reflux during infancy. *Gastroenterology 84*, 741–746.

Langer, J. C., Wesson, D. E., Ein, S. H., Filler, R. M., Shandling, B., Superina, R., & Papa, M. (1988). Feeding gastrostomy in neurologically impaired children: Is an antireflux procedure necessary? *Journal of Pediatric Gastroenterology & Nutrition, 7*(6), 837–841.

Molitt, D. L., Golladay, S., & Seibert, J. (1985). Symptomatic gastroesophageal reflux following gastrostomy in neurologically impaired patients. *Pediatrics 75*(6), 1124–1126.

Murphy, M. S. (1990). Constipation. In W. A. Walker, P. R. Durie, J. R. Hamilton, J. A. Walker-Smith, & J. B. Watkins (Eds.), *Pediatric gastrointestinal disease*. Edinburgh: Blackwell Scientific Publications.

Nanayakkara, C. S., & Paton, J. Y. (1985). Sandifer syndrome: An overlooked diagnosis? *Developmental Medicine and Childhood Neurology, 27*, 816–818.

Orenstein, S. R. (1991, May/June). Gastroesophageal reflux. *Current Problems in Pediatrics*, pp. 193–241.

Rappaport, L. A., & Levine, M. D. (1986). The prevention of constipation and encopresis: A developmental model and approach. *Pediatric Clinics of North America, 33*, 859–869.

Rode, H., Millar, A. J. W., Brown, R. A., & Cywes, S. (1992). Reflux strictures of esophagus in children. *Journal of Pediatric Surgery, 27*(4), 462–465.

Ross, M. N., Haase, G. M., Reiley, T. T., & Meagher, D. P. (1988). The importance of acid reflux patterns in neurologically damaged children detected by four channel esophageal pH monitoring. *Journal of Pediatric Surgery, 23*(6), 573–576.

Roy, C. C., & Silverman, A. (Eds.). (1975). *Pediatric clinical gastroenterology* (2nd ed., pp. 134–152). St. Louis, MO: C. V. Mosby.

Sondheimer, J. M., & Morris, B. A. (1979). Gastroesophageal reflux among severely retarded children. *Journal of Pediatrics, 90*, 710–714.

Spitz, L., & Kirtane, J. (1985). Results and complications of surgery for gastroesophageal reflux. *Archives of Diseases of Childhood, 60*, 743–747.

Tam, P. K. H. (1986). An immunochemical study with neurospecific enolase and substance P of human enteric innervation. The normal developmental pattern and abnormal deviations in Hirschsprung's disease and pyloric stenosis. *Journal of Pediatric Surgery, 21*, 227–232.

Vanderhoof, J. A., Rappaport, P. J., & Paxson, C. L. (1978). Manometric diagnosis of lower esophageal sphincter pressure incompetence in infants: Use of a small single lumen perfused catheter. *Pediatrics, 62*, 805–808.

Warren, J. R. & Marshall, B. J. (1983). Unidentified curved bacilli on gastric epithelium in active chronic gastritis. *Lancet, 1*, 1273–1275.

Werlin, S. L., Dodds, W. J., & Hogan, W. J. (1980). Mechanism of gastroesophageal reflux in children. *Journal of Pediatrics, 97*(2), 244–249.

Wesley, J. R., Coran, A. G., Sarahan, T. M., Klein, M. D., & White, S. J. (1981). The need for evaluation of gastroesophageal reflux in brain damaged children referred for feeding gastrostomy. *Journal of Pediatric Surgery, 16*(6), 866–871.

Wilkinson, J. D., Dudgeon, D., & Sondheimer, J. M., (1991). A comparison of medical and surgical treatment of gastroesophageal reflux in severely retarded children. *Journal of Pediatrics, 99*(2), 202–205.

Williams, T. A., Tsukada, J. T., & Boyle, J. T. (1989). Mechanism of GER in recumbent neurologically impaired children. *Gastroenterology, 96*(5), A547.

CHAPTER

13

Surgical Management of Gastroesophageal Reflux in Children

MARK A. HOFFMAN, M.S., M.D., F.A.C.S., F.R.C.S. (C.)
AND ARTHUR J. ROSS, III, M.D., F.A.C.S.

CONTENTS

- **Surgical Overview of Gastroesophageal Reflux**
- **Fundoplication**
- **Pyloroplasty**
- **Gastrostomy**
- **Alternatives to Antireflux Procedures**
- **Summary**
- **References**

Over the past decade, procedures for the relief of gastroesophageal reflux have become commonly performed operations in large pediatric surgical centers. Whether this reflects an actual increase in the prevalence of gastroesophageal reflux, a greater clinical awareness of the problem, or an increase in the percentage of children with reflux who are now being referred for surgical management, is unclear. The majority of children requiring antireflux procedures exhibit some degree of congenital

Over the past decade, procedures for the relief of gastroesophageal reflux have become commonly performed operations in large pediatric surgical centers. Whether this reflects an actual increase in the prevalence of gastroesophageal reflux, a greater clinical awareness of the problem, or an increase in the percentage of children with reflux who are now being referred for surgical management, is unclear. The majority of children requiring antireflux procedures exhibit some degree of congenital

283

or acquired neurologic impairment spanning a varied and heterogeneous group of etiologies. Improvements in the care of this particular group of children and the well-recognized association between neurologic dysfunction and gastroesophageal reflux account for much of the dramatic increase in antireflux surgery (Cadman, Richard, & Feldman, 1978; Holmes, 1971; Sondheimer and Morris, 1979; Tovar, Morras, Garay, & Tapia, 1986). The frequent accompaniment of co-morbid and secondary medical and surgical conditions so frequently encountered in this group of patients amplifies the enormous challenge in overall management, and mandates an individually tailored, comprehensive, and multidisciplinary approach to the pre- and postoperative evaluation and care. Likewise, strict attention to intra-operative management and operative detail are necessary to optimize results and achieve the best possible outcome.

The large and ever-increasing volume of surgery for gastroesophageal reflux does not reflect consensus on this topic. If the indications for antireflux surgery were at all times well defined, the operative procedures strictly standardized, the complication rates uniformly low, and the results unquestionably excellent, then there would be little need for debate. None of these conditions for general agreement, unfortunately, have been realized, and broad areas of controversy involving all aspects of antireflux surgery exist and remain unresolved. These controversies become particularly cogent when the surgical management of gastroesophageal reflux in children with neurologic impairment and developmental disabilities is discussed. These patients comprise a well-recognized "high-risk" group for failure of both medical and surgical therapy (Guggenbichler & Menardi, 1985; Spitz & Kirtane, 1985). A surfeit of early and late postoperative complications are exceedingly common in this patient population, whereas antireflux procedures in otherwise normal

children more closely approximate the excellent results seen in adults (DeMeester, Bonavina, & Albertucci, 1986).

This chapter focuses on the surgery for gastroesophageal reflux in children with neurologic and developmental disabilities. Three general areas are addressed. First, the problem of gastroesophageal reflux in the child with neurological dysfunction is examined in detail from a surgical prospective, and the overall efficacy of the more commonly employed operative procedures is evaluated. The role of gastric emptying procedures in the management of gastroesophageal reflux is also discussed. Second, the issue of gastrostomy in the child with neurological impairment, with or without routine "protective" antireflux procedure, is critically reviewed, and a management scheme outlined. And third, alternative surgical strategies for the management of gastroesophageal reflux are presented.

Surgical Overview of Gastroesophageal Reflux

Gastroesophageal reflux may be classified as physiologic, uncomplicated, and complicated (Boix-Ochoa, 1986; 1987). Physiologic gastroesophageal reflux persists beyond the neonatal period into the first few months of life, and subsequently subsides with maturation of the lower esophageal sphincter mechanism. Uncomplicated gastroesophageal reflux implies the presence of reflux in the absence of adverse sequelae. Both the physiologic and uncomplicated forms rarely come to surgical attention, and antireflux procedures, for the most part, are advocated for the management of complicated gastroesophageal reflux which fails more conservative therapeutic measures. Surgery, therefore, is regarded as a second line of management under usual circumstances.

Complicated gastroesophageal reflux implies a deficit or breakdown in the lower esophageal sphincter mechanism, with the addition of adverse sequelae (Table 13–1) arising from this functional derangement (Edwards, 1982; Katz & Castell, 1987; Ramenofsky, 1986; Skinner, 1985; Sondheimer, 1988). These adverse consequences of gastroesophageal reflux comprise the indications for surgical correction. In general, three prerequisites should be satisfied prior to recommending antireflux surgery: (1) the presence of gastroesophageal reflux should be demonstrated by any of the variety of available methods (Jonsell & De Mestier, 1984); (2) the complications of gastroesophageal reflux must be documented; and, (3) failure of conservative treatment should be established.

The physiology of the intrinsic protective mechanisms which combat gastroesophageal reflux under normal circumstances are inherently complex, centering around a score of anatomic, neural and neuroendocrine, hormonal, and pharmacologic factors and agents (Katz & Castell, 1987). The multifactorial nature of gastroesophageal integrity renders a

Table 13–1. Complications of gastroesophageal reflux.

Nutritional
    failure to thrive
    rumination

Respiratory
    aspiration
    recurrent upper respiratory infection
    asthma
    apnea
    respiratory distress
    "near-dying" spells

Esophagitis
    stricture
    anemia
    dysphagia
    pain

Other
    "torticollis" (Sandifer's syndrome)

---

simple explanation of the association between central nervous impairment and gastroesophageal reflux difficult. Several animal models have correlated depressed lower esophageal sphincter pressure with increased intracranial pressure and acute and chronic brain injury (Vane et al., 1982). Abnormalities in gastric motility have also been noted (Matthews et. al, 1988). The validity of these models and the interactions of acute and chronic cortical and subcortical injury with the myriad of other factors responsible for lower esophageal sphincter competency await further definition.

The role of pyloro-antral and esophageal dysmotility syndromes in the pathogenesis of gastroesophageal reflux and its complications is poorly understood. Although it appears intuitively correct that delayed gastric emptying would predispose to reflux, and abnormal esophageal peristalsis would invite prolonged periods of acid exposure within the esophagus, it is difficult to judge the interplay of these factors within the total framework of complicated gastroesophageal reflux. Some children with gastroesophageal reflux exhibit a global esophagogastric motor abnormality, described as the "gastroesophageal reflux syndrome" (Fonkalsrud, Ament, & Berquist, 1985; Fonkalsrud, Berquist, Vargas, Arment, & Foglia, 1987). This includes gastroesophageal reflux, delayed gastric emptying and esophageal dysmotility in its full expression. The child with corrected esophageal atresia, in particular, demonstrates poor lower esophageal motility, and gastroesophageal reflux is the most common ongoing problem encountered after correction of the atresia (Johnson & Beasley, 1991). The phenomenon is also noted in the presence of severe reflux esophagitis, where a cause or effect relationship is difficult to discriminate.

Delayed gastric emptying is more frequently noted in children with neurologic impairment, and there appears to be an inconsistent relationship of gastric motor dysfunction to central nervous system injury. Quantitative assessment of gastric emptying is usually performed using radiolabelled solid food or liquid formula, with the percent of labelled material retained in the stomach represented as a function of time (McCallum 1990; Papaila et. al, 1989;). A "correction factor" may be applied when gastroesophageal reflux is present to account for gastric escape of the radioactive tracer into the esophagus. Functional impairment of esophageal motility is delineated by multi-channel manometric measurements.

The considerations and format of any antireflux procedure rely on functional restoration of the antireflux barrier by anatomic means, in the sense that existing anatomic relationships are manipulated or altered to augment deficient function. Several operations (Table 13–2) have evolved for the treatment of gastroesophageal reflux in both children and adults. Many of these procedures are strictly of historical interest, and are

Table 13–2. Operative procedures for the management of gastroesophageal reflux.

Allison repair

Total fundoplication (Nissen)

Partial fundoplication (Thal)

Posterior gastropexy (Hill)

Anterior gastropexy (Boerema)

Angelchick antireflux prosthesis

Belsey-Mark IV procedure

Collis gastroplasty with Belsey or Nissen fundoplication

Uncut Collis gastroplasty with Nissen fundoplication

Toupe procedure

---

rarely performed today. All, however, represent an effort to reinforce the barrier to reflux by improving the valvular activity of the lower esophageal sphincter mechanism, thereby encouraging esophageal clearance into the stomach without backwash. In the pediatric age group, the Nissen fundoplication (complete wrap) and Thal operation (partial wrap) have thus far emerged as the most commonly utilized procedures, while a third procedure, the uncut Collis-Nissen fundoplication, is presently being studied at the Children's Hospital of Philadelphia. The role of laparoscopic fundoplication awaits further definition within the pediatric age group.

Fundoplication

The Nissen fundoplication, described by Professor Rudolf Nissen from the University of Basel, Switzerland in 1956, has emerged as the "gold standard" procedure for the correction of gastroesophageal reflux in infants and children (Bettex & Oesch, 1983). The operation was popularized in the United States for the treatment of complicated gastroesophageal reflux in children by Dr. Judson Randolph at the Children's National Medical Center in Washington, DC. Randolph (1983) reported his 15 year experience with the Nissen fundoplication in 72 infants. Excellent results were achieved: 94% of patients had a good result with follow-up extending from 1 to 13 years. There were six (8.3%) operative failures. No mention of the neurologic status of these patients was made in this report, and the most common indications for surgery were failure to thrive (48.6%), chronic pulmonary infection (33.3%), and choking or apnea spells (11.1%).

The essential components of Nissen's operation (see Figure 13–1) involve: (1) extensive mobilization of the esophagus at

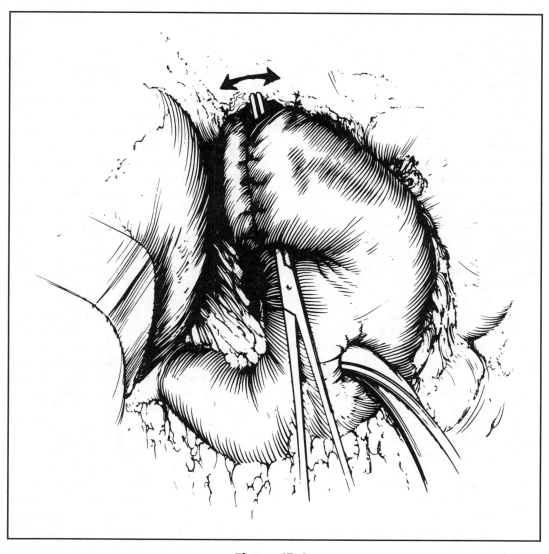

Figure 13–1.

The Nissen fundoplication. A loose 360° or complete wrap of the fundus of the stomach is performed around the lower segment of the esophagus. (From Ross, A. J. [1993]. Nissen fundoplication. In D. D. Sabiston [Ed.], *Atlas of general surgery* [pp.316–322], Philadelphia, PA: W. B. Saunders Co., p. 322, with permission.)

the esophageal diaphragmatic hiatus for restoration of the intraabdominal esophagus; (2) crural tighten; (3) mobilization of the fundus of the stomach by division of the short gastric vessels and splenic attachments; and, (4) a 360° wrap of the fundus around the lower esophageal segment (Johnson, 1985; Johnson, 1986; Randolph, 1983; Rouse, Guzzetta, & Randolph, 1989). The procedure is far from standardized (Jamieson & Duranceau, 1984), and various additional maneuvers have been added including pledgetted crural and fundic approximation (Robie and Pearl, 1991), multiple point suturing of the fundic wrap (Ferraris, Martinez, & Burrington 1985), tacking of the wrapped fundus to the diaphragm and esophageal hiatus, and posterior gastropexy (Boix-Ochoa, 1987). These variations in technique make series comparisons difficult, as the term "Nissen fundoplication" has become a generic designation embracing a variety of modified procedures.

Concerns with the Nissen fundoplication have focused upon the issues of "gas-bloat" syndrome and the unpredictable capacity to vomit after a complete wrap (Bettex & Oesch, 1983; Negre, 1983). The "gas-bloat" syndrome describes postprandial discomfort secondary to aerophagia, gastric distention, and an inability to belch (Polk, 1984). As both belching and vomiting are normal childhood events, the Thal (Thal, 1968) partial fundoplication (see Figure 13–2) has become the current major alternative procedure because of its consistent preservation of these functions. The Kansas City group (Ashcraft, 1986; Ashcraft et al., 1978) have been major advocates of this operation.

Although the adult experience with antireflux procedures for the management of hiatus hernia and gastroesophageal reflux has yielded excellent results (DeMeester, Bonavina, & Albertucci, 1986), several problems have plagued the application of these operations to the pediatric age group.

The incidence of serious complications, particularly postoperative small bowel obstruction, is considerably higher than would be anticipated after elective laparotomy (Tunell, Smith, & Carson, 1983; Wilkins & Spitz, 1987). Jolley, Tunell, Hoelzer, and Smith (1986) have reported a 6.2% incidence of small bowel obstruction in 210 pediatric patients undergoing Nissen fundoplication. When the Oklahoma group combined their data with the antireflux surgery experiences from Salt Lake City, London, Toronto, and Kansas City, the overall incidence of small bowel obstruction after Nissen or Thal fundoplication was 5.5% (24/436). The predominant cause of obstruction was adhesive, although postoperative intussusception was not uncommon. Pearl et al. (1990), reporting combined a combined experience from the Hospital for Sick Children in Toronto and the Walter Reed Army Medical Center in Washington, DC, found an early postoperative small bowel obstruction rate of 4.2% in 233 children undergoing antireflux operations (178 Nissen and 55 Thal fundoplications). The overall complication rate for the series was 27.4%. Of particular note, when the neurologically impaired group of 153 patients was examined separately, the incidence of postoperative small bowel obstruction was 6.5%, and the early and late postoperative complication rate was 33.3%. The postoperative small bowel obstruction rate was 1.2%, and the postoperative complication rate was 16% in the group of children who were neurologically normal. Dedinsky et al (1987) from the University of Indiana and Turnage, Oldham, Coran, and Blane (1989) from the University of Michigan report instances of postoperative small bowel obstruction in 4.2% and 8.7% of patients undergoing Nissen fundoplication in their respective series. The Michigan group reported an overall postoperative complication rate of 45%. The high risk nature of their patient population is reflected in the fact that 57% of

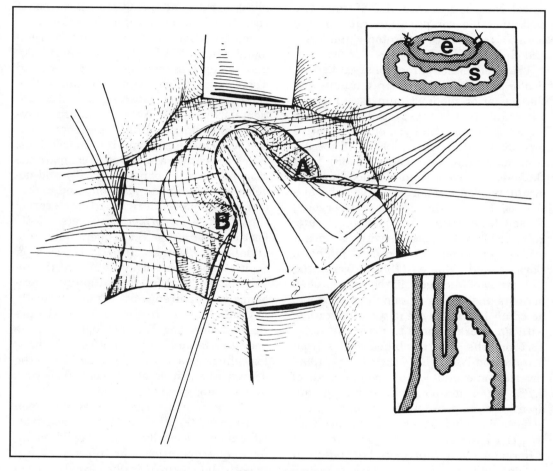

Figure 13–2.
The Thal fundoplication. A 180° or partial wrap of the fundus is performed anteriorly around the lower esophageal segment (From Ashcraft, K.W. [1986]. Thal fundoplication. In K. W. Ashcraft, K. W. & T. M. Holder [Eds.], *Pediatric esophageal surgery* [pp. 209–216], Orlando, FL: Grune & Stratton, Inc., p. 213, with permission.)

their patients had significant neurologic impairment, while 80% of patients had at least one additional medical problem. The series from Indianapolis showed a complication rate of 16%, with 69% of patients exhibiting some degree of neurologic dysfunction. These figures are inordinately high considering the postoperative small bowel obstruction rate of 0.8% and the postoperative complication rate of less than 5% for elective laparotomy in infancy and childhood.

The incidence of paraesophageal herniation or prolapse of the wrapped fundus into the posterior mediastinum (see Figures 13–3 and13–4) is substantial, accounting for most failures and remedial operative procedures (Pearl et al., 1990). Alrabeeah, Giacomantonio, and Gillis (1988) from Dalhousie University in Halifax found an overall incidence of paraesophageal herniation of 17% in 89 children undergoing Nissen fundoplication. The highest rate, 20%, was found in patients with significant mental dysfunction. Turnage, Oldham, Coran, and Blane (1989) from the University of Michigan, in their series of 46 patients undergoing Nissen fundoplication, noted an 11% incidence of wrap migration, with an average time to presentation of 13.1 months. The combined series from Toronto and Walter Reed (Pearl et al., 1990) revealed an overall wrap herniation rate of 7.7%. When neurologically impaired children were compared with the neurologically normal group in this series, the incidence was 11.1% versus 1.2%, a highly significant difference. Paraesophageal herniation or prolapse of the wrap into the posterior mediastinum accounts for 35% to 100% of reoperations after fundoplication (Pearl et al., 1990), although this finding does not necessarily mandate remedial surgery in the absence of recurrent reflux (Blane, Turnage, Oldham, & Coran, 1989).

While it would be hoped that the significant rate of complications for the Nissen and Thal fundoplications would be offset by

excellent long-term results, this has proven to be an unrealized expectation. Recurrent symptoms of gastroesophageal reflux secondary to wrap herniation, slippage, or disruption occur with a predictable frequency, and there is an apparent direct relationship between the percentage of neurologically impaired children, the postoperative complication rate, and the ultimate incidence of operative failure in most large series.

In the report from Indianapolis (Dedinsky et al., 1987), 38 of 429 patients (8.8%) undergoing Nissen fundoplication required a second antireflux operation because of recurrent symptoms. Of this group of 38 patients, 29 patients (76%) had severe neurologic impairment, while 5 patients (13%) had associated congenital malformations. When the data are analyzed to compare the reoperative rate for neurologically and developmentally impaired as opposed to otherwise normal children, the reoperative rate was 10% for former group versus 0.8% for the latter group. Subsequent data from Oklahoma (Tuggle, Tunell, Hoelzer, & Smith, 1988) specifically examined the results of the Thal fundoplication in neurologically impaired versus neurologically normal children. In the series of 116 patients undergoing Thal fundoplication, the operative failure rate was 3% in 68 neurologically normal children versus 17% in the 48 patients with significant central nervous system impairment.

The combined series from Walter Reed and Toronto (Pearl et al., 1990) demonstrated that neurologically impaired children underwent reoperation four times more frequently than neurologically normal children for recurrent reflux (19% versus 5%), and concluded that neurologic status was a major predictive factor of operative success in the control of reflux for both the Nissen and Thal fundoplications. In the Ann Arbor series of 46 infants and children undergoing Nissen fundoplications, 11.4% required reoperation for recurrent symptoms. All reoperated patients suffered either neurolog-

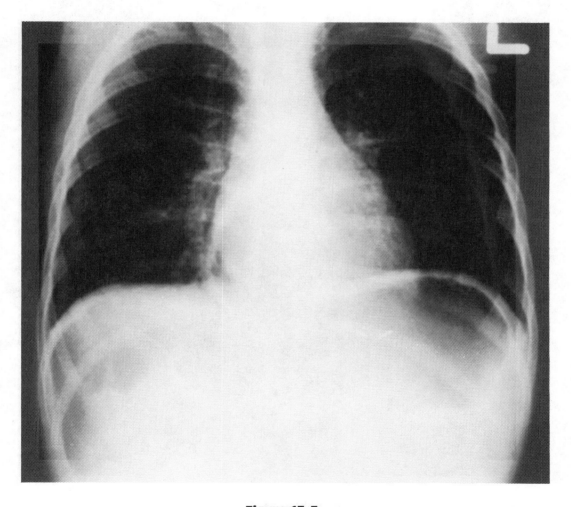

Figure 13–3.
Chest x-ray of a patient with recurrent symptoms of gastroesophageal reflux 1 year after a Nissen fundoplication. The wrap has migrated into the posterior mediastinum.

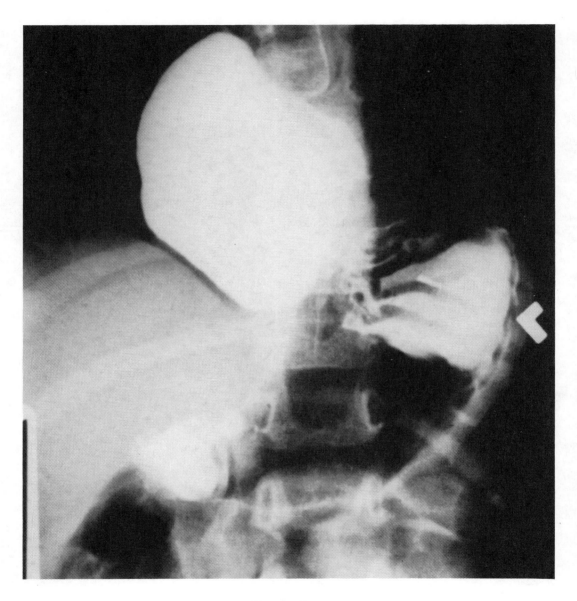

Figure 13–4.
Upper gastrointestinal barium contrast examination of a patient with recurrent symptoms of reflux after a Nissen fundoplication. The wrap has slipped down around the body of the stomach, and the fundus has migrated into the posterior mediastinum.

ic impairment or a developmental anomaly (esophageal atresia).

The overall picture that emerges from the extensive experience with the Nissen and Thal fundoplication is one of significant disparity between the complication rate and outcome in normal versus developmentally and neurologically impaired children. General discontent with these results lends itself to three related lines of inquiry: (1) What risk factors are inherently present in the neurologically and developmentally impaired patient population that cause such a high failure rate of these procedures? (2) Are there elements of these operations that adversely interact with these risk factors and prejudice the results in these patients? And, (3) is there a better designed operation which might improve the outcome?

A number of consequences and conditions (see Table 13–3) associated with neurologic and developmental impairment exist which confound any surgical attempt to reinforce the antireflux barrier and jeopardize the fundoplication (Orringer, 1989).

Table 13–3. Risk factors for recurrent gastroesophageal reflux following fundoplication.

Factors that jeopardize esophageal sutures
   reflux esophagitis
   periesophagitis

Factors that place tension on the repair
   esophageal shortening
   excessive esophageal mobilization
   deformity
   spasticity

Factors that "stress" the fundoplication
   chronic pulmonary disease
   contipation/straining
   seizure activity
   chronic singulus
   retching
   aerophagia

These factors clearly inter-relate, and pose a multi-pronged challenge to the integrity of the wrap and its maintenance within the abdominal environs. In a report from the Ohio State University (Caniano, Ginn-Pease, & King, 1990) which examined the risk factors responsible for 21 failures of fundoplication (20 Nissen and 1 Thal fundoplications), forceful emesis was associate with 29% of the wrap disruptions. Major primary preoperative factors included chronic respiratory symptoms, vomiting, and corrected esophageal atresia. In a group of 36 failures of Nissen fundoplication reported by Wheatley, Coran, Wesley, Oldham, and Turnage (1991) from the University of Michigan, 31 of the 36 failures (81%) were in neurologically impaired children, and a movement or seizure disorder was documented in 21 patients (58%).

A recent report from the Medical University of South Carolina (Smith, Otherson, Gogan, & Walker, 1992) examined the results of antireflux surgery in 35 children with profound neurologic disability. Operative failure was documented in 20% of patients, and a secondary procedure to correct recurrent reflux was required in 17% of patients. Nine patients developed paraesophageal herniation of the wrap into the posterior mediastinum, and this complication accounted for 83% of the reoperative procedures. Of particular note in this series, 23 patients (66%) had a seizure disorder, 18 patients (51%) exhibited muscular spasticity, and 17 patients (49%) had pulmonary disease. These conditions are known risk factors for operative failure. These authors conclude that "the Nissen fundoplication in our series of patients with profound neurologic disability confirms the experience of others who report increased risks of death, recurrence of symptoms, paraesophageal hernia, and small bowel obstruction in these children as compared with neurologically normal patients. Further refinements in diagnostic and treatment strategies are needed to improve patient selection and reduce risks in this markedly impaired group of children" (p. 657).

Hoffman, Stylianos, and Jacir (1990) have reported a preliminary experience with the uncut Collis-Nissen fundoplication (see Figure 13–5) in 55 patients, 91% of whom had significant neurologic impairment. This procedure is being critically studied at the Children's Hospital of Philadelphia. The components of this operation have several theoretical advantages over the standard Nissen and Thal fundoplications: (1) there is minimal dissection within the esophageal hiatus, with no attempt to "restore" or lengthen the intra-abdominal esophagus by displacing the mediastinal segment downwards; (2) the esophagus is lengthened within the abdomen by tubularizing a variable length of the lesser curvature of the stomach with an intestinal stapling device; (3) a fixed, acute angle of His is developed at the staple line; (4) no sutures are placed within the tenuous esophageal musculature, but rather, the fundic wrap is sutured to the neo-esophagus composed of tubularized stomach; and (5) the wrap is anchored to the neo-esophagus at two points: the staple line along the left lateral border, and the suture line anteriorly (Hoffman, Stylianos, & Jacir, 1990; Piehler, Payne, Cameron, & Pairolero, 1984). The long-term outcome of this procedure in children awaits further definition.

Pyloroplasty

Disordered gastric motility has frequently been observed in infants and children with gastroesophageal reflux, and the effectiveness of prokinetic medications in the medical management of reflux highlights this problem as a contributory factor in the pathogenesis of complicated reflux (Jolley, Tunell, Leonard, Hoelzer, & Smith, 1987;

McCallum, 1990). An association between failed antireflux operation and delayed gastric emptying has also been suggested (Maddern, Jamieson, Chatterton, & Collins, 1986).

Fonkalsrud, Berquist, Vargas, Ament, and Foglia (1987) from the University of California, Los Angeles reported a series of 352 children with complicated gastroesophageal reflux referred for surgical management. All children were studied preoperatively with radionuclide gastric emptying scans, in addition to 24-hour pH probe, esophageal manometry, and barium swallow examination. Of the total group, 32 patients required either simultaneous antireflux procedure with pyloroplasty (26 patients) or subsequent pyloroplasty after an antireflux operation (6 patients). Another group of six patients required pyloroplasty alone to successfully manage the reflux. The preoperative findings in this small group consisted of significantly delayed gastric emptying with a mildly abnormal pH probe result and normal lower esophageal sphincter pressure. Of note, 121 patients (34%) in the total series demonstrated some degree of central nervous system dysfunction, and 22 (18%) of these patients required pyloroplasty. This incidence represented twice the percentage of those with no central nervous system abnormalities who required a gastric emptying procedure. Another view of these data reveals that 69% of children requiring pyloroplasty were neurologically impaired, whereas only 4% of neurologically normal children had a similar requirement. Interestingly, experimental evidence has also implicated central nervous system injury with disordered gastric motility. Mathews et al (1988) have demonstrated alterations in the migrating myoelectric complexes (MMC) in the antral and prepyloric areas under conditions of acute brain injury in a feline model of elevated intracranial pressure and suggest that this may, in part, explain the require-

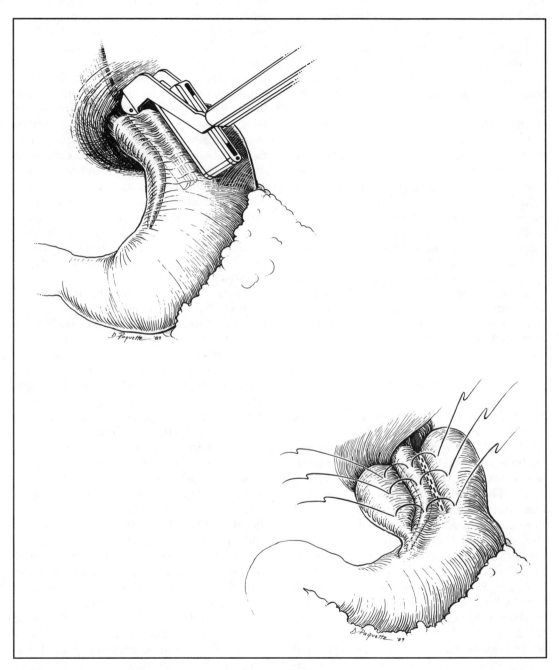

Figure 13–5.
The uncut Collis-Nissen fundoplication. The essential features include esophageal lengthening along the lesser curvature of the stomach and a loose 360° wrap of the fundus around the neo-esophagus. (From Hoffman, M. A., Styianos, S., & Jacir, N. N. [1990]. Technique of the transabdominal uncut Collis-Nissen fundoplication. *Pediatric Surgery International*, *5*, 471–472, with permission).

ment for pyloroplasty in as many as a third of children with neurologic disorders who demonstrate gastroesophageal reflux.

Papaila et al. (1989) from the Riley Hospital for Children in Indianapolis evaluated 99 infants and children with symptomatic gastroesophageal reflux by radionuclide gastric emptying scans. In 28 patients (28.2%), the scan demonstrated significant delay in gastric transit. Seventy-five percent of these patients had severe neurological dysfunction. Twenty-one of these patients underwent pyloroplasty at the time of initial fundoplication, and an additional 5 patients required pyloroplasty as a secondary procedure because of clinically significant delayed gastric emptying manifested as early satiety, postprandial pain, "gas-bloat," and gagging. This group advocates the preoperative evaluation of gastric emptying in all patients prior to fundoplication, with the addition of pyloroplasty when indicated by a significantly abnormal result.

Gastrostomy

Surgical gastrostomy remains a cornerstone in the nutritional support of patients in whom oral alimentation is not feasible and sustained nasogastric intubation is not possible or practical (Rempel, Colwell, & Nelson, 1988). The introduction and refinement of endoscopic techniques for gastrostomy tube placement has added a further dimension to the topic, and this procedure has demonstrated a wide applicability with low morbidity in skilled hands (Gauderer, 1991; Gregoire, Morin, Rousseau, & Lacerte, 1989; Ponsky & Gauderer, 1989; Ponsky, Gauderer, Stellato, & Aszodi, 1985). Infants as small as 2.5 kilograms have undergone successful gastric intubation with this technique, and the reported morbidity is less than 3% in experienced centers (Gauderer, 1991).

Although the universal caveat: "if the gut works, use it" is sensible from a physi-

ologic perspective, it must be interpreted with caution in the setting of gastroesophageal reflux, where the digestive functions of the gut are indeed preserved, but the protective mechanisms are faulty. Gastrostomy tube feeding under these circumstances may become a frustrating and futile exercise secondary to vomiting or lead to the sequelae of aspiration pneumonitis or worsening malnutrition. The danger is especially salient in the child with defective oropharyngeal protective mechanisms (Mollitt, Golladay, & Seibert, 1985; Stringel et al., 1989). This has spawned a controversy regarding routine or "protective" antireflux procedures at the time of gastrostomy in all children with neurologic impairment, even in the absence of gastroesophageal reflux.

Wesley, Coran, Sarahan, Klein, and White (1981) have demonstrated the need for thorough evaluation of the child with central nervous system dysfunction referred for gastrostomy tube placement and underscored the scope to this problem. In a group of 22 children with neurologic impairment referred to the surgical service for gastrostomy tube placement at the University of Michigan, 19 patients demonstrated significant gastroesophageal reflux on barium swallow examination. The majority of these patients presented with symptoms of either vomiting and failure to thrive (73%) or episodic aspiration pneumonitis (23%). All patients in this series underwent concomitant Nissen fundoplication, with 18 of 22 (82%) patients rendered symptom-free and tolerant of gastrostomy tube feedings. This report highlights the importance of the preoperative evaluation of the neurologically impaired child being considered for gastrostomy tube placement. Few pediatric surgeons would disagree with this admonition, nor the need for an antireflux procedure in conjunction with gastrostomy when gastroesophageal reflux is documented.

The focal point of debate centers on whether an antireflux procedure should be routinely coupled to the placement of a gastrostomy in all children with neurologic impairment, irregardless of the presence or absence of gastroesophageal reflux on preoperative evaluation. Jolley, Smith, and Tunell (1985) from Oklahoma reported 32 children, 28 of whom (88%) had central nervous system disease, who were referred for feeding gastrostomy and studied preoperatively with barium swallow and extended pH probe monitoring. Of these patients, 23 (72%) had demonstrable gastroesophageal reflux, and 22 of these patients underwent combined gastrostomy and antireflux operation. The 9 patients without demonstrable reflux underwent gastrostomy alone. In the latter group, 6 of the 9 patients developed significant gastroesophageal reflux on postgastrostomy extended pH probe study, and persistent vomiting with gastrostomy tube feedings developed in four patients (three required an antireflux procedure and one died from unspecified causes). Thus, 29 of the 32 patients (91%) were considered to be potentially "at risk" for the development of gastroesophageal reflux, either pre- or postgastrostomy tube placement. The conclusion drawn from the data is a need for a "protective" antireflux operation in children with central nervous system impairment referred for feeding gastrostomy. Although this report appears compelling, the group of particular interest was patients without preoperative gastroesophageal reflux who subsequently developed significant reflux after gastrostomy. Less than half (44%) of the children without reflux prior to gastrostomy followed a progression to symptoms severe enough to warrant an antireflux operation.

Langer et al. (1988) from the Hospital for Sick Children in Toronto reported a similar finding in 50 neurologically impaired children undergoing gastrostomy alone in the absence of preoperative gastroesophageal reflux. In this group, 22 patients (44%) subsequently developed symptomatic reflux, with 17 patients (34%) requiring an antireflux procedure subsequent to gastrostomy. Wheatley, Wesley, Tkach, and Coran (1991) from the University of Michigan reported a group of 43 children with neurologic impairment and negative evaluation for gastroesophageal reflux who underwent gastrostomy alone. Only 6 children (14%) from this group went on to develop significant reflux.

Although a consensus is difficult to reach on this topic, the experience thus far supports the conclusion that routine antireflux procedure in conjunction with feeding gastrostomy should not be contemplated in the absence of demonstrable gastroesophageal reflux in children with neurologic impairment. Although it has been shown experimentally that gastrostomy placement appears to decrease lower esophageal sphincter pressure (Canal, Vane, Goto, Gardner, & Grosfeld, 1987), the significance of this finding from a clinical vantage point is only partially substantiated and not uniformly noted (Grunow, Al-Hafidh, & Tunell, 1989).

Recently, Stringel (1990) has advocated lesser curvature gastrostomy to obviate the adverse physiologic effects of the standard greater curvature intubation. In nine neurologically impaired patients in which this technique was performed, none developed clinical evidence of gastroesophageal reflux. It is proposed that this method prevents the development of gastroesophageal reflux by increasing the length of the intraabdominal esophagus and the acuity of the angle of His, thereby reinforcing the antireflux barrier. Although these early results are encouraging, a larger series is required before definite recommendations can be made.

A unified approach (see Figure 13–6) to the management of gastrostomy tube placement in the child with central nervous system dysfunction includes a thor-

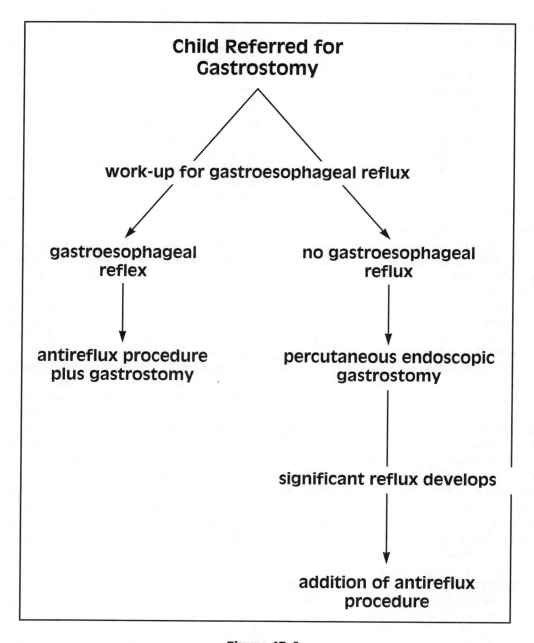

Figure 13–6.
Algorithm for the management of the child referred for gastrostomy tube placement.

ough work-up for gastroesophageal reflux. In the absence of reflux, a percutaneous gastrostomy is the simplest method of gastric intubation. If close follow-up reveals symptomatic and refractory gastroesophageal reflux, then antireflux operation should be performed.

Alternatives to Antireflux Procedures

On occasion, a child will present with complicated gastroesophageal reflux and feeding dysfunction for whom an antireflux procedure is not appropriate. The circumstances that may contraindicate the performance of an antireflux procedure in the setting of clinically significant gastroesophageal reflux, while not absolute, generally include: (1) a patient whose general medical condition is so poor that only the simplest and expeditious procedure, generally under a local anesthetic, would be reasonable; (2) a patient who continues to exhibit significant gastroesophageal reflux despite multiple failed antireflux procedures; and (3) a patient with an extremely limited life expectancy.

Although total parenteral nutrition via central venous access represents one option, the risks and complications of line placement, the long-term problems of line maintenance and sepsis, and the high cost of this mode of nutritional support render it an unattractive alternative when some form of enteral feeding is possible (McArdle, Palmason, Morency, & Brown, 1981). Likewise, prolonged utilization of nasoduodenal/jejunal feeding catheters can be cumbersome, and entail the requirement for tube placement under radiologic or endoscopic guidance, the problems of inadvertent tube displacement or dislodgment, and particulate occlusion and tube fatigue necessitating replacement. As a

general rule, patients whose projected requirement for tube feedings exceeds 3 months should be considered for surgical or percutaneous enteric intubation (Moore & Greene, 1985). In the setting of significant gastroesophageal reflux, when an antireflux procedure is deemed inappropriate, the surgical alternatives revolve around some form of jejunostomy. Several options exist: (1) Witzel or Stamm jejunostomy; (2) Roux-en-Y (Maydl) or "small-stoma" isoperistaltic tube jejunostomy; (3) "continent" Roux-en-Y jejunostomy; (4) open transpyloric jejunostomy; (5) simultaneous endoscopic transpyloric gastrostomy/jejunostomy; and, (6) fluoroscopically guided jejunal catheter placement via a surgically or endoscopically created gastrostomy tube tract. The major differences in each of these techniques are the anesthesia required to perform them, the presence or absence of a permanent jejunal stoma, and the ease with which reintubation can be performed should tube dislodgment occur.

The most basic techniques of long-term jejunostomy are the Witzel or Stamm jejunostomy techniques, in which a catheter is placed into a proximal loop of jejunum, either through concentric purse-string sutures (Stamm) or within a short serosal tunnel (Witzel), and brought out through the abdominal wall (Liu & Walker, 1991). Either technique may easily be performed through a limited incision under local anesthesia. The major drawback is the inconsistent ability to replace the tube should inadvertent dislodgment occur, and the occasional obstructive effect of the Witzel jejunostomy.

The Maydl Roux-en-Y jejunostomy requires a general anesthetic to perform, and has the added relative disadvantage of an intestinal anastomosis, making the procedure more time consuming. The proximal end of a 40 centimeter Roux limb is matured to the skin, allowing for "blind" reintubation. However, the tube must be advanced well into the Roux limb to prevent reflux of the feedings out of the stoma, and it often becomes necessary to perform this under fluoroscopic guidance to prevent kinking of the tube during the intubation process. Other problems with this technique include skin excoriation and stomal prolapse. The "small stoma" isoperistaltic jejunostomy is created by fashioning a small "tube" of antimesenteric full-thickness jejunal wall beginning in the caudad direction using the GIA stapling device (Bernstein, Brunicardi, Seymour, & Stillman, 1989). The proximal portion of this tubularized portion of jejunal wall is then matured to the skin as a stoma, which is easily reintubated. The procedure may be performed under a local anesthetic. Experience with this technique in pediatric patients is minimal, and it is unlikely that small children would be suitable candidates for this method because of the limited diameter of the small intestine.

A continent feeding jejunostomy in children has been described by Azizkhan, Lacey, and Herbst (1989) from the University of North Carolina, Chapel Hill, and consists of a short Roux-en-Y limb with an intussuscepted "nipple-valve" constructed near the proximal end, just below the abdominal wall (Herbst, 1980). The technique has several attractive features. The stoma is easily reintubated, and it requires a much shorter length of tubing for successful intubation and feeding. The valve mechanism eliminates seepage of intestinal contents or feedings onto the abdominal wall. The Chapel Hill group has also found that bolus feedings were well tolerated via this form of jejunostomy. Intermittent catheterization rather than a chronic indwelling catheter is therefore feasible, as the stoma is easily accessed. The procedure requires a general anesthetic to perform. A potential problem of nipple-valve disruption exists, with resultant loss of continence of the jejunostomy in the face of a very short Roux limb. This would result in considerable leakage of intestinal contents onto the abdominal wall and the need for early revision.

The final three forms of jejunostomy are permutations of the concept of jejunal intubation through a surgically or endoscopically placed gastrostomy tract. This may be performed either at the time of initial gastrostomy formation or as a delayed procedure. An advantage of these procedures is that simultaneous gastric drainage and jejunal feeding may be accomplished, thereby venting the stomach to discouraging reflux, while at the same time providing enteral nutrition "downstream."

In general, all forms of long-term jejunal feeding represent a compromise, from a surgical perspective, to the correction of the underlying problem of gastroesophageal reflux and gastrostomy tube placement. By bypassing the stomach, regulatory parameters of digestion are short-circuited, and problematic diarrhea, gastric bacterial overgrowth, and gastric atrophy are encouraged.

Summary

Procedures for the correction of complicated gastroesophageal reflux are commonly performed operations in most pediatric surgical centers, and the majority of children requiring these procedures exhibit some degree of neurologic impairment or developmental disability. Unfortunately, there is an apparent dichotomy when the results in this group of children are compared to those in otherwise normal children. This appears to hold true for both of the standard operations, the Nissen and Thal fundoplications, and has led to a general sense of frustration and dissatisfaction within the pediatric surgical community. Clearly, operative procedures that are appropriate to one group of children may not be reasonable for another, and further investigation and refinement of operative design and technique represent a fertile area for surgical clinical research.

References

Alrabeeah, A., Giacomantonio, M., & Gillis, D. A. (1988). Paraesophageal hernia after Nissen fundoplication: A real complication in pediatric patients. *Journal of Pediatric Surgery, 23*, 766–768.

Ashcraft, K. W. (1986). Thal fundoplication. In K. W. Ashcraft & T. M. Holder (Eds.), *Pediatric esophageal surgery* (pp. 209–216). Orlando, FL: Grune & Stratton.

Ashcraft, K. W., Goodwin, C. D., Amoury, R. W., McGill, C. W., & Holder, T. M. (1978). Thal fundoplication: A safe and simple operative treatment for gastroesophageal reflux. *Journal of Pediatric Surgery, 13*, 643–647.

Azizkhan, R. G., Lacey, S. R., & Herbst Jr., C. A. (1989). Continent feeding jejunostomy in children. *Pediatric Surgery International, 4*, 288–290.

Bernstein, M. O., Brunicardi, F. C., Seymour, N. E., & Stillman, R. M. (1989). A technique for feeding jejunostomy. *Surgery, Gynecology & Obstetrics, 168*,173–174.

Bettex, M. & Oesch, I. (1983). The hiatus hernia saga. Ups and downs in gastroesophageal reflux: Past, present, and future perspectives. *Journal of Pediatric Surgery, 18*, 670–680.

Blane, C. E., Turnage, R. H., Oldham, K. T., & Coran, A. G. (1989). Long-term radiographic follow-up of the Nissen fundoplication in children. *Pediatric Radiology, 19*, 523–526.

Boix-Ochoa, J. (1986). Address of honored guest: The physiologic approach to the management of gastric esophageal reflux. *Journal of Pediatric Surgery, 21*, 1032–1039.

Boix-Ochoa, J. (1987). Children and reflux. In T. R. DeMeester & H. R. Matthews (Eds.), *International trends in general thoracic surgery: Benign esophageal disease* (Vol. 3, pp. 205–218). St. Louis, MO: C.V. Mosby.

Cadman, D., Richard, J., & Feldman, W. (1978). Gastro-esophageal reflux in severely retarded children. *Developmental Medicine and Child Neurology, 20*, 95–98.

Canal, D. F., Vane, D. W., Goto, S., Gardner, G. P., & Grosfeld, J. L. (1987). Reduction of lower esophageal sphincter pressure with Stamm gastrostomy. *Journal of Pediatric Surgery, 22*, 54–57.

Caniano, D. A., Ginn-Pease, M. E., & King, D. R. (1990). The failed antireflux procedure: Analysis of risk factors and morbidity. *Journal of Pediatric Surgery, 25*, 1022–1026.

Dedinsky, G. K., Vane, D. W., Black, T., Turner M. K., West, K. W., & Grosfeld, J. L. (1987). Complications and reoperation after Nissen fundoplication in childhood. *American Journal of Surgery, 153*, 177–183.

DeMeester, T. R., Bonavina, L.,& Albertucci, M. (1986). Nissen fundoplication for gastroesophageal reflux disease: Evaluation of primary repair in 100 consecutive patients. *Annals of Surgery, 204*, 9–20.

Edwards, D. A. W. (1982). The anti-reflux mechanism, its disorders and their consequences. *Clinics in Gastroenterology, 11*, 479–496.

Ferraris, V. A., Martinez, L., & Burrington, J. D. (1985). Modified fundoplication technique for correction of gastroesophageal reflux in children. *Surgery, Gynecology & Obstetrics, 161*, 379–380.

Fonkalsrud, E. W., Ament, M. E., & Berquist, W. (1985). Surgical management of the gastroesophageal reflux syndrome in childhood. *Surgery, 97*,42–48.

Fonkalsrud, E. E., Berquist, W., Vargas, J., Ament, M. E., & Foglia, R. P. (1987). Surgical treatment of the gastroesophageal reflux syndrome in infants and children. *American Journal of Surgery, 154*, 11–18.

Gauderer, M. W. L. (1991). Percutaneous endoscopic gastrostomy: A ten-year experience with 220 children. *Journal of Pediatric Surgery, 26*, 288–294.

Gregoire, R. C., Morin, J., Rousseau, B., & Lacerte, M. (1989). Percutaneous endoscopic gastrostomy made easier. *Surgery, Gynecology & Obstetrics, 168*, 171–172.

Grunow, J. E., Al-Hafidh, A. S., & Tunell, W. P. (1989). Gastroesophageal reflux following percutaneous endoscopic gastrostomy is children. *Journal of Pediatric Surgery, 24,* 42–45.

Guggenbichler, J. P. & Menardi, G. (1985). Conservative treatment of gastroesophageal reflux and hiatus hernia. *Progress in Pediatric Surgery, 18,* 78–83.

Herbst Jr., C. A. (1980). Continent feeding jejunostomy. *Surgery, Gynecology & Obstetrics, 151,* 555–556.

Hoffman, M. A., Stylianos, S., Jacir, N. N. (1990). Technique of the transabdominal uncut Collis-Nissen fundoplication. *Pediatric Surgery International, 5,* 471–472.

Holmes, T. W. (1971). Chalasia, peptic esophagitis, and hiatal hernia. A common syndrome in patients with central nervous system disease. *Chest, 60,*441–445.

Jamieson, G. G., & Duranceau, A. (1984). What is a Nissen fundoplication? *Surgery, Gynecology & Obstetrics, 159,* 591–593.

Johnson, D. G. (1985). Current thinking on the role of surgery in gastroesophageal reflux. *Pediatric Clinics of North America, 32,* 1165–1179.

Johnson, D. G. (1986). The Nissen fundoplication. In K. W. Ashcraft & T. M. Holder (Eds.), Pediatric esophageal surgery (pp. 193–208). Orlando, FL: Grune & Stratton.

Johnson, D. G. & Beasley, S. W. (1991). Gastrooesophageal reflux. In S. W. Beasley, N. A. Myers, & A. W. Auldist (Eds.), *Oesophageal atresia* (pp. 341–358). London: Chapman & Hall Medical.

Jolley, S. G., Smith, E. I., & Tunell, W. P. (1985). Protective antireflux operation with feeding gastrostomy. Experience with children. *Annals of Surgery, 201,* 736–740.

Jolley, S. G., Tunell, W. P., Hoelzer, D. J.,& Smith, E. I. (1986). Postoperative small bowel obstruction in infants and children: a problem following Nissen fundoplication. *Journal of Pediatric Surgery, 21,* 407–409.

Jolley, S. G., Tunell, W. P., Leonard, J. C., Hoelzer, D. J.,& Smith, E. I. (1987). Gastric emptying in children with gastroesophageal reflux. II. The relationship to retching symptoms following antireflux surgery. *Journal of Pediatric Surgery, 22,* 927–930.

Jonsell, G., & De Mestier, P. (1984). Comparison of diagnostic methods for selection of patients for antireflux operations. *Surgery, 95,* 2–5.

Katz, P. O. & Castell, D. O. (1987). Function of the normal human esophagus. In T. R. DeMeester & H. R. Matthews (Eds.), *International trends in general thoracic surgery: Benign esophageal disease,* (Vol. 3, pp. 3–15). St. Louis, MO: C. V. Mosby Co.

Langer, J. C., Wesson, D. E., Ein, S. H., Filler, R. M., Shandling, B., Superina, R. A., & Papa, M. (1988). Feeding gastrostomy in neurologically impaired children: Is an antireflux procedure necessary? *Journal of Pediatric Gastroenterology and Nutrition, 7,* 837–841.

Liu, K. J. M. & Walker, F. W. (1991). Surgical procedures on the small intestine. In G. D. Zuidema & L. M. Nyhus (Eds.), *Shackelford's Surgery of the alimentary tract,* (Vol. 5, 3rd ed., pp. 264–285). Philadelphia, PA: W. B. Saunders.

Maddern, G. J., Jamieson, G. G., Chatterton, B. E., & Collins, P. J. (1986). Is there an association between failed antireflux procedures and delayed gastric emptying? *Annals of Surgery, 202,* 162–165.

Matthews, D. E., Heimansohn, D. A., Papaila, J. G., Lopez, R., Vane, D. W., & Grosfeld, J. L. (1988). The effect of increased intracranial pressure (ICP) on gastric motility. *Journal of Surgical Research, 45,* 60–65.

McArdle, A. H., Palmason, C., Morency, I., & Brown, R. A. (1981). A rationale for enteral feeding as the preferable route for hyperalimentation. *Surgery, 90,* 616–623.

McCallum, R. W. (1990). Gastric emptying in gastroesophageal reflux and the therapeutic role of prokinetic agents. *Gastroenterology Clinics of North America, 19,* 551–564.

Mollitt, D. L., Golladay, S., & Seibert, J. J. (1985). Symtomatic gastroesophageal reflux following gastrostomy in neurologically impaired patients. *Pediatrics, 75,* 1124–1126.

Moore, M. C. & Greene, H. L. (1985). Tube feeding in infants and children. *Pediatric Clinics of North America, 32,* 401–417.

Negre, J. B. (1983). Post-fundoplication symptoms—Do they restrict the success of Nissen fundoplication? *Annals of Surgery, 198*, 698–700.

Orringer, M. B. (1989). The collis-Nissen operation for reflux esophagitis. In L. M. Nyhus & R. E. Condon (Eds.), *Hernia* (pp. 653–667). Philadelphia, PA: J. B. Lippincott.

Papaila, J. G., Wilmot, D., Grosfeld, J. L., Rescorla, F. J., West, K. W., & Vane, D. W. (1989). Increased incidence of delayed gastric emptying in children with gastroesophageal reflux. *Archives of Surgery, 124*, 933–936.

Pearl, R. H., Robie, D. K., Ein, S .H., Shandling, B., Wesson, D. E., Superina, R., Mctaggart, K., Garcia, V. F., O'Connor, J. A., & Filler, R. M. (1990). Complications of gastroesophageal antireflux surgery in neurologically impaired versus neurologically normal children. Journal of *Pediatric Surgery, 25*, 1169–1173.

Piehler, J. M., Payne, W. S., Cameron, A. J., & Pairolero, P. C. (1984). The uncut Collis-Nissen procedure for esophageal hiatal hernia and its complications. *Problems in General Surgery, 1*, 1–14.

Polk, H. C. (1984). Operations for reflux esophagitis. Indications, techniques, and misadventures. In J. S. Najarian & J. P. Delaney (Eds.), *Advances in gastrointestinal surgery* (pp. 57–63), Chicago, IL: Year Book Medical Publishers.

Ponsky, J. L. & Gauderer, M. W. L. (1989). Percutaneous endoscopic gastrostomy: Indications, limitations, techniques, and results. *World Journal of Surgery, 13*, 165–170.

Ponsky, J. L., Gauderer, M. W. L., Stellato, T. A., & Aszodi, A. (1985). Percutaneous approaches to enteral alimentation. *American Journal of Surgery, 149*, 102–105.

Randolph, J. (1983). Experience with the Nissen fundoplication for correction of gastroesophageal reflux in infants. *Annals of Surgery, 198*, 579–584.

Ramenofsky, M. L. (1986). Gastroesophageal reflux: Clinical manifestations and diagnosis. In K. W. Ashcraft & T. M. Holder (Eds.), *Pediatric Esophageal Surgery* (pp. 151–179). Orlando, FL: Grune & Stratton.

Rempel, G. R., Colwell, S. O., & Nelson, R. P. (1988). Growth in children with cerebral palsy fed via gastrostomy. *Pediatrics, 82*, 857–862.

Robie, D .K. & Pearl, R. H. (1991). Modified Nissen fundoplication: Improved results in high-risk children. *Journal of Pediatric Surgery, 26*, 1268–1272.

Ross, A. J. (1994). Fundoplication for gastroesophageal reflux in infants and children. In D. C. Sabiston (Ed.), *Atlas of general surgery* (pp. 316–322). Norwalk, CT: Appleton & Lange.

Rouse, T. M., Guzzetta Jr., P. C. & Randolph, J. (1989). Gastroesophageal reflux in infants and children. In L. M. Nyhus, L. M. & R. E. Condon (Eds.), *Hernia* (pp. 614–622). Philadelphia, PA: J. B. Lippincott.

Skinner, D. B. (1985). Pathophysiology of gastroesophageal reflux. *Annals of Surgery, 202*, 546–556.

Smith, C. D., Otherson, H. B., Gogan, N. J., & Walker, J. D. (1992). Nissen fundoplication in children with profound neurologic disability: High risks and unmet goals. *Annals of Surgery, 215*, 654–659.

Spitz, L., & Kirtane, J. (1985). Results and complications of surgery for gastro-oesophageal reflux. *Archives of Disease in Childhood, 60*, 743–747.

Sondheimer, J. M. (1988). Gastroesophageal reflux: Update on pathogenesis & diagnosis. *Pediatric Clinics of North America, 35*, 103–116.

Sondheimer, J. M. & Morris, B. A. (1979). Gastroesophageal reflux amoung severely retarded children. *Journal of Pediatrics, 94*, 710–714.

Stringel, G. (1990). Gastrostomy with antireflux properties. *Journal of Pediatric Surgery, 25*, 1019–1021.

Stringel, G., Delgado, M., Guertin, L., Cook, J. D., Maravilla, A., & Worthen, H. (1989). Gastrostomy and Nissen fundoplication in neurologically impaired children. *Journal of Pediatric Surgery, 24*, 1044–1048.

Thal, A. P. (1968). A unified approach to surgical problems of the esophagogastric junction. *Annals of Surgery, 168*, 542–550.

Tovar, J. A., Morras, I., Garay, J.& Tapia, I. (1986). Etude fonctionnelle du reflux gastro-oesophagien chez les enfants encephalopathes. *Chirgury Pediatrique, 27,* 134–137.

Tuggle, D. W., Tunell, W. P., Hoelzer, D. J. & Smith, E. I. (1988). The efficacy of Thal fundoplication in the treatment of gastroesophageal reflux: The influence of central nervous system impairment. *Journal of Pediatric Surgery, 23,* 638–640.

Tunell, W. P., Smith, E. I. & Carson, J. A. (1983). Gastroesophageal reflux in childhood. The dilemma of surgical success. *Annals of Surgery, 197,* 560–565.

Turnage, R. H., Oldham, K. T., Coran, A. G. & Blane, C. E. (1989). Late results of fundoplication for gastroesophageal reflux in infants and children. *Surgery, 105,* 457–464.

Vane, D. W., Shiffler, M., Grosfeld, J. L., Hall, P., Angelides, A., Weber, T. R. & Fitzgerald, J. F. (1982). Reduced lower esophageal sphincter (LES) pressure after acute and chronic brain injury. *Journal of Pediatric Surgery, 17,* 960–964.

Wesley, J. R., Coran, A. G., Sarahan, T. M., Klein, M. D., & White, S. J. (1981). The need for evaluation of gastroesophageal reflux in brain-damaged children referred for feeding gastrostomy. *Journal of Pediatric Surgery, 16,* 866–871.

Wheatley, M. J., Coran, A. G., Wesley, J. R., Oldham, K. T, & Turnage, R. H. (1991). Redo fundoplication in infants and children with recurrent gastroesophageal reflux. *Journal of Pediatric Surgery, 26,* 758–761.

Wheatley, M. J., Wesley, J. R., Tkach, D. M. & Coran, A. G. (1991). Long-term follow-up of brain-damaged children requiring feeding gastrostomy: Should an antireflux procedure always be performed? *Journal of Pediatric Surgery, 26,* 301–305.

Wilkins, B. M., & Spitz, L. (1987). Adhesion obstruction following Nissen fundoplication in children. *British Journal of Surgery, 74,* 777–779.

CHAPTER

14

Dental Treatment

EDWARD M. SONNENBERG, D.D.S.

CONTENTS

The typical dental school curriculum often lacks exposure to either didactic or clinical care for individuals with disabilities. Disabling conditions are never adequately presented as a group of problems (both medical and dental) that require special care in performing even routine dental procedures, and there is currently no textbook in print on dentistry for the disabled. To understand the "hows" of dental care for children with developmental disabilities, the dentist must first have an adequate understanding of developmental disabilities and the specific dental conditions routinely associated with specific disabilities. The purpose of this chapter is to define developmental disabilities from a dental perspective and describe techniques of dental treatment for children with developmental disabilities.

The Triad of Treatment

When performing dental treatment on children with developmental disabilities, three people are involved: the child (patient), the parent (guardian or caretaker), and the dentist.

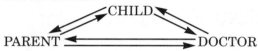

The Child

Children with developmental disabilities, like all children, can react to dental personnel and treatment with attitudes ranging from benign acceptance to violent refusal. The child may enjoy the attention from the dentist and the stimulation of the vibrating cleaning cup; at the opposite extreme, opening his or her mouth and keeping it open might be perceived by some children with developmental disabilities as a life-threatening action. The extent of a child's physical compromise (e.g., cardiac lesions, susceptibility to recurrent infections also can limit his or her facility in cooperating with treatment. Depending on the extent of care needed and the child's ability to cooperate, regular, routine dental care is possible for many children with developmental disabilities.

The Parent

Depending on the self-help ability of the child with developmental disabilities, he or she may have to rely on someone else for varying degrees of care. Some parents reject the disabled child; others overprotect the child. Both attitudes can compromise good dental care. If dental evaluation is avoided by an overprotective parent, optimal care is not possible; early decay can go untreated.

The parent (guardian or caretaker) is best able to disclose the child's level of cooperative ability and impart the child's abilities and limitations to the professional (e.g. brushes own teeth, wears hearing aids, glasses, or dentures). Parents of children with developmental disabilities will go through three general stages in dealing with the identification of their children's disabilities:

1. Disorganization: The parent will seek out many specialists (doctors, psychologists, therapists) to treat the child and try to find a miracle cure.
2. Reintegration: The parent will try to work with the child on his or her own to overcome the disability.
3. Mature Adaptation: The parent finally will accept the child's problem and cope with it constructively.

The Dentist

In a busy practice, it can be difficult to regularly "mainstream" patients with developmental disabilities into the everyday group of patients. It can take longer to complete procedures on some patients with developmental disabilities. Making an office accessible by design (hallways, doorways, corners) may be difficult with limited office space. Federal regulations must be known and adhered to in construction today.

Nondisabled patients may feel uncomfortable sharing reception room space with a disabled patient. If this proves to be a problem, time can be set aside on a regular basis and reserved for treatment of children with disabilities. Appointments may be broken with greater frequency due to medically compromising conditions or physical constraints (e.g., wheelchairs don't go in snow). Extensive care may require the dentist to deal with various agencies (e.g., Association for Retarded Citizens, United Cerebral Palsy, Division of Guardianship of the respective state, federal agencies), expanding the post-doctoral education of the dentist into previously unknown areas.

Developmental Disabilities

Mental Retardation

Mental Retardation (MR) is defined as significantly below-average general intellectual functioning existing concurrently with deficits in adaptive behavior and manifested during the developmental period. Approximately 3% of the population is retarded. Below average intellectual functioning is measured as an IQ below 70. The American Association of Mental Deficiency (AAMD) classifies the retarded into four groups (Capute, 1974):

1. Mildly or Educable Retarded (EMR): IQ 55–69
2. Moderately or Trainable Retarded (TMR): IQ 40–54)
3. Severely Mentally Retarded (SMR): IQ 25–39
4. Profoundly Mentally Retarded (PMR): IQ below 25

The child who is EMR often is diagnosed only after he or she starts school. The child's level of impairment may be mild enough so that his or her intellectual limitations go unnoticed. Optimally, individuals in the EMR range function at the third- to sixth-grade level (9–12 years of age). Approximately 80% of the EMR attain employment. With proper habilitation, 20% of those employed work in skilled occupations.

Children with IQs in the TMR range function at a mental age of 4–8 years and are routinely identified in early childhood. A significant developmental lag will exist in attainment of developmental milestones and in language development. The goal for children in the TMR range is enhancement of self-help skills, social and communication skills for living, and working in a sheltered environment. Children with IQs in the TMR range will need supervision and/ or assistance in daily living activities. Factitious illness (self-induced trauma) can be a persistent problem for some with IQs in the TMR range.

Many children with IQs in the SMR ranges have biochemical or genetic disorders and demonstrate several features characteristics into syndromes. Some common features include hirsutism (hairiness), microcephaly (small head), and dysplastic (malformed) teeth. Children in the SMR and PMR ranges are more limited than those in the TMR range, and their self-help, communication, and social skills should be maximized so that their interactions and care can remain optimal either at home or other care facilities. Other than the technical aspects of repairing a specific tooth or cleaning a certain mouth, children who are retarded may present a problem based on communication. Adverse reaction to dental treatment is often the result of communication that is misread by the retarded patient. If a child's behavior deteriorates, behavior management is the key. (Behaviorally oriented care is explained in the section on Dental Care).

Down Syndrome

Down syndrome is the most common pattern of genetic malformation in humans. It was first identified by John Hayden Down in 1866 (Nowak, 1976). Trisomy 21, the genetic cause of Down syndrome, is seen in 1:660 live births, and its presence is associated with advancing maternal and paternal age. The common findings associated with Down syndrome include a flattened forehead, brachycephaly (reduced head anterior-posterior dimension), eczema, hypoplasia of frontal sinus, a small nasal bridge, oblique slant of eyes, narrow palpebral fissures, epicanthal folds, ear anomalies, simean crease of the palm, a short, thick neck (a potential problem with general anesthesia), cardiac anomalies, and leukocyte aberrations. Dental abnormalities include scrotal tongue, relative macroglossia, palatal abnormalities, hypoplastic maxilla, occlusal disharmonies, reduced tooth number, delayed tooth eruption, dysplastic teeth, and rapidly progressing periodontal disease. The periodontal disease is so aggressive, that if left untreated will cause significant tooth loss early in life (Barnett, Press, Friedman, & Sonnenberg, 1986). The IQ of children with Down syndrome rarely is above 50, but their social performance is routinely higher. Some children with Down syndrome also can display a stubborn and obstinate attitude that can present problems with dental care.

Other Syndromes

Other chromosomal and inherited syndromes of mental retardation also have characteristic systemic and oral manifestations. Some of these include Hunter's and Hurler's syndromes, Tay Sachs syndrome, Cri du Chat, Rubinstein Taybi syndrome, Lesch-Nyan syndrome. Other than Down syndrome, the dentist might be familiar only with the Lesch-Nyan syndrome due to its characteristic self-mutilation activities.

Physical Handicaps

Physical disabilities in children can present some of the most frustrating cases to treat because the barrier to care is not one of the understanding; instead, the patient's disability produces a "physical barrier" to care.

Cerebral Palsy

Cerebral Palsy (CP) is a general term used to describe a group of nonprogressive muscle and nerve disorders caused by brain damage that occurred either prenatally, during birth, or during the postnatal period before the central nervous system reaches maturity (Nowak, 1976). The incidence of cerebral palsy is 1–2 per 1,000 births (Capute, 1974). Motor disabilities arising from spinal cord injuries are excluded from the definition of CP as are progressive neuromuscular diseases.

The causes of CP include anoxia, intracranial hemorrhage, trauma, premature birth, infection, toxemia of pregnancy, Rh incompatibility, and developmental anomalies. Many children who have CP also have an additional disability such as a seizure disorder, mental retardation, or complicating behavioral or emotional disorders (Nowak, 1976). Approximately 50% have normal intelligence. The physiologic (motor) classification of CP includes spasticity, athetosis, rigidity, ataxia, tremor, atonia, and mixed types. The most common types are spastic (50%) and athetoid (25%). The topographical classification includes monoplegia, paraplegia, hemiplegia, triplegia, quadriplegia, and double hemiplegia.

Dental findings in children with cerebral palsy include bruxism; a narrow, high palate; a high incidence of malocclusion (from swallowing and speech patterns) and periodontal disease (from poor oral hygiene); and hypoplastic enamel defects (formation defects). Involuntary movements and exaggerated bite reflexes present challenges and hazards for both patient and doctor. Severe wear of teeth can produce bite changes that could initiate temporo-mandibular-dysfunction and pain (TMJ).

Congenital Defects

Oral facial defects have been noted throughout history in many cultures. In the past, individuals were stigmatized or eliminated because of their malformations in some cultures; whereas in other cultures the defect was treated as a sign of divine intervention (Nowak, 1976). The attitudes of contemporary society lies some where between the extremes of earlier cultures. These defects result from genetic conditions or environmental factors. Faulty development can occur in different parts of the head and its bones and in some syndromes creates a characteristic appearance. Children with Crouzon's or Apert's syndrome (cranio-facial dysostosis with premature closure of cranial sutures), for example, demonstrate underdeveloped middle face with an exophthalmic appearance. Pierre Robin Syndrome is associated with hypoplasia of the mandible, glossoptosis, posterior displacement of the tongue, and isolated clefts of the hard palate. Life-threatening neonatal respiratory problems can occur as the mandible's small size can force the tongue against the posterior pharyngeal wall. Often the mandible will experience catch up growth after the newborn period, and the microgenia usually disappears during the preschool years.

Dental considerations for the patient with congenital craniofacial defects range from routine dental care to treatment of the malformation. If the child with the congenital defect is also retarded, the child may be very difficult to treat.

Mandibulo-facial dysostosis (Treacher Collins syndrome) is a syndrome related to the development of the head and neck structures referred to as branchial arches in embryonic life. Different facial structures are affected; in addition to mental retardation, children with mandibulo-facial dysostosis also demonstrate mandibular

hypoplasia, zygomatic hypoplasia, anti-Mongolian eye slants, external ear defects, a fish-like mouth, a highly arched or cleft palate, and a high frequency of malocclusion and dysplastic, displaced teeth (Nowak, 1976). Skin tags may exist on the face between the ear and the mouth.

Cleft Lip and/or Cleft Palate

Clefts on the lips and/or palate are the most frequently seen orofacial defect. Clefting occurs in approximately 1:1,000 births, but its incidence is greater in different ethnic groups, more common in Japanese, less common in Blacks or Jews (Nowak, 1976). Parental age has little influence on incidence. Clefts can be of just the lip, the lip and primary palate (unilateral or bilateral), a midline cleft of the posterior palate, a through and through cleft of the lip, or include both the primary and posterior palate.

Problems associated with cleft lip and/or palate include psychologic, speech, otologic, and swallowing difficulties. Dental problems associated with cleft lip and/or palate include mouth growth and development, tooth number, malposed teeth, fused teeth, delayed eruption, and super eruption of teeth.

Soft tissue surgery for lip closure and nostril symmetry can be done at almost any age, but is usually performed when the baby is 3 months old. Many surgeons use the "rules of 10s," that is, that the child weighs at lest 10 pounds, has a hemoglobin of at least 10 grams, has a white count no higher than 10,000, and is at least 10 weeks of age. Generally, the primary cleft palate surgery can be performed before 2 years of age. It is desirable to repair the palate early enough to permit the child to develop normal speech, while avoiding adverse affects on growth and development of the maxillary arch and midface. Alveolar bone repair via grafts should be performed at the age of 9 years or older to avoid inhibition of the antero-posterior growth of the maxilla.

Sensory Disabilities

Blindness and deafness are the most common handicaps. Most sensory handicaps are the result of prenatal exposure to disease or congenital malformations that cause development of sensory handicaps. Because the child's cognitive ability is not affected, treatment must first be based on developing good methods of communication. The child who is deaf often can read lips (it is rare to understand more than half of what is lip read) but may communicate better in sign language. A significant concurrent problem of deafness is impairment of language development. Due to hearing problems and language deficiency, children who are deaf are sometimes misdiagnosed as mentally retarded.

Children who are blind may develop a greater acquity of other senses (hearing, smell) to compensate for the lack of vision. Blindness is one of the most easily noticed handicaps. With both blindness and deafness, the dentist must learn the level of the child's independence and dependence to provide appropriate treatment

Other Developmental Disabilities of Interest to Dentists

Autism

In 1944, Kanner described a group of patients who demonstrated a syndrome of an "inborn autistic disturbance of affective contact" (Kopel, 1977). Some of the characteristics of children who are autistic include delayed developmental milestones, mental retardation, neurologic immaturity, retarded bone age, feeding difficulties, self-stimulating behavior, overactivity, delayed language onset, problems with behavior and socialization, poor eye contact, resistance to being held, and inappropriate affect. Two thirds of children with autism achieve some functional speech, but parents often believe that their child has a hearing loss because they "act as though they were deaf." Echolalia (the repeating of a word or phrase spoken by the child) is another common finding. The autistic child is a behavioral challenge to the entire dental setting. From the fear of lying down to the intrusive examination of the mouth, the autistic child may struggle throughout the entire course of care. Continuous physical restraint by dental personnel and parents may be necessary just to examine the teeth.

Convulsive Disorders

Convulsive disorders may be the result of cerebral damage or insult before, during, or soon after birth. Many types of seizure conditions exist in children. Convulsions can occur at any age, but are most common during the first 2 years of life (Nowak, 1976). Some seizures are short-lived and have little effect on appearance (petit mal), whereas others can last several minutes and involve considerable body and head movements (grand mal). During a seizure the patient can inflict significant trauma to himself and can even experience the arrest of all respiratory movement. Drug Therapy can significantly improve a convulsive disorder. Some of the drugs used include Valium®, Phenobarbital®, Dilantin®, Depakane®, Tegretol®, and Mysoline®.

The combination of retardation and seizures creates a significantly difficult patient with potentially poor cooperation and the ever present concern of a possible seizure during treatment. High tooth decay rates and periodontal disease are common. Characteristic Dilantin® hyperplasia is the most commonly treated condition associated with seizure-prone patients (see Figunes 14–1 and 14–2). Overgrowth of

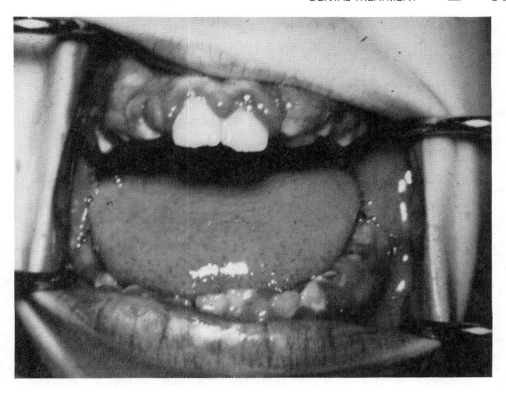

Figure 14–1.
Generalized mild Dilantin hyperplasia of the maxillary and mandibular gingiva of a seizure-prone patient.

gum tissue can be so severe that teeth disappear under the overgrowing tissue.

Attention Deficit Hyperactivity Disorder, Learning Disabilities, and Neurological Impairment

This is an interesting group of disabilities that present similarly in child behavior in the dental setting. Children with these disabilities demonstrate behavior problems (e.g., a short attention span), neurologic problems (e.g., asymmetric reflexes), psychologic problems (e.g., scattering of mental functioning), and auditory and visual perception disabilities. Children with these disabilities often behave as if they have a problem with processing certain input information.

It is estimated that up to 10% of school-age children demonstrate some type of cerebral dysfunction (Capute, 1974). Dyslexias comprise between 0.5 and 3% of children with an equal number demonstrating neurological impairment. Males are affected significantly more frequently than females.

Concerns in dental treatment for these patients include regular preventive/restorative care. Accomplishing this can, at times, be a challenge. Reaction to the sensation of local anesthesia or to the sound of the drill can provoke unwanted reactions. Impulse control can create problematical situations throughout treatment.

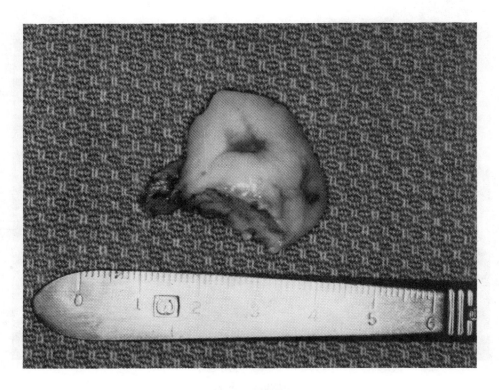

Figure 14–2.
A piece of hyperplastic gingiva that had caused a temporary blockage of the trachea of a seizure-prone patient. This tissue was removed as part of the gum reduction (gingivectomy) surgery performed on this patient in the operating room under general anesthesia.

Dental Care

Behavior

The behavior of a child with developmental disabilities in the dental setting is similar to that of any child. The setting should be structured so the child receives appropriate support from parents and dental personnel. The use of appropriate behavioral management techniques is critical. Treatment should be directed at the child's mental not chronological age. Usually this information is available from the child's social worker or psychologist or from school records. Once this information is at hand, appropriate techniques can be designed.

Mental Age Less Than 1 to 3 Years

Behavior techniques have little use here. Children with limited understanding may perceive even a dental examination as an unwanted intrusion. If the patient weighs over 100 pounds, the dispute over treatment can lead to frustration for all parties concerned. Depending on the extent of a child's dental care needs and the limitations of the child's attention span, treatment (fillings, gum treatment, extractions) may best be done with the patient sedated or under general anesthesia.

Mental Age 3 to 6 Years

With this group the most basic behavioral techniques show success. The goal should be elimination or reduction of negative behavior and support and promotion of positive behavior. The "tell, show, do" technique is the simplest behavioral technique to initiate. The patient is told what is to be done, then shown by example how it is done, and then the procedure is done. The goal is to prevent "tell, show, don't."

Voice control (the modulation of tonal quality of the voice) also is an effective tool to gain a child's attention.

Practicing the "hands down" exercise with an autistic child is a form of voice control. In the hands down exercise, the parent rehearses with the child at home before the scheduled visit so that the child will not reach and grab the hands of the dentist during treatment (Kopel, 1977). Extending voice modulation to whispering in a child's ear can prove just as effective as using a loud voice in gaining a child's attention. It is appropriate to follow the voice control with a supportive comment if the patient complies to promote positive behavior.

Other techniques that can be met with success include systematic desensitization and modeling. In the former, anxiety-provoking stimuli are gradually introduced to the patient to reduce acting out behavior in the dental setting. In modelling, a cooperative individual is shown to the patient so that future care can be modeled after successful care. This technique works well utilizing siblings and friends. The use of positively reinforced behavior often is successful in working with children with autism.

If behavioral techniques do not work satisfactorily, the use of sedative agents should be considered. Nitrous oxide relative analgesia can be of tremendous value if the child is willing to accept the mask and the physical sensations of the gas. If trust has already been established between doctor and patient, nitrous oxide can be attempted successfully. Nitrous oxide also is appropriate for children with cerebral palsy because it relaxes them and reduces rigidity and unwanted movement or mouth closure (a mouth prop or gag should routinely be used when treating a patient with an uncontrollable bite reflex).

Sedation should be the next level to be considered in treatment of children with developmental disabilities. Oral or intramuscular sedation can be used to facilitate dental care. However, the use of premedicating agents should not be attempted without special training. Proper noninvasive monitoring should be the only acceptable level of care. Including the onset, duration, and wear-off time, the premedicated patient will be sedated for up to 6 hours. During the time of treatment the practitioner should have no distractions so that full attention can be paid to the patient and all treatment can be completed in one visit. Following proper medical evaluation, safe treatment can even be done routinely under general anesthesia. Limitations including health of the child's mouth, type of procedure, and skills of the practitioner determine the plan of treatment for any patient.

Mental Age 6 Years and Older

By this stage any patient should be workable based on skills and desires of the dentist. A 6-year-old usually can be reasoned with and might need at most nitrous oxide to complete most routine dental treatment. It would be unusual to hospitalize a child for treatment under general anesthesia due to the level of this patient's understanding. When communicating with a child of school-age level or above, routine discussions should be appropriate for the child's age and not too infantile.

Dental Treatment

A total dental care program for children with developmental disabilities is made up of many components, the most basic of which—and the one with potentially the greatest impact—is prevention. Ideally, the patient should be the preventive practitioner when not at the dentist; however, if a child's mental or physical constraints prevent him or her from performing the preventive procedures, a parent, guardian, or caregiver must perform these duties. The use of a task analysis approach to evaluating oral hygiene ability is appropriate with these children (Figure 14–3). Included in a child's total preventive program should be brushing, flossing, fluoride toothpaste, and disclosing agents to expose plaque. Of course, the dentist must provide other components of prevention such as sealants, cleanings, scalings, topical fluoride applications and nutritional counseling (Sonnenberg & Shey, 1979). Eating properly is necessary for proper general development, including tooth development. All primary teeth (baby, milk, deciduous) begin formation prenatally, and only one cusp tip (point on a back tooth) of one secondary (permanent, succedaneous) molar begins formation prenatally. Therefore, primary tooth formation will be affected by the pregnant mother's nutrition, whereas permanent teeth will be under the control

CHART I

TOOTHBRUSHING PROGRESS SHEET

	Teacher provided NO CUES Student's performance was:		Teacher provided VERBAL CUES Student's performance was:		Teacher provided VERBAL AND VISUAL CUES Student's performance was:		Teacher provided VERBAL, VISUAL AND PHYSICAL CUES Student's performance was:	
	CORRECT	INCORRECT	CORRECT	INCORRECT	CORRECT	INCORRECT	CORRECT	INCORRECT
1. Pick up toothbrush								
2. Palmar grasp								
3. Brush outside surfaces-left								
4. Brush outside surfaces-right								
5. Brush inside surfaces-left								
6. Brush inside surfaces-right								
7. Brush biting surfaces-left								
8. Brush biting surfaces-right								
9. Rinse brush								
10. Rinse mouth (optional)								
11. Wipe mouth (optional)								
12. Put equipment away								
13. Discard disposables								

Figure 14–3.
The Task Analysis of Toothbrushing chart can be used with children with developmental disabilities to evaluate their ability to self-care. Deficient brushing can be evaluated, corrected, and reevaluated to determine effectiveness of training.

of post-natal nutrition. Teeth, unlike bone, do not have the general capacity for self-repair. If insult occurs, the tooth is permanently affected. The shape of the tooth and the color of the tooth are both susceptible to change from nutritional influences. Of course, it is easy say that a developmentally disabled child should get the same amounts of proper foods from the food groups that any child deserves. But a child with neuromuscular disorders who is unable to chew or swallow or feed himself may never get the optimal amount of food regularly. Once a child reaches adolescence, food choice will affect decay rate, and good oral hygiene becomes an even more critical factor. Physical disabilities can affect access to food, food preparation, feeding, digestion, and absorption. Dietary counseling for the child with developmental disabilities must focus on both decay control and weight control.

The dental examination must be performed to examine the extent of disease and the level of the child's dental care needs. Most practitioners have their own examination techniques and format. The parent (guardian or caregiver) is most important in completing the examination component of a child's care. Parents can relate the child's past history of care and inform the dentist of any special precautions that should be followed. Assisted restraint by the parent can help all participants in care both physically and emotionally (some parents, however, can be obstructive. The dentist must identify problem parents and create a working situation where treatment occurs.)

Taking dental x-rays can be a challenge with any patient. The child with developmental disabilities may make this an even greater challenge Again, utilization of the parent is critical. The parent can hold the x-ray film, the child's head, or both if the patient is unable to stay still with the film in his or her mouth. Other modifications to the usual techniques can be helpful. A Snap-A-Ray holder can provide an ignitable extra "pair of fingers" to hold the film between the child's teeth (Figure 14–4). Cross arch radiographs (Figure 14–5), although lacking in contrast at times, produce excellent views of both teeth and other hard tissues. Film size, utilizing this technique, can range from small intraoral x-rays to 8×10 inch head plates (Figures. 14–6 to 14–9).

As part of the medical history, a child's medication history must be ascertained, including past and present medications, and any unusual drug reactions the child has experienced. Many drugs can affect the teeth. The vehicle used in liquid medications can build up on the teeth and potentially cause either extrinsic discoloration or even decay. Tetracyclines have been known to cause intrinsic discoloration if administered during the ages when teeth are forming. Besides Dilantin®, calcium channel blockers (Nifetipine®, Procardia®) can cause gingival overgrowth. Cyclosporins can affect gingival health as can birth control pills. Besides diagnostic and preventive care, the dentist should provide all aspects of total patient care including aesthetic composite fillings, silver amalgam fillings, and crowns for badly decayed teeth. Ideally, replacement of missing teeth should be performed, if at all, with fixed bridges (cemented onto teeth) to eliminate concerns about removing or losing replacements. Full or partial dentures (false teeth) are contraindicated in people with insufficient muscle control or mental capabilities to enable then to wear the teeth.

Periodontal (gum) disease is ubiquitous to both disabled and nondisabled populations. Individuals with Down syndrome demonstrate a rapidly progressing form of periodontal disease that is more advanced than in both the non-Down syndrome retarded and the non-disabled populations. As early as the teenage years, the patient with Down syndrome may show advanced

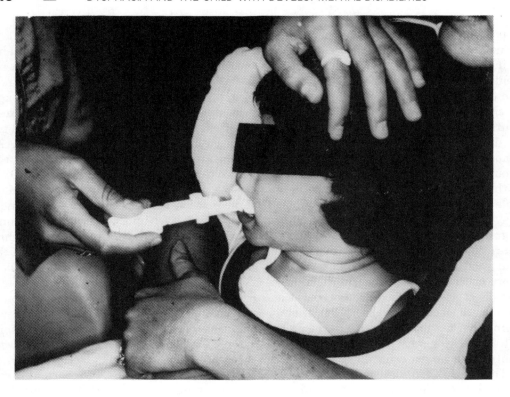

Figure 14–4.
Two parents hold the child in the chair for an x-ray. One parent is holding the Snap-A-Ray holder in the child's mouth with the x-ray film in place.

gum disease comparable to that of some-one 30 years older (Barnett et al., 1986). To date no demonstrable cause, other than lo-cal factors, has been associated with this aggressive form of gum disease.

Other modalities of dental care for chil-dren with developmental disabilities are based on the dentist's ability to provide and the patient's level of need and ability to co-operate. Replacement of missing teeth in pa-tients with cleft palate or anomalies of the maxilla or mandible is definitely possible.

Usually, in complex cases, a maxillofacial prosthondotist is best able to do the tooth re-placement. Obturator fabrication can begin just after birth to facilitate feeding and or-thopedic retention following lip closure. Tooth replacement in the obturator can occur later,

when appropriate and necessary for function. Other treatments include oral surgery, en-dodontics (root canals), and orthodontics.

Federal law dictates that individuals who are disabled be given equal considera-tion for employment and health care as persons who are not disabled. Structural barriers to treatment such as narrow hall-ways or doorways are not a problem in newer buildings; these barriers have been eliminated. In the best of all possible worlds, dental care is just one component of total health care for children with developmen-tal disabilities. Ideally, medical and dental treatment for these children would occur at a single facility housing all health care personnel (Ziring et al., 1988). In such a setting questions or concerns about the

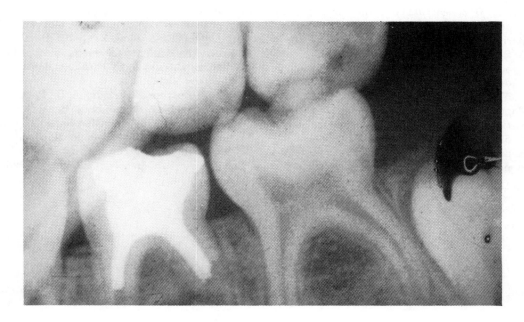

Figure 14–5.
A cross-arch intraoral bite-wing decay detection x-ray. The film did not touch the child's tongue (something that stimulates the gag reflex readily).

child's ability or inability to undergo treatment could be discussed and worked out in a multidisciplinary setting. With physician, dentist, and other health care personnel working together, the best course of treatment can be determined.

Summary

Regular dental treatment is a civil right of all citizens, including children with developmental disabilities. When considering a comprehensive health care program for a child with developmental disabilities, dentistry is often a difficult service to acquire. Dental care for children with developmental disabilities usually falls under the aus-

pices of pediatric or hospital based dentists. However, with exposure to children with developmental disabilities, a confidence-building phenomenon can occur. Dentistry for the disabled involves skills beyond quality preventive/restorative care. Comprehensive dental care for children with mild developmental disabilities is within the skill range of almost any dentist. The ability, not the disability, of the patient must be addressed.

References

American Dental Association, Council on Community Health, Hospital, Institutional and Medical Care. (1991, May). *Oral health guide-*

lines for patients with physical and mental disabilities. Chicago: American Dental Association.

Barnett, M. L., Press, K. P., Friedman, D., & Sonnenberg, E. (1986). Prevalence of periodontitis and dental caries in a Down's syndrome population. *Journal of Periodontology*, 57, 288–293.

Capute, A. J. (1974). Developmental disabilities. *Dental Clinics of North America, 18*(3), 557–577.

Kopel, H. (1977). The autistic child in dental practice. *Journal of Dentistry for Children*, *44*, 302–309.

Nowak, A. J. (1974). *Dentistry for the handicapped patient*. St. Louis: C. V. Mosby.

Sonnenberg, E., & Shey, Z. (1979). Review of preventive dentistry for the handicapped individual. *Journal of Clinical Preventive Dentistry, 1*, 16–20.

Ziring, P., Kastner, T., Friedman, D., Pond, W., Barnett, M. L., Sonnenberg, E., & Strassburger, K. (1988). Provision of health care for persons with developmental disabilities living in the community. *Journal of the American Medical Association, 260*, 1439–1444.

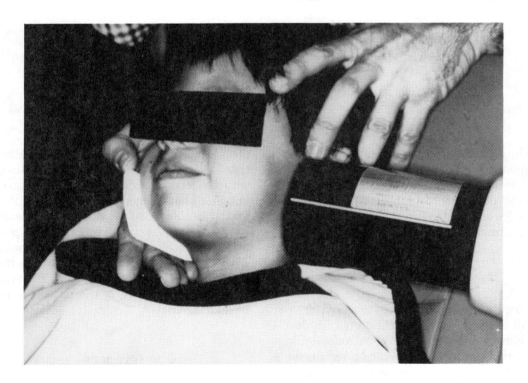

Figure 14–6.
The parent is holding a large 2$^{1}/_{2}$ × 3 inch piece of film on the child's cheek to get a view of developing teeth and jaws (lateral oblique view).

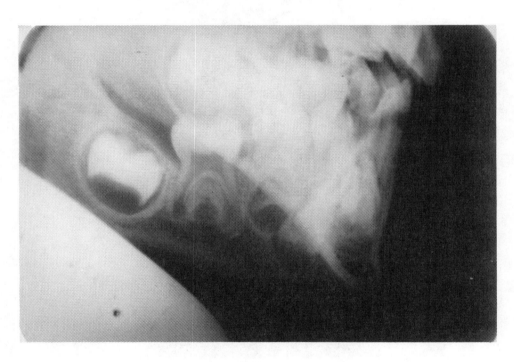

Figure 14–7.
The lateral oblique view of the teeth and jaws.

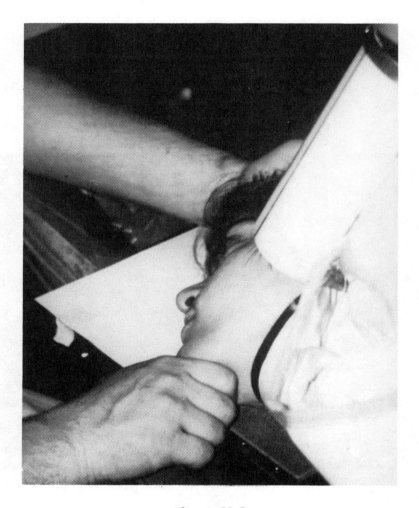

Figure 14–8.
A parent holds the head of a child with developmental disabilities enabling the dentist to obtain a large extraoral view of the jaws and developing teeth. Depending on the sharpness of the radiograph, even evaluation of decay is possible.

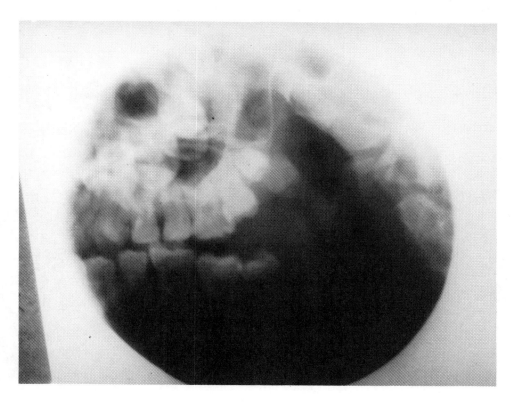

Figure 14–9.
The radiograph taken in Figure 14–8.

CHAPTER

15

Dental Care

ALAN B. ROSENTHAL, D.M.D.

CONTENTS

Oral health and function is universally accepted as essential to overall good health and the well-being of the developing child. It is important not to compromise the value of proper oral hygiene; routine maintenance; access to routine and emergency dental treatment, supervision, and continuing education of children with development disabilities.

To effectively deal with and provide proper dental care for an individual who occasionally or permanently deviates from the "norm," many factors must be considered: patient cooperation; physical handicaps; social, academic, family, and home environment; technical difficulties; and possibly one's own negative attitudes or prejudices toward the disabled. The physician, dentist, and oral hygienist, as well as other support personnel, need to work together as an interdisciplinary team to focus on and identify the child's special health care needs.

Treatment plans for dental care for the child with developmental disabilities and dysphagia must be made on an individual basis. The primary dental health care provider must understand the child's specific medical history, dental history, and behavioral and physical parameters.

Premedication is undeniably a valuable adjunct in dentistry. However, patience and proper training on the part of the dentist may be more effective in creating a cooperative environment than drug administration.

The approach to oral hygiene and dental treatment will vary depending on the individual's disability. The following sections discuss variations in dental care for individuals with Down syndrome, cerebral palsy, seizure disorders, autism, and blindness.

Characteristics of Specific Disabilities

Down Syndrome

General Features

The physical appearance of a patient with trisomy 21 may include microcephaly, with prominence of the forehead; a round flat face; iris anomalies; protruding of the tongue; and broadened and shortened hands, feet, and digits (Stewart, Barber, Troutman, & Wei, 1982; Thompson & Thompson, 1973). The level of intelligence of children with Down syndrome ranges from mild to severe retardation. Life expectancy can be curtailed by congenital heart disease and respiratory tract infections (Nelson et al., 1969).

Dental Treatment and Management

There are several dental anomalies that the dental practitioner should recognize as

being associated with Down syndrome: congenitally missing teeth, pointed incisors and canines, severe gingival and periodontal disease, delayed eruption of permanent teeth, and a protruding lower jaw (Class III malocclusion) with an underdeveloped maxilla. Dental abnormalities include scrotal tongue, hypoplasia of the frontal sinus, hypoplastic maxilla, reduced tooth number, dysplastic teeth, and palatal abnormalities. There also appears to be a correlation between the degree of mental retardation and the incidence of dental caries. Although the tongue may appear larger than normal, this is actually due to insufficient development of the mouth.

The incidence of cardiac disease reported in Down syndrome patients ranges from 24 to 35% (Cohen, 1975; Holmes et al., 1972; Thompson & Thompson, 1973). There is a high incidence of atrioventricular septal defects, along with atrioventricular valve insufficiency. It is imperative that antibiotic prophylaxis be given to patients with cardiac anomalies following the American Heart Association (1994) guidelines before beginning dental treatment.

Depending on the degree of retardation, dental treatment should be a nonthreatening experience for these patients. Children with Down syndrome are generally cooperative. With children who present extreme behavior problems, a dentist may elect to use a mild premedication or, in rare situations, general anesthesia.

Cerebral Palsy

General Features

The manifestations of cerebral palsy include motor function aberrations, paralysis, muscular weakness, seizures, and mental retardation (Nelson et al., 1969). Children with cerebral palsy may exhibit spasticity (40–70%), athetosis (25%), ataxia (10%), rigidity (5%), tremors (5%), speech defects (50–75%), severe mental retardation (45%), visual defects (20–50%), deafness (10–30%), seizures and convulsions (35–60%), and severe physical handicaps (25%) (Stewart et al., 1982).

Communication with the patient is the key to proper management when providing dental care. With a proper understanding of the above characteristics and recognition of the limitations of the individual, communication will be more attainable.

Dental Management

The most serious reasons for peridontal disease and caries in children with cerebral palsy are neglect, faulty nutrition, and prolonged exposure of the teeth to food. Many specific characteristics that may affect provision of dental care are observed with treating children with cerebral palsy, including limited head movement, spasms of facial muscles, spastic tongue thrusting, drooling, malocclusion

secondary to abnormal swallowing and speech movements, mouth breathing, bruxism (grinding of the teeth), poor swallowing, lack of sensation, and tremor-like head movements. Dental abnormalities include high narrow palate, peridontal disease, and hypoplastic enamel defect.

Cooperation from the patient can be achieved with proper preparation, understanding, and patience. Several adjuncts in the dental armamentarium may facilitate treatment: (1) A *rubber mouth block* may be used to hold the mouth open (see Figures 15–1 to 15–3). (2) *Restraints* may be used to help keep the patient with involuntary muscle movements still. Before using these restraints, the need for them should be explained to the patient and the parents. The dentist should also always cradle the child's head for support. It should always be clarified that this is not a form of *punishment* but rather *protection* for the patient.

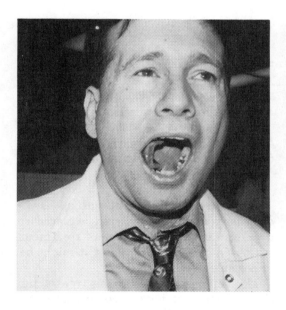

Figure 15–1.
Rubber mouth blocks come in three sizes: small child, child, and adult.

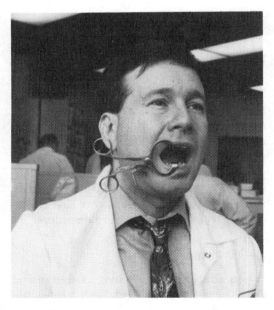

Figure 15–2.
A Molt mouth gag prop in place.

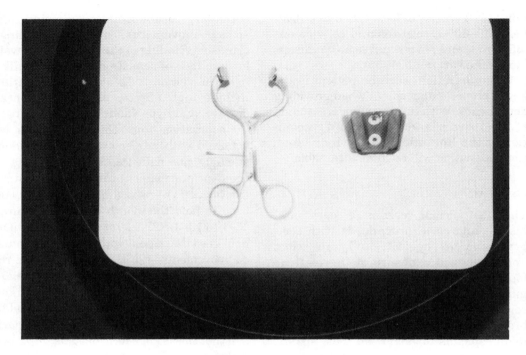

Figure 15–3.
Molt mouth gag prop (left), rubber mouth block (right).

Seizure Disorders

General Features

Several medications used to treat seizure disorders have an impact on dental treatment, including phenytoin (Dilantin®), phenobarbital, mephobarbital (Mebaral®), primidone (Mysaline®), and ethosuximide (Zarotin®) (Silver et al., 1973). High decay rates and peridontal disease are side effects of drug treatment for seizure disorders.

Dental Treatment

When the health provider is delivering dental care to a patient with a possible seizure disorder, several questions should be asked:

1. What kind of seizure disorder is believed to occur?
2. Is there an aura (warning)?
3. What type of medication is the patient taking and did he or she take it today?
4. Is there a specific time of day it occurs?
5. When was the last time a seizure occurred?

Before treating a patient with a seizure disorder, a mouth prop should be placed as a preventative measure before treatment starts. Once a seizure begins, it might be impossible to place this prop.

If a seizure begins during treatment, the following actions need to be taken: (1) Ensure that the patient does not fall out of the chair; (2) Maintain the mouth prop; (3) Loosen the patient's clothing; (4) If a rubber dam is being used, immediately remove it; (5) Constantly maintain the patient's safety and continue to observe; (6) After the seizure has subsided, the patient is usually sedated or unconscious. At this time, place the temporary restoration.

If a patient with a seizure disorder is undergoing prosthetic treatment, it is preferable to use a fixed appliance, rather than a removable one, for safety.

One of the most common dental characteristics of patients with seizures is gingival hyperplasia from Dilantin®. The incidence of this hyperplasia is 10–30%, with an emphasis on the anterior regions (Bhasker, 1977). The increased amount of gingival tissue is a focus of infection because it creates an uncleanable environment. Inflammation around the teeth becomes rampant due to an accumulation of plaque and calculus. Unfortunately, a series of surgical procedures (gingivectomies) is the only treatment to remove this excess tissue and create a cleanable area. Good oral hygiene is extremely important with these individuals. The hyperplasia in edentulous (toothless) individuals does not seem to be as prevalent, but when it does occur, it can cause problems with dentures.

The dental health care provider needs to have a good understanding of the pharmacology involved and the side effects of drugs. If there is a need to prescribe antibiotics to control infection, pain medication, or sedation, the synergistic or antagonistic relationship of the drugs used with seizure medications needs to be known.

Blindness

General Features

Legal blindness is defined as 20/200 vision after correction (Hathaway, 1959). This disability does not negate the approach and methods of teaching children normal oral hygiene. A slow approach to any physical violation of the mouth or face should be taken. The age at which blind children begin to successfully learn oral hygiene techniques is 8–10 years old. A child is not to be pushed or pressured, but rather allowed to follow an individual pace. Goal setting is important. *Life size* plastic and rubber models of teeth can be a tremendous aid. During the instruction of oral hygiene, these models provide an opportunity for the child to feel the difference between primary and permanent teeth, eruption of teeth, and the alignment of teeth.

When teaching either brushing or flossing, a slow progression of easy steps should be followed:

1. Placing the brush, with the health provider's hand over the patient's, on the teeth;
2. Slowly moving and brushing one area of the mouth;
3. Letting go, and letting the patient brush alone;
4. Having the patient do the entire procedure alone.

A floss-aid may assist the patient with flossing of the teeth. Successful oral hygiene education helps give these children a strong sense of independence.

When dealing with the family or guardian of a child with disabilities, there may be obstacles. One must first have a good understanding of the child's personal and social background, intelligence, and specific disabilities and limitations. Although families mean well, parents are sometimes so overwhelmed with the child's medical problems that the child's dental health is neglected. Unfortunately, family members who are fearful of dentists themselves sometimes will influence their children with these fears.

Oral Hygiene

The degree of attention and assistance needed for instruction of oral hygiene can be classified into three groups: (1) self-care, 92) partial care, and (3) total care (Bensburg et al., 1969).

Individuals in the *self-care* group may need some modifications in the toothbrush handle (see Figure 15–4) due to physical limitations, but can usually become independent in oral hygiene. It is very important to standardize the techniques of oral hygiene and the methodology of teaching it. The dentist, hygienist, parents and aids should schedule regular meetings to reinforce and standardize the information given to the patient. Motivation and positive reinforcement are important teaching tools.

The *partial care* group is classified as moderately disabled and needs more direct assistance. Encouragement is necessary in performing comprehensive dental care. An empirical approach in expressing avoidance of pain by brushing is sometimes helpful because long-term goals are difficult for these patients to grasp. Patience is the key in working with this group of individuals.

During the training sessions, it may be helpful to proceed with an easy step-by-step procedure: (1) Hold the toothbrush with the patient; (2) Put the brush in the mouth; (3) Put the toothbrush on the

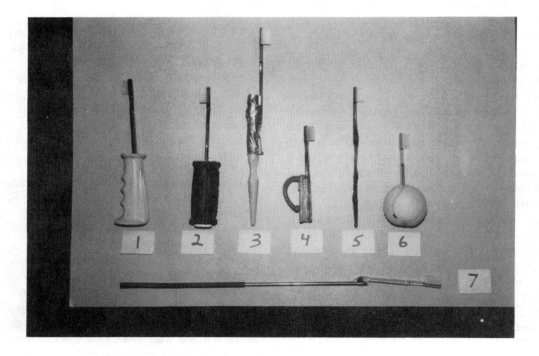

Figure 15–4.
Examples of modified toothbrushes. 1. Bicycle handle filled with plaster. 2. Foam rubber handle filled with plaster. 3. Hairbrush handle with bristles cut off and a taped-on toothbrush. 4. Nail brush handle with tape. 5. Brush handle heated and stretched for longer reach. 6. Tennis ball with brush. 7. Spoke of bicycle wheel for longer reach.

teeth; (4) Brush the teeth; (5) Let the patient try the entire cycle himself; (6) Repeat. Positive reinforcement is always beneficial, whether it is a smile, a hug, or a verbal compliment. Being creative, patient, and catering to individual needs is of key importance. For example, it may be necessary to repeat demonstrations many, many times before the patient will comprehend and grasp the learned pattern.

The *total care* group is the most difficult in which to develop a self-care routine. This is primarily due to the severity of their disabilities. Studies have shown that an electric toothbrush is very advantageous in helping these children care for their teeth. In this group, unlike the self-care and partial care groups, the provider usually maintains and ensure proper oral health.

Dental Treatment

When delivering care, several positions facilitate proper treatment and ensure safety for the provider and patient: (1) Standing, while cradling the patient's head in one arm and holding the jaw; (2) Sitting on a couch with the patient's head in the provider's lap; (3) Sitting on the floor and restraining the child by holding him or her between the provider's legs. Patients in wheelchairs or patients who are bedridden can be maintained using these positions.

Whether or not a patient is disabled, fears about having dental work done are to be expected. Some people fear needles or the noise of the drill. Others may have had a bad experience in the past, feel uncomfortable lying down in a vulnerable position in front of a stranger, or simply not like having something put in their mouth. Fear is unpredictable, although many studies have shown that maternal anxiety has a major influence on children's behavior (Johnson & Baldwin, 1969).

Behavior modification can be enhanced by good communication. Developing a relationship with the patient in a nonthreatening role, such as a friend, not that of a dentist or other health provider, may help subdue some children's fears.

Studies have shown that up to 75% of dentists in the United States refuse to treat disabled children for the following reasons (Robert Wood Johnson Foundation, 1979; Willard & Nowak, 1981):

1. Staff not properly trained;
2. Disruption of office routine;
3. Need for special equipment;
4. Reluctance of families to bring handicapped child into a public place;
5. Physical limitations of office accessibility.

One of the saddest facts about this is that, not only are most of the obstacles easily overcome, but approximately 10% of these dentists do not refer these children to dentists or facilities that do treat individuals with disabilities.

One of the most difficult tasks of the provider is deciding when to allow the child to express his or her emotions and when to adopt an authoritarian role. Without training, the dentist must use his or her best judgment, based on experience, in allowing the individual to express his or her feelings while maintaining and promoting a self-supportive role.

Positive reinforcement is an excellent technique for behavior modification (Macillan & Forness, 1970). The health provider is playing a role as a teacher and therefore is responsible not only for maintaining the individual's oral hygiene but also fostering the child's cognitive skills without constant reinforcement.

When the child first visits the office, it is recommended that a slow, methodical, confident approach be taken. The child's first visit might just include walking through the office. If the child shows no reluctance, an oral examination radiographs, and dental prophylaxis with fluoride, in that order, can be included. A properly trained assistant is an invaluable adjunct when dealing with the child with developmental disabilities. The assistant is responsible for ensuring the child's safety and comfort, while the dentist or other health provider is primarily responsible for actually treating the child.

Definitive procedures need to be completed in the shortest amount of time: stainless steel crowns should be used instead of amalgam; endontics rather than pulp capping should be used; absorbable suture material should be employed; and any decalcifications need to be excavated and filled.

Most importantly, the dentist must do no harm and realize that sometimes the best treatment is no treatment. The dentist can help the child with developmental disabilities and dysphagia develop the skills necessary to be more self-sufficient in dental hygiene.

Summary

Children with developmental disabilities experience significant and unfortunate benign neglect with their dental care. Even though the more pressing needs of these individuals are medical rather than dental related, the responsible health provider will recognize the importance of their basic dental needs.

It is important to have a general understanding of a particular syndrome, which include classical and identifiable oral sequelae. The oral manifestations that may be seen with developmental disabilities include dental caries, peridontal disease, defective tooth development, abnormal craniofacial growth, and a variety of habitual oral reflex aberrations. This author emphasizes that chronic oral pathology may inhibit the progress of a favorable medical prognosis. Therefore, cooperation between the dentist and physician will assure a more holistic approach to a child's total health.

The dignity of these children must also be considered. Too often we are blinded by the confines of our profession and become oblivious to our obligation of social responsibility.

Prevention of dental disease and maintenance of good oral health were discussed in this chapter, with excellent references provided for readers interested in more information on this subject.

References

Bensberg, G. J., et al. (1969). *Dental care for the mentally retarded*. Birmingham: Center for Developmental Learning Disorders, University of Alabama.

Bhaskar, S. M. (1977). *Synopsis of oral pathology* (5th ed.). St. Louis: C. V. Mosby.

Cohen, M. M., Sr. (1975). Chromosomal disorders. *Dental Clinics of North America, 19*(1), 87.

Hathaway, W. (1959). Education and health of the partially seeing child (4th ed.). New York: Society for the Prevention of Blindness.

Holmes, L. B., Moser, H. W., et al. (1972). *Mental retardation: An atlas of diseases and associated abnormalities*. New York: Macmillan.

Johnson, R., & Baldwin, D. C., Jr. (1969). Maternal anxiety and child behavior. *Journal of Dentistry for Children, 36,* 87.

Macillan, D. L., & Forness, S. R. (1970, December). Behavior modification: Limitations and liabilities. *Exceptional Children,* pp. 291

Nelson, W. E., et al. (Eds.). (1969). *Textbook of pediatrics* (9th ed.). Philadelphia: W. B. Saunders.

Robert Wood Johnson Foundation. (1979). Dental care for handicapped Americans: A national problem (Special Report No. 2). Princeton, NJ: Author.

Silver, H., et al. (1973). *Handbook of pediatrics*. Los Altos, CA: Lange Medical Publications.

Stewart, R. E., Barber, T. K., Troutman, K. C., & Wei, S. H. Y. (1982). *Pediatric dentistry*. St. Louis: C. V. Mosby.

Terhune, J. A. (1973). Predicting the readiness of elementary school children to learn an effective dental flossing technique. *Journal of the American Dental Association, 86,* 1332.

Thompson, J. S., & Thompson, M. W. (1973). *Genetics in medicine*. Philadelphia: W. B. Saunders.

Willard, D., & Nowak, A. (1981). Communicating with the family of a child with a developmental disability. *Journal of the American Dental Association, 102,* 647.

CHAPTER

16

Nursing Assessment and Management

MARY LOTZE, P.N.P., M.S.

―――――― **CONTENTS** ――――――

Parent-Child Interactions and Feeding Problems

Feeding is a reciprocal process that depends on the abilities and characteristics of both the parent and the child (Satter,

1992). Feeding problems impinge on the relationship between parents and their children, particularly when children have developmental disabilities. It is estimated that 1 to 2% of infants and children suffer severe and prolonged feeding problems that impinge on growth (Dahl, 1987), and that 25 to 33% of children exhibit common difficulties such as food refusal and overeating (Linscheid, 1985). Feeding problems established early in life can persist and generalize into other areas of development. Struggles with feeding can result in difficulty with a child's ability to eat not only a variety of foods but to regulate body weight and achieve appropriate growth (Satter, 1992). Dahl and Kristiansson (1987) found significantly higher frequencies of infections and behavior problems among 2-year-old children who had early feeding problems. Feeding interactions during the first year of life which are of positive quality tend to be consequently linked to the child's subsequent cognitive and linguistic abilities and even have been credited with an increase in secure attachments to major caregivers (Barnard et al., 1989). According to Humphrey (1991), feeding an infant is a two person process in which parent and infant coordinate their behaviors to accomplish a basic and essential activity of daily living. Feeding is a face to face interaction that is bi-directional. The quality of interaction may range from positive and growth enhancing for both parent and infant to negative and destructive. Because feeding is a major activity that is repeated several times a day, it offers the infant and caregiver valuable learning experiences as they coordinate actions to meet the infant's nutritional needs. The parent-child interactions that occur during the feeding process contribute to the developing parent-child relationship. When developing feeding programs for children with dysphagia, professionals must consider the relationship between the child and the various family members for a successful feeding program to be implemented. As Humphrey points out (1991), in using the transactional model as a basis for feeding programs, the strength of one family member in the dyad can compensate for a difficulty experienced by another family member. Thus, the infant with special needs may be less influenced by biological risk factors when an adult can compensate and provide the modifications during those interactions.

When developing feeding programs for children with developmental disabilities, Bax (1989) suggests that implications of the feeding program on the other aspects of the child's development and its relationship to family functions must be considered. Brizee, Sophos, and McLaughlin (1990) also point out that a child's feeding difficulty can create problems for the parent-child interaction. Humphrey (1991) states that the experiences of parent-infant interactions during the feeding process become an integral part of their developing relationship.

What, then, are some of the areas that professionals working with children with dysphagia need to keep in mind when developing a feeding program? One important determinant of how a parent and infant will interact is the child's developmental level and the competencies that infant exhibits in various interactions with parents and other family members. Sucking is a mechanism in infants that helps regulate state organization and relieves stress (Campos, 1989). Infants with dysphagia who cannot suck may be missing an important ability to self-regulate (Humphrey, 1991). Although difficulty in sucking frequently represents an underlying neurological deficit, sucking is viewed as a naturally occurring behavior by most parents. This can affect the infant's social interactions with other family members, and valuable learning opportunities may be lost.

Infants with motor problems have been shown to need additional response time during feeding and also may use alternative means of signaling. Parents of children with motor handicaps, cerebral palsy in particular, have been known to become quite proficient in identifying these alternate signals which professionals may often miss. Infants may use a number of signals such as eye contact, facial expression, and body movements to influence the feeding behavior of the adult (Humphrey, 1991). On the other hand, some studies have shown an increase in the frequency of commands used by mothers when the child had a handicapping condition. The parents' increased amount of directiveness appeared to be linked to the presence of a handicapping condition rather than a motor problem. This observation led researchers to ponder the question of whether the increased directiveness on the part of mothers was a result of seeing the feeding episode as an instruction and teaching therapy session rather than a relaxed social interaction such as occurs in children without feeding problems (Mahoney, Fors, & Wood, 1990).

Another factor that can impact on the infant-caregiver relation is the physical appearance of the infant. Researchers examining the relationship between children with craniofacial anomalies and their mothers found that these infants touched their mothers and smiled less and looked away more than infants who did not have such anomalies (Bardon, Ford, Jensen, Roger-Salyer M., & Roger-Salyer K. C., 1989). Of interest, however, is that the parents of these infants in these studies reported more satisfaction in parenting. Premature infants, because of their small and fragile appearance, present special problems. Magyary (1984) found premature infants were less responsive and more disorganized than full-term infants, and Minde (1984) found that they tended to develop feeding difficulties. Parents of infants born prematurely also frequently failed to adapt food selection and feeding methods to the infants nutritional needs and developmental level (Ernst et al., 1983).

Changing parenting practices and family routines has become a main focus in early intervention when the child's feeding problem cannot be eliminated; however, most professionals do not know how families acquire parenting skills such as feeding an in-

fant. Humphrey (1991) suggests that feeding offers opportunities for the development of the adult caregiver role. Feeding the infant is seen as a tangible part of the nurturing process, and weight gain is often viewed as evidence of success in the parenting role. Thus, growth in the child promotes psychosocial development in the parent. Consequently, if an infant does not gain weight, it can affect the parent's developing self-concept and parenting skills. Humphrey (1991) suggests that parental caregiving behaviors are not automatic but are acquired as part of a developmental process. Thus, each parent's internal model of parent-infant relationships influences how he or she interacts with a difficult to feed infant. This relationship is examined in closer detail in the chapter on nonorganic failure to thrive (NOFTT) (Chapter 7).

The parents' current social and cultural situation will determine where they will turn to learn more about parenting or child development (Hopkins & Westra, 1989). Recognition of the sources of influences on parenting practices is critical. Unfortunately, in the hospital situation, many professionals assume that they are the primary source of information on feeding infants, and if parents do not fulfill the program, they may be viewed by professionals as noncompliant (Trostle, 1988). Professionals need to appreciate parents as partners and attempt to understand what parents know about child development, particularly feeding, and realize their knowledge and beliefs shape their parenting behaviors (Miller, 1988).

Professionals working with the child and family with dysphagia also need to consider cultural factors: How is the role of the mother viewed in this family? Is it a matriarchal versus a patriarchal system? How does a family view the development of independence versus dependence? How is the family influenced by opinions of other family members? What is the role of extended family members, particularly grandparents, nieces, nephews, aunts, and uncles? How does the family view seeking help from professionals? Is it seen as a weakness or is it viewed as a helping behavior (Lotze, 1988)? How food and eating are viewed as a part of family function is very important when put in the cultural context of various ethnic backgrounds.

When developing a feeding program for the baby with dysphagia, the mother is usually the first family member to be taught the program by professionals. However, it is important to consider the roles of all family members within the family's cultural and ethnic context to gain ultimate cooperation in making a child's feeding program successful. Finally, as Humphrey (1991) explains, using a transactional model to address feeding problems promotes parent-infant interaction, and a strong parent-infant relationship has potential for maximal compensation for medical and developmental problems that occur in dysphagia in infants.

Evaluation of Newborn Feeding Interactions

Evaluation of newborn feeding interactions can be accomplished through use of the Nursing Child Assessment Feeding Scale (NCAFS) (Barnard, 1979). The NCAFS is designed to assess the contributions and characteristics unique to the feeding interactions of both parents and children during the first year of life. It examines six key areas that are important to the interaction adaption process between parent and child (Barnard, 1979). The NCAFS consists of 76 behavioral items to observe during feeding. The six areas include four parent behavior items: sensitivity to infant cues, response to infant distress, social-emotional growth fostering behaviors, and cognitive growth fostering behaviors. The two infant behavior items are clarity of infant cues and responsiveness to parent. Through the use of this tool, professionals are able to identify be-

haviors that indicate a parent's sensitivity to the child's cues during feeding. The tool also helps identify behaviors that indicate a parent is providing growth fostering situations for the infant socially and intellectually during feeding, as well as child behaviors that indicate the child is giving clear cues and is responsive to the parent. Finally, the scale identifies parent and child roles and responsibilities that facilitate a positive feeding interaction (Barnard, 1979). This scale, or similar scales, can be a significant help to professionals in providing a method for objectively observing parent-child interactions which can be validated by others and delineating clear areas for intervention and strategies for working with children with dysphagia and their families.

Introduction of Solid Foods and Breast-feeding

Infants are normally physiologically ready to take solid foods when the extrusion reflex is no longer present, the swallowing reflex is sufficiently coordinated so that solid foods can be swallowed easily without choking, and the gastrointestinal tract has matured enough so that foods can be eaten without danger of producing allergy (Marlow & Redding, 1988).

Infants are developmentally ready to eat solid foods when they can balance their heads well in sitting, can turn away from foods they dislike or foods offered after their appetites have been satisfied, and have begun the process of teething (Marlow & Redding, 1988). Thus, it is generally recommended that solid foods not be introduced to infants before 4 to 6 months (Committee on Nutrition, 1980). In the normal infant, the accepted advantages of waiting until the infant is 4 to 6 months old to introduce solids are commonly acknowledged to be to avoid allergies, to avoid overweight or obesity, and the development of a more mature swallowing pattern. However, infants with dysphagia may need thickened feedings for increased calorie intake, need to reduce weight loss and improve energy. Thus, the use of thickened feedings is frequently an integral part of a feeding program as recommended by a dysphagia team. This aspect of feeding is covered more intensively in Chapter 3, Clinical Evaluation and Treatment, and Chapter 4, Nutrition Support.

Breast-feeding

Although mothers of normal babies are encouraged to breast-feed, the same encouragement is often not given to mothers of babies with developmental disabilities, particularly babies with dysphagia, but the advantages for both remain the same. The breast-fed baby rarely develops allergies to mother's milk and is much less apt to suffer from allergies later in life. Breast milk is well tolerated even by immature babies (Meier & Anderson, 1987), and nursing itself helps develop good tongue and jaw development. The stimulation received from the mother's closeness and from actual suckling can also aid respiratory functions and, consequently, the oxygenation of the blood. The social-emotional advantages of breast-feeding have long been recognized as facilitating bonding and the parent-child interaction. Most sick or disabled babies can be breast-fed according to Jones (1985), even children with a cleft lip and a small cleft palate (Arvedson & Brodsky, 1993). If the baby is in the hospital, the nursing staff and physicians need to be alerted to the fact that the mother wishes to nurse the baby. If an infant cannot be taken out of an incubator or if the mother cannot always be with the baby, and there are times when the baby must be fed by a bottle, a mother can express her milk so that the baby receives human milk and she keeps up her milk supply so she can nurse the baby at home. The local La Leche League can be a useful resource for mothers to begin developing skills in nursing their infant with feeding problems. A book written by Dorothy Brewster (1979) entitled *You Can Breastfeed Your Baby Even in Special Situations* also offers helpful suggestions for nursing babies with a variety of disabilities and shows how most physically disabled and ill babies can be breast-fed. If a mother must supplement what her child gets from nursing, it must be kept in mind that bottle feeding provides such an easy means of sucking that a baby could reject the breast. An alternative to the bottle for a nursing mother with a baby who is slow to feed or has a weak suck is use of a supplemental feeding device such as Lact-aide. The Lact-aide is a system with a feeding tube coming from a container hung around the mother's neck and filled with breast milk. When nursing, the mother can tape the tube to her nipple so when the baby sucks, the infant stimulates the mother's milk supply and gets some of the breast milk supplemented by milk from the tube (Arvedson & Brodsky, 1993).

Problems encountered in breast-feeding the child with dysphagia include hypotonia, which may result in a weak suck with poor closure, and hypertonia, which may result in arching, making it difficult for the baby to mold to the mother. Either of these patterns must be explained to the mother in understandable terms so the mother does not become frustrated and the baby does not get overtired. Babies with extreme extensor patterns are sometimes felt by mothers to be rejecting because of elicitation of the asymmetrical tonic neck reflex when the baby turns its head to nurse at the nipple. Another parent perception that can make breast-feeding the child with the developmental disabilities and dysphagia difficult is if the mother perceives the baby is not getting enough milk to meet nutritional needs. Monitoring the baby's weight gain can allay this concern.

Breast-feeding the Child with Cleft Lip/Cleft Palate

As mentioned previously, the child with cleft lip or mild cleft palate may be breast-fed

(Arvedson & Brodsky, 1993). In the infant with a cleft lip, breast-feeding is often successful with minimal modification according to Wolf and Glass (1992). They report that infants with cleft lip generally have adequate oral mechanics to produce compression of the nipple for milk delivery. Although suction to form and position the nipple may be compromised, the soft tissue of the breast may work better than an artificial nipple to fill the cleft and allow the development of suction for nipple positioning. The size and shape of the mother's breast may facilitate or limit this process.

In the case of the infant with a cleft palate, the infant may develop adequate suction to form and position the nipple if the cleft is small. When the infant cannot produce adequate suction for nipple positioning, Wolf and Glass (1992) recommend that the mother manually assist the infant in the nipple creation and positioning. Feeding when the breast is full and rigid combined with hand expression of milk may also be successful. If the cleft is large, however, it will be difficult to achieve proper nipple positioning, and compression may also be compromised by the lack of an opposing surface. When a large cleft is present, breast-feeding in the normal manner is generally not successful. Wolf and Glass (1992) recommend the use of such feeding tube devices as Medela, Supplemental Nursing System (SNS), or Lact-aide as described previously.

When a cleft lip and palate are present, the cleft is generally quite large. Palatal obturators are used by some centers with varying degrees of success. They are used to block the cleft and allow development of compression and possibly suction. However, breast-feeding is unlikely to be successful in the infant with a cleft lip and palate. There is no suction to form and position the nipple adequately, and compression may be compromised by the lack of an adequate opposing surface. Wolf and Glass (1992) recommend the breast-feeding experience may be possible using a feeding tube device, again such as the Medela, SNS, or Lact-aide.

Nursing Interventions

Appropriate interventions on the part of the nursing staff and dysphagia team can promote healthy parent-child interaction. The nurse can support the breast-feeding mother in maintaining adequate nutrition for the baby through proper breast-feeding techniques. In cases where the baby is nutritionally at risk, breast-feeding can be used as a supplemental activity. The nurse can teach the parents to read the infant's cues using such tools as the Nursing Child Assessment Feeding Scale, as discussed previously and encourage the use of "en face" position in which there is direct eye contact between the mother and the baby. This will facilitate parent-child interaction which is essential for continued healthy relations.

Coyner (1983) states the following advantages of breast-feeding a handicapped or atypical infant:

1. Added time for physical closeness, bringing with it the numerous tactile, visual, olfactory, and social experiences thought to benefit both the infant and mother.
2. Development of a natural suckling pattern as opposed to the suck pattern necessitated by most artificial nipples. The optimal development of oral-facial musculature is facilitated by the act of suckling milk from the breast.
3. Provides the handicapped infant with the immunologic benefits available from human milk.
4. Prevents the adverse affects of deficiencies and excesses noted with artificial feeding that are known to stress the developing systems of the infant as well as affect the infant's future nutritional status.

Coyner (1983) concludes that teaching and assisting a mother to breast-feed her handicapped infant is no more time and energy consuming than attaining nutrition with formula and bottle feeding.

Clothing

Many children with developmental disability and dysphagia have problems with both heavy perspiration and excessive drooling. This combination can cause problems of being wet over the chest and other areas of the body. The state of being wet can render the child more susceptible to rashes as well as being uncomfortable and unappealing socially. Dressing the child in multiple layers of lightweight, porous clothing such as tops, sweaters, and bottoms are options that can minimize this problem.

Bibs

Children with developmental disabilities tend to have excessive salivation which, in turn, can cause irritation of the skin around the mouth and chin area and the neck and the chest. Therefore, vinyl-backed bibs are often used with these children, and it is important to observe these areas for irritation. Gentle washing of the skin with soap and water and application of a mild cream can help maintain the skin in good integrity. The use of terry cloth bibs, which can be changed frequently and washed easily, is another suitable alternative.

Assessment of Utensils for Feeding

Types of Feeding Utensils

The appropriate selection of equipment that enhances a child's feeding abilities depends on understanding the purpose and selection criteria for that equipment (Morris & Klein, 1987). Certain criteria apply to all equipment; other criteria are applicable to specific characteristics of the individual child with

a feeding problem. When developing a feeding program for infants and young children, it is important for professionals to not only use the right equipment but to help parents learn how to obtain those utensils for use in the home. Among the items used by professionals in feeding therapy programs are nipple straws, special nipples including premie nipples, spoons with curved handles, cups with cut-outs, and a variety of bottles. This section will review some of the criteria for selecting various utensils and equipment to use in the feeding program as outlined by Morris and Klein (1987).

Pacifiers

Because babies are born with a strong physiological need to exercise through sucking, which provides pleasure and self-quieting, most babies can benefit from a pacifier. However, some caution is needed in the way in which a pacifier is used. A pacifier can be used with infants who show a tight suck, no tongue thrust, and enjoy it. If the infant spits the pacifier out or still shows a tongue thrust or bite, use of a pacifier at that time is not recommended (Morris & Klein, 1987).

A pacifier should have an outer shield molded to the shape of the lips to provide sustained contact and stimulation for lip closure. The pacifier should also fit the size and shape of the child's mouth and be well constructed so it does not come apart when the baby sucks or chews on it.

Nipples

The holes in the nipple should not be artificially enlarged, and they should not allow an uncontrolled flow of liquid into the infant's mouth. The nipple should fit the size and shape of the infant's mouth and provide an adequate stiffness or resistance to the infant's sucking pattern. A softer nipple, such as a premie nipple, may be more appropriate for an infant whose suck is weak or who tends to tire easily. The nipple should not collapse with the infant's sucking. As discussed earlier, babies with developmental disabilities may have a weak suck and may need to supplement the flow of milk from breast-feeding with a supplemental mechanism. The liquid from the nipple of the breast-feeding mother is assisted by tubing that does not interfere with the nursing process and provides the infant with the additional required nutrients. Supplemental nursing systems include such products as SNS, Medela, and Lact-aide. These are all commercially available for nursing mothers who have children with a weak or ineffective suck.

Bottles

There are many kinds of nursing bottles on the commercial market, and any one of a number can be appropriate for the infant. The criteria for an effective bottle include that the bottle is easy for the infant to hold and fits the size and shape of the feeder's hand. One bottle on the market is constructed so the milk will fill the nipple as the bottle empties (the anti-colic bottle by Correcto).

Cups

Introduction of cup drinking is a major milestone in a feeding program for children with dysphagia. The criteria for an effective cup include that the cup can be tipped up to get liquid at the bottom without tipping the child's head back, it should not shatter or break if the child bites the edge, and it should allow the feeder a clear view of the child's mouth. This has lead to the popularity of the cut-out cup so frequently used in early intervention feeding programs. The cup also should provide a thick or rolled lip for extra stability, and the cup should provide a mechanism for greater control of the liquid flow in the instance where the ability to handle a large volume of liquid is poor. Finally, the cup should be of appropriate

physical shape and allow for developmentally appropriate holding of the cup for the child who is initiating self-feeding (Morris & Klein, 1987).

Straws

As recommended earlier, feeding in the semi-upright to upright position is the position of choice. This is facilitated in many children through the use of a nipple straw which snaps into the base of the nipple. These straws, which are readily available in most supermarkets, draw formula from the base of the bottle, making it possible to feed the child with the head in a more flexed position without ingesting air along with the formula. The criteria for choosing an effective straw include that the straw should be able to be cut, bent, or adjusted to be used to achieve a mature straw drinking pattern and should not break or shatter if the child bites it. The straw should be usable with other adaptive equipment to provide needed support or control for the lips and provide a mechanism for greater control of the liquid flow for the child whose ability to handle a large volume of liquid is poor (Morris & Klein, 1987).

Spoons

Although parents and professionals can frequently use kitchen utensils, adaptive spoons or special vinyl-coated spoons may be indicated in certain instances based on the child's special needs. Criteria for choosing an effective spoon include that the bowl of the spoon should be relatively flat so that food can be removed easily by the child's upper lip, and the spoon should not shatter or break if the child bites on it. The bowl of the spoon should fit the size of the child's mouth. This is an important feature. Metal spoons should be covered or coated or have a plastic bowl if an infant is hypersensitive to temperature or taste or has a bite reflex. This may be also indicated in the child who has a tendency towards seizure if they are not under good control. The length of the handle should be appropriate to the size of the feeder's hand, and the specialist on the dysphagia team can make that judgment most appropriately. Frequently, spoon handles must be built up or adapted to the infant's grasp. This can be accomplished through the use of materials such as velcro, triangle finger grip material, foam, and even frequently found items around the house. One parent in a recent issue of *Exceptional Parent* developed an inexpensive adaptive spoon through the use of velcro, a triangle pencil grip, and a bicycle handlebar grip (Pilegard, 1992).

Bowls

Although any bowl can usually be used to initiate feeding items such as cereal and pureed fruits and vegetables, the use of a scooper bowl or scooper plate is often helpful in getting the proper amount onto the spoon, particularly when the baby is being encouraged to initiate self-feeding.

Positioning

In developing a feeding program for infants with developmental disabilities and dysphagia, positioning is critical. The upright position facilitates the normal sucking pattern. The position of choice is one with the child upright with hip and head flexion. This pattern facilitates break-up of the extensor pattern and will decrease abnormal tongue thrust. Another advantage of the upright position is that it facilities direct "en face" contact between the infant and the caregiver. The upright position is instrumental in facilitating prespeech and language development (Coyner & Zelle, 1983). In implementing a program for parents, professionals should help them avoid the tendencies to tip the child backward while feeding (Finnie, 1975). Nipple straws will allow a bottle to be held while maintaining the child in the upright position for feeding.

The baby's head should not be tilted backward during drinking, because this makes initiation of swallow more difficult and may predispose the infant to aspiration. This method does not permit the infant to develop normal suckle-swallow or learn to coordinate breathing and swallowing. More detailed information on explicit feeding positions and strategies are found in Chapter 8.

Tone can affect posture and must be carefully evaluated (Connor, Williamson, & Siepp, 1978). The child with hypotonia, or low tone, may need more head control or more body support. Infants with hypotonia must be observed for evidence of stridor. Stridor can be caused by intrinsic or extrinsic blockage of the upper airway. Intermediate inspiratory stridor, which can be caused by a slackness of muscle tone, needs medical attention to differentiate it from continuous stridor, which warrants immediate medical intervention (Haynes, 1983). For the child with hypertonia, a nipple straw in the bottle may make it possible for the child to sit in the semi-upright position and maintain the head slightly forward.

Finding the position that is most comfortable for parent and baby may take several tries. All parents should be cautioned about laying the baby down and propping bottles. This may cause the baby to choke. Additionally, propping a bottle does not allow feeding to be the emotional interaction time between parent and child that is considered important for fostering positive parent-child relations.

Gastrostomies and Parent Education

Gastrostomy tube placement is becoming increasingly common in children with developmental disabilities according to Nelson and Hallgren (1989). Following surgery, it is important that an appropriate program be developed to assist the family with gastrostomy management at home. These management plans should include the type of gastrostomy catheter to be used, guidelines for formula preparation and feeding, method of gavage to be used, and techniques for stoma and catheter care.

Type of Catheter

The dePezzer, Malecot, and Foley, until recently, were the most commonly used types of gastrostomy catheters. However, during the last 10 years, designer gastrostomy tubes and skin level feeding devices that meet the special needs of children have become available. The first tube designed exclusively for gastrostomy feedings was developed by Medical Innovations Corporations (MIC). This short or more aesthetically appealing gastrostomy tube with an internal balloon and external anchoring device addressed the limitations encountered when using Foley catheters (Huddleston & Ferraro, 1991). The first skin-level feeding device, the button, originally made available from Bard, included several advantages such as greater comfort for the infant, decreased incidence of tube migration, and less accidental removal. Families also reported perceiving this device as more normal, and that it did not interfere with the child's mobility.

Skin Care

The gastrostomy stoma should be inspected daily for signs of leakage, bleeding, and skin irritation. Families should be instructed to cleanse the area daily with soap and water. If a button is in place, keeping the skin dry may be difficult. A clean piece of gauze, like a tracheostomy dressing, can be placed under the wings to facilitate this. If skin breakdown does occur, a stoma adhesive powder and a skin barrier such as duoderm are usually sufficient. Parents should be instructed that small amounts of fluid draining around the gastrostomy tube are not uncommon or harmful. Silver nitrate applications

may be helpful to control granulation tissues that may form around the gastrostomy opening (Nelson & Hallgren, 1989).

Feeding Techniques

The equipment used will depend on whether the feeding is bolus or continuous. The feeding tube should be rinsed with warm water after each feeding, and at least once a day the tube should be washed with hot soapy water and rinsed thoroughly. Huddleston and Palmer (1990) have found that food occlusions are best treated with tap water irrigation if discovered early. However, enzyme solutions may be required for occlusions that have remained in the tube for longer periods. Occlusions secondary to medication have been successfully removed with warm tap water. If the tube becomes coated with formula, it should be flushed with warm water. If this is unsuccessful, it may be flushed with a diet soft drink, cranberry juice, or seltzer.

If the child is on fatty supplements or oil-based medications, the tube may become occluded. In this case, a 1/4 teaspoon of pancreatic enzyme can be added to 5 ccs of water to facilitate the residual fat breakdown in the tube. Families should be reminded to wash their hands before starting a feeding or handling equipment. Following feeding, the system should be flushed. Water flushes need to be recorded as intake. A more detailed description on gastrostomies and GI buttons is presented in Chapter 12 on gastrointestinal problems in children with developmental disabilities.

How to Set Up a Gastrostomy Training Program for Families

It is imperative that families receive instruction about gastrostomy feedings before taking their children home. Setting up a training program for parents requires cooperation of the nursing department, the nutrition department, the speech and hearing department, the occupational therapy department, the surgeon, the gastroenterologist, and the dysphagia team. Whether the child is an inpatient or the procedure is done as an outpatient will determine where the training takes place. It is important that instructions be given to families in written format and in manageable sessions. Families should be allowed time to demonstrate their skills with the techniques to professionals, for example using dolls, before attempting these techniques on their own children. Training families of children with a gastrostomy should be an integral part of discharge planning. There may be follow-up in the community with a variety of community agencies such as a visiting nurse association, home care program, an early intervention program, or the hospital itself may have a follow-up feeding clinic. If the child is fortunate enough to be in a tertiary center with a dysphagia team, it will be important for the family to keep appointments on an outpatient basis with the team to monitor such areas as adjustment of the gastrostomy device; management of common complications such as skin breakdown, overgrowth tissue, leaking, vomiting, and diarrhea; advancement of feedings; evaluation of the child's nutritional status; and assessment of oral feedings and oral development. With appropriate professional guidance, families can become quite proficient in providing gastrostomy feedings and care to their children with developmental disabilities.

Prevention of Aspiration and Asphyxiation from Foods and Liquids

Infants with neuromotor problems frequently have feeding difficulties associated with an abnormal suckle-swallow reflex. This, in turn, can cause the infant to be tense, even impatient and irritable. The caregiver in these cases is sometimes tempted to enlarge the hole of the nipple, tilt the baby back, and let the liquid trickle down the back of the throat. This is dangerous, because it can cause choking and puts the child in jeopardy of aspiration of fluid into the lungs. As explained earlier, the position of choice for feeding therapy, and also to prevent aspiration and asphyxiation, is upright.

Saliva may be more viscous in children with developmental disabilities. If a child aspirates saliva, it is harder for the child to cough up. For this reason, a supine position is not recommended. The prone position or sidelying for rest or play with absorbant, nonirritating material placed under the mouth area is the position of choice. Bolsters and wedges may be used for play for infants so disabled they cannot sit, stand, or move.

Children with developmental disabilities and dysphagia may have difficulty in achieving mouth closure and in coping with drooling. Oral motor therapy should include oral hygiene as part of a well-rounded program. In general, a normal saline solution made by dissolving a half teaspoon of salt in 8 oz of water is a good cleansing agent. The infant or the child's mouth may be cleansed by wrapping gauze around an adult finger, dampening it in the saline solution, and cleansing the mouth manually. Care should be taken to ensure that the gauze does not slip down the child's throat. It is not advisable to use cotton swabs, because the cotton tip can fall off and choke the child. Excess salivation can also cause irritation of the skin around the mouth, chin area, and the neck and the chest of the child if appropriate layering is not provided. Good skin hygiene includes mild cleansing with a gentle soap followed by application of a mild water repellant cream to protect the skin around these areas. As noted earlier, the child should be observed closely for any evidence of continuous stridor. Continuous stridor with retraction of the ribs is an indication of blockage of the airway and requires immediate medical attention.

In babies and children up to age 5, the airway is significantly smaller than in adults; thus, foods that can lead to a child choking or suffocating should be avoided. According to McClannahan (1987), four kinds of food cause the most hazard:

1. Foods that are small, thin, smooth, or slick when wet. These foods may slip through and block the throat.
2. Hard or tough foods. These foods may block the throat.
3. Foods that are round or cylindrical and pliable or compressible. These foods can easily form a plug in the airway.
4. Foods that are highly viscous, thick and sticky foods. These mold to the airway.

Thus, the following foods should be avoided for children under the age of 5, regardless of the problem with feeding, to avoid asphyxiation (McClannahan, 1987):

■ hot dog-like products unless chopped or diced
■ grapes unless cut up
■ popcorn
■ peanuts and other nuts
■ sunflower and other seeds
■ candy, both soft and hard
■ chewing gum
■ raw carrots
■ apple pieces, especially for children under 2
■ cookies and biscuits, especially for children under 2

Obstructed Airway Procedure

In initiating a feeding program for children with developmental disabilities, it is important for both professionals and parents alike to recognize symptoms of choking and to initiate the Obstructed Airway Procedure or CPR, if necessary (Longo, 1983; Rehm, 1983).

Caution: Written material alone does not constitute training in obstructed airway procedure. To gain the appropriate skills, it is necessary to practice under the guidance of certified instructors.

The following are symptoms of a choking child in distress (Thompson, 1983):

1. The child cannot breath, speak, or cry out.
2. The child turns pale, becomes cyanotic.

3. The child collapses due to loss of consciousness.

Action must be taken quickly as soon as any of these symptoms are observed. If a child is coughing, the airway is only partially obstructed; leave the child alone. If the child has complete airway obstruction, no air can be expelled and the child will be unable to make a sound (American Heart Association, 1988).

Obstructed Airway: Conscious Infant (Under 1 Year Old)

The obstructed airway procedure must be modified in an infant. It is implemented in the following manner. If the infant is unable to cry or cough effectively, deliver four back blows.

1. Support the infant's head and neck with one hand held firmly holding the jaw.
2. With the adult forearm supported on the thigh, straddle the infant face down with the head lower than the trunk.
3. With the heel of the adult free hand, deliver four back blows forcefully between the infant's shoulder blades. (The blows along with the pressure of the adult's thigh on the infant's abdomen simulate the subdiaphragmatic thrust of the Heimlich Maneuver.)

If this does not dislodge the obstruction, deliver four chest thrusts:

1. Hold the infant in the lap between the adult's arms with the infant turned on his or her back and the head lower than the trunk.
2. Place the index and middle finger of one hand against the infant's abdomen above the navel and approximately one finger's width below the point between the two nipples on the infant's chest.
3. With the index and middle fingers in position, deliver four thrusts in the midsternal region with a quick upward thrust.

4. After locating the position for chest thrusts, be sure the adult's fingers are not on the tip of the sternum.

Alternate these maneuvers in rapid sequence: four back blows, then four chest thrusts. Repeat sequence until the object is expelled.

It is important that this procedure be used in infants and toddlers, because it controls the force of the thrust. This is necessary to prevent damage to the abdomen, abdominal viscera, especially the liver and spleen, and rib cage (American Heart Association, 1988).

Obstructed Airway: Unconscious Infant (Under 1 Year Old)

The procedure for the infant with an obstructed airway who is unconscious is a combination of back blows, chest thrusts, and mouth to mouth resuscitation. It is implemented in the following manner:

1. Turn the infant on his or her back as a unit being careful to support the head and neck.
2. Use the head-tilt/chin-lift maneuver to position the infant's head in a neutral position.
3. Open the airway and determine the infant is not breathing.
4. Make a tight seal over the infant's mouth and nose and give two rescue breaths.
5. Reposition the infant's head and try to give rescue breaths again.
6. Position infant as described previously for back blows and deliver four back blows.
7. Next position infant for chest thrusts and deliver four chest thrusts.
8. Perform tongue-jaw lift by turning the infant's head up, and open mouth by placing thumb in the infant's mouth over tongue. Lift the tongue and jaw forward with fingers wrapped around the infant's lower jaw. Remove the obstruction only if it is visible.

9. Otherwise, reposition the infant's head using the head-tilt/chin-lift maneuver and give two rescue breaths.
10. If the airway remains obstructed, alternate back blows, chest thrusts, obstructed object check, open airway, and rescue breathing in rapid sequence (American Heart Association, 1988).

Obstructed Airway: Conscious Child (1 to 8 Years Old)

The Heimlich Maneuver for children is carried out in the same manner as for adults; however, the nurse simply lessens the force of the subdiaphragmatic thrust on the child. The Heimlich Maneuver for a conscious child is performed as follows:

1. Stand behind the child and wrap your arms around the child's waist.
2. Make a fist with one hand and place the thumb side against the child's abdomen slightly against the naval and below the rib cage.
3. Grasp your fist with your other hand and press into the child's abdomen with a quick upward thrust. Repeat thrusts several times if necessary (American Heart Association, 1988).

The Heimlich Maneuver may also be performed on the conscious child in the sitting position according to Thompson (1983). If the child is sitting, the nurse stands or kneels behind the child's chair and performs the maneuver in the same manner as described as the child was standing. The back of the chair acts as support for the child's back and appears to augment the effect of the subdiaphragmatic thrust. It should be noted that the Heimlich Maneuver is not a bear hug. Compress only with your hands, not with your arms, or damage to the rib cage or internal abdominal organs can result. With children age 1 to 8 years old, the force of the thrust should be less than that for an adult.

Obstructed Airway: Unconscious Child (1 to 8 Years Old)

The procedure for the child with an obstructed airway who is unconscious is a combination of mouth to mouth resuscitation and subdiaphragmatic thrusts. It is implemented in the following manner:

1. Turn the child on his or her back as a unit with support to the head and neck.
2. Implement the head-tilt/chin-lift maneuver to position the child's head in a neutral position.
3. Observe chest and feel for breath.
4. Pinch nostrils and make a tight seal over the child's mouth.
5. Give two rescue breaths.
6. Reposition the child's head, pinch nostrils, and give rescue breaths again.
7. Next, kneel at the child's feet or stand at child's feet if child is on a table.
8. Place the heel of one hand on the child's abdomen at midline slightly above the navel and below the tip of the sternum.
9. Place the second hand directly on top of the first hand and press into the abdomen with quick upward thrusts.
10. Give 6 to 10 subdiaphragmatic abdominal thrusts.
11. Perform tongue jaw lift as described previously. Remove the obstruction only if it is visible.
12. Reposition the child's head using the head-tilt/chin-lift maneuver and give two rescue breaths.
13. If the airway remains obstructed, alternate abdominal thrusts, obstructed object check, open airway, and rescue breathing in rapid sequence (American Heart Association, 1988).

Thompson (1983) notes that in addition to acting quickly to save an infant who is choking, another area of nursing responsibility lies in educating parents to prevent choking. This education can take place in the hospital, in the physician's office, or in an early intervention program (Long, 1992). Nurses can teach parents the following:

1. Do not force feed infants or prop bottles.
2. Introduce solid foods at a time when the baby has teeth for proper chewing or as designated by the dysphagia team.
3. Check toys for small removable parts such as buttons, snaps, and so forth. Babies are completely dependent on their parents for survival.
4. Remove small objects from a child's reach.
5. Prevent children under age 6 who do not have their molar teeth from eating hard candy, popcorn, raw carrots and celery, or fish with bones.
6. Cut children's food, especially meat, into small portions.
7. Set a good example for children by not putting objects in your mouth.

CPR for Infants and Young Children

This life-saving procedure consists of two techniques that should be used concurrently, mouth to mouth resuscitation and external cardiac massage. Mouth to mouth resuscitation should be started and continued at the same time that closed cardiac massage is administered by another person. If the infant or child is in respiratory arrest, the nurse should immediately auscultate for a heartbeat and palpate for the carotid, brachial, or femoral pulse. In an infant, the brachial pulse is palpated.

Caution: Written material alone does not constitute a CPR course. To gain the skills of CPR, it is necessary to practice on manikins, with certified instructors as guides.

Mouth to Mouth Resuscitation

The child's head should be tilted back only slightly to prevent obstruction of the airway. The technique of mouth to mouth resuscitation in young children is similar to that for adults except that both the nose and the mouth are covered. The jaw should be brought forward slightly, as described previously, so that the tongue is not obstructing the airway. Breathe into the infant's nose and mouth or the child's mouth two times with complete filling of the adult's lungs after each breath. In older children, only the mouth is covered and the nostrils are firmly pinched so they are airtight. Small breaths are given for 1 to 1½ seconds per inflation. The mouth is removed to permit the child to exhale. The child should be observed for thoracoabdominal respiratory movements when giving mouth to mouth resuscitation. If there is no pulse, external cardiac massage must be initiated. In the absence of a brachial pulse, breathe for the infant at a rate of 20 times per minute or one breath every 3 seconds. In the absence of a carotid pulse, breathe for the child at a rate of 15 times per minute or one breath every 4 seconds (American Heart Association, 1988).

External Cardiac Massage

In external cardiac massage, the heart is compressed between the sternum and the vertebrae.

The method and identification of external landmarks for compression differ for the infant and child. To locate landmarks on the infant, the nurse draws in imaginary line between the nipples and places the index finger farthest from the head of the infant under the intermammary line at the point where it intersects with the sternum. The area of compression is located one finger width's below this intersection or at the location of the middle and ring fingers. The tips of the index and middle fingers are used to apply chest compression to a depth of 0.5 to 1 inch done at least 100 times a minute in the infant. Chest compression downward 1 to 1½ inches at a rate of 80-100 times per minute is used in the child (American Heart Association, 1988). The heel of the hand is utilized in the child at a point just above the tip of the sternum. During external cardiac massage, the back of the infant or child should be supported on a firm surface. The sternum should be compressed firmly and smoothly and the pressure released immediately so that cardiac filling can occur adequately. Caution should be used to avoid vigorous compression, because this can result in fracture of the sternum and mild cardiac injury. With effective cardiopulmonary resuscitation, femoral, carotid, and brachial pulses should become palpable. The color of the mucous membranes should improve, and the pupils should constrict. During cardiopulmonary resuscitation, the infant or child should be kept warm, because chilling causes pulmonary vasoconstriction and increases the need for oxygen (American Heart Association, 1988).

Many hospitals are now offering expectant parents courses in CPR (Wagner & Braun, 1992). It is advisable that this become a routine part of training for expectant parents, because choking can precipitate a life or death situation in the child with developmental disabilities and dysphagia. If early intervention programs are conducting feeding therapy, at least one team member should be currently certified in CPR and the Obstructed Airway Procedure. Many early intervention programs routinely offer CPR training to parents through the American Red Cross and other voluntary agencies. However, asphyxiation and aspiration can be avoided through management of a good feeding program and appropriate education of parents and other family members.

Families and Intervention Strategies

Role of the Family

Family members must be viewed as essential team members in any feeding program for infants with dysphagia. Professionals must allow families to define themselves as they may not reflect traditional families. Nuclear families are generally thought to consist of mothers and fathers, siblings, aunts and uncles, and grandparents. Families can also consist of extended family members, friends, and the community. Families today are much more likely to consist of single parents, blended families, and non-traditional families. Family settings for children with developmental disabilities can also consist of foster care, residential placement, and other custodial situations.

Family Assessment

The foundation of an intervention plan for feeding difficulties must start with a family assessment according to Bailey and Simeonsson (1988) and Turnbull and Turnbull (1986). The meaning of a child's behavior around mealtime needs to be explored with the parents or primary caregivers. Parents should also identify to professionals sources of advice on parenting practices such as grandparents, extended family members, and friends. This will let professionals know how parents are developing their philosophy and practice for feeding behaviors with their infant. Professional recommendations consistent with the family's social network that influences feeding practice will increase the probability of family application (Humphrey, 1991).

Implementation

Feeding difficulties may be a source of parent-professional stress (Humphrey, 1991). Parenting is influenced by a number of factors, and professional input may not be weighed as heavily as advice from others in the parents' social network. Teamwork of families and professionals is needed in all aspects of early intervention. Intervention programs are most effective when families participate as partners with professionals (Phillips & Brostoff, 1989). Feeding a child with a developmental disability may take several hours a day, and the family may decide to use an alternate option that they feel is best for family function. Therapeutic feeding suggestions need to be evaluated in re-

lation to how much time the particular activity will take and its consequent impact on other aspects of family-child interactions according to Morris (1987). Strategies that enhance the family's feeling of control over some aspects of the child's intervention is important. Professionals must work with families on strategies that are not simply child focused, but emphasize parent-child interaction. Programs that have specifically supported optimal parent-child interactions have been successful in reducing the amount of physical directiveness and increasing the responsiveness of parents according to Hanzlik (1989) and Mahoney and Powell (1988). A healthy family-child relationship can foster maximum support for compensation for the problems that result from dysphagia in children with developmental disabilities

Experiences with feeding influence the developmental progress of the parent and infant. Interactive behaviors of the dyad may be directly or indirectly affected by characteristics of the underlying problem in the infant associated with the dysfunction (Humphrey, 1991). As stated previously, research on individual differences among families suggest they will influence reactions to an infant's difficulty in feeding. The impact of the family system on the parent-child subsystem and the reciprocal impact of the dyad on general family functioning needs to be acknowledged by professionals. If feeding issues compromise the general quality of the parent-child relationship, the child may be at risk for a less than optimal long-term outcome, even when nutritional status is improved (Humphrey, 1991).

Role of Siblings

Siblings play an important role in the families of children with dysphagia. In the instance of an older sibling, a great deal of responsibility may be given to that child to help with the care of the younger sibling, particularly feeding and dressing. There may be resentment on the part of the older sibling for this added responsibility if not approached properly. Younger siblings of the child with dysphagia may find less time and attention devoted to them and consequently may either act out or withdraw. Professionals need to be sensitive to the needs of all family members as they develop the child's feeding program. A visit to the home when other family members, particularly siblings, are present is an opportunity for professionals to evaluate family relationships and encourage family members to be a part of the total program.

Role of Grandparents and Other Extended Family Members

Because other family members are an extension of the nuclear family, it is important for professionals to recognize the role that grandparents and other family members play in the family system. If there is no opportunity during the home visit to interface with other family members, they may be invited to participate in a feeding session with the parent and the professional or at least be encouraged to be a part of the discharge planning process. The more family members are involved and supportive of the feeding program, the more supports the parents will have and the more competent they will consequently feel in implementing the program that is best suited for their child and family.

Family Training to Help with Feeding

As stated throughout this chapter, feeding is a critical social activity that helps children develop appropriate developmental skills as well as provide appropriate nutrition. Important developmental skills that the infant must acquire are regulation of state and attachment as well as the development of separation and individuation (Satter, 1992). The groundwork for these skills should begin at approximately 6 months of age in the infant. Parent feeding behaviors that support homeostasis and attachment on the one hand and separation and individuation on the other are critical for promotion of healthy psychosocial development. Tables 16–1 and 16–2 outline parent behaviors, as defined by Satter (1992), that support these phases.

Although these principles were developed for feeding behavior with the normal developing child, they apply to feeding therapy with modifications for the child with dysphagia and developmental disabilities. Children need appropriate supports from parents to manifest their eating capability. A synchronous relationship between the child and parent will support effective feeding. Finally, the focus in feeding should not always be on getting food into the child. Such emphasis puts stress on the parent-child relationship. The focus of a feeding program should also be on the feeding relationship and helping the child learn eating skills and positive eating behaviors (Humphrey, 1991).

Summary

Nurses are in a key position to play an integral role in the assessment and management of the child with dysphagia, as well as working with the family. Evaluating parent-child interactions during feeding, helping parents choose appropriate feeding methods and utensils, and encouraging all family members to participate in the program are critical. Parent education programs on breast-feeding, gastrostomies and their care, prevention of aspiration and asphyxiation, and CPR and obstructed airway procedures are all essential components of a comprehensive service. When families and their children experience success in the feeding process through carefully planned and coordinated nursing intervention, the parent-child relationship is enhanced.

Table 16–1. Parent Behaviors that Support Homeostasis and Attachment.

Follow the baby's signals about what time to feed.

Feed promptly when the baby is hungry before the baby becomes aroused from heavy crying.

Hold the baby so you can look at each other during feeding.

Hold the baby securely but not restrictively.

When using a bottle, hold it still at an appropriate angle and don't move the bottle or the baby.

Be sure the nipple flows at appropriate speed.

Stimulate the rooting reflex by touching the baby's cheek.

Touch the nipple to the baby's lips and let the baby open his or her mouth before feeding.

Let the baby decide how much to have and at what tempo.

Let the baby pause, rest, socialize, and go back to eating.

Talk and smile but don't overwhelm the baby with attention.

Burp only if the baby seems to need it. Don't disrupt feeding with unnecessary burping and wiping.

Stop the feeding when the baby refuses the nipple or indicates satiety and lack of interest in eating by turning away, refusing to open the mouth, or arching the back.

Source: From "The Feeding Relationship" by E. Sattler, 1992, p. 2. *Zero to Three, 12*(5), 1–9, with permission.

Table 16–2. *Parent Behaviors that Support Separation and Individuation.*

Feed when the child wants to eat, but gradually evolve a time structure that is appropriate for everyone in the family.

Seat the child upright and facing forward.

Sit directly in front of the child.

Hold the spoon so the child can see it.

Be engaging but not overwhelming. Take care not to overload the child with talking or behavior.

Talk in a quiet and encouraging manner.

Wait for the child to open up and pay attention before feeding.

Let the child touch the food and eat with fingers.

Let the child self-feed when ready.

When the child is self-feeding, remain present in the situation, don't take over.

Let the child decide how fast to eat.

Let the child decide how much to eat.

Respect the child's food preferences.

Respect the child's caution about new foods.

Remember, all children learn to eat eventually.

Source: From "The Feeding Relationship" by E. Sattler, 1992, p. 3. *Zero to Three, 12*(5), 1–9, with permission.

References

American Heart Association. (1988). *Textbook of pediatric basic life support.* Dallas, TX: American Heart Association.

Arvedson, J., & Brodsky, L. (1993). *Pediatric swallowing and feeding, assessment and management.* San Diego, CA: Singular Publishing Group.

Bailey, D., & Simeonsson, R. (1988). *Family as assessment in early intervention.* Columbus, OH: Merrill.

Bardon, R. C., Ford, M. E., Jensen, A. G., Roger Salyer, M., & Roger-Salyer, K. C. (1989). Effects of cranio-facial deformity in infancy on the quality of mother-infant interaction. *Child Development, 60,* 781–792.

Barnard, K. (1979). *Nursing Child Assess-ment Feeding Scale.* (Available from NCAST Publications, Mail stop WJ 10, University of Washington, Seattle, WA 98195.)

Barnard, K., & Erickson, M. (1976). *Teaching children with developmental disabilities.* St. Louis, MO: C. V. Mosby.

Barnard, K., Hammond, M. A., Booth, C. L., Bee, H., Mitchell, S., & Spieker, S. (1989). Measurement and meaning of parent-child interaction. In F. Morrison, C. Lord, & D. Keating (Eds.), *Applied developmental psychology* (Vol. 3, pp. 40–76). New York: Academic Press.

Bax, M. (1989). Eating is important. *Developmental Medicine and Child Neurology, 31,* 285–286.

Brewster, D. (1979). *You can breastfeed your baby...even in special situations.* Emmaus, PA: Rodale Press.

Brizee, L. S., Sophos, C. M., & McLaughlin, J. F. (1990). Nutrition issues in developmental disabilities. *Infants and Young Children, 2,* 10–21.

Campos, R. G. (1989). Soothing pain-elicited distress in infants with swaddling and pacifiers. *Child Development, 60,* 781–792.

Committee on Nutrition, American Academy of Pediatrics. (1976). Commentary on breast-feeding and infant formulas, including proposal standards for formulas. *Pediatrics, 5,* 278–285.

Committee on Nutrition, American Academy of Pediatrics. (1980). On the feeding of supplemental food to infants. *Pediatrics, 65,* 1178–1181.

Connor, F., Williamson, G., & Siepp, J. (1978). *Program guide for infants and toddlers with neuromotor and other developmental disabilities.* New York: Teachers College Press.

Coyner, A. (1983). Meeting health needs of handicapped infants. In R. Zelle & A. Coyner (Eds.), *Developmentally disabled infants and toddlers* (pp. 1–59). Philadelphia: F. A. Davis.

Coyner, A., & Zelle, R. (1983). Habilitative approaches to facilitate more adaptive oral motor patterns related to eating and expressive language. In R. Zelle & A. Coyner (Eds.), *Developmentally disabled infants and toddlers* (pp. 443–455). Philadelphia: F. A. Davis.

Dahl, M. (1987). Early feeding problems in an affluent society: III. Follow-up at two years: Natural course, health, behavior and development. *Acta Pediatrica Scandinavia, 76,* 872–880.

Dahl, M., & Kristiansson, B. (1987). Early feeding problems in an affluent society: IV. Impact on growth up to two years of age. *Acta Pediatrica Scandinavia, 76,* 884–888.

Davis, B., & Steele, S. (1991). Case management for young children with special health care needs. *Pediatric Nursing, 17*(1), 15–19.

Ernst, J. A., Bull, M. J., Rickard, K. A., Brady, M. S., Schreiner, R. L., Gresham, E. L., & Lemans, J. A. (1983). Feeding practices of the very low-birthweight infant within the first year. *Journal of the American Dietetic Association, 82,* 158–162.

Finnie, N. (1975). *Handling the young cerebral palsied child at home.* New York: E. P. Dutton.

Hanzlik, J. (1989). The effect of intervention on the free-play experience for mothers and their infants with developmental delay and cerebral palsy. *Physical and Occupational Therapy in Pediatrics, 9,* 33–51.

Haynes, U. (1983). *Holistic health care for children with developmental disabilities.* Baltimore, MD: University Park Press.

Hopkins, B., & Westra, T. (1989). Maternal expectations of their infants development: Some cultural differences. *Developmental Medicine and Child Neurology, 31,* 384–390.

Huddleston, K., & Ferraro, A. (1991). Preparing families of children with gastrostomies. *Pediatric Nursing, 17*(2), 153–158.

Huddleston, K., & Palmer, K. (1990). A button for gastrostomy feedings. *Maternal and Child Nursing, 15*, 315–319.

Humphrey, R. (1991). Impact of feeding problems on the parent-infant relationship. *Infants and Young Children, 3*(3), 30–38.

Jones, M. (1985). *Home care for the chronically ill or disabled child*. New York: Harper & Row.

Linscheid, J. (1985). Feeding disorders during infancy and early childhood. *Feelings and their medical significance, 27*(3). Columbus, OH: Ross Laboratories.

Longo, A. (1983). Teaching parents CPR. *Pediatric Nursing, 9*(6), 445–448.

Long, C. (1992). Teaching parents infant CPR—Lecture or audiovisual tape? Maternal and Child Nursing, 17, 30–32.

Lotze, M. (1988). Developmental disabilities. In D. Marlow & B. Redding (Eds.), *Textbook of pediatric nursing* (pp. 971–982). Philadelphia: W. B. Saunders.

Magyary, C. (1984). Early social interactions: Preterm infant-parent dyads. *Issues in Comprehensive Pediatric Nursing, 7*, 233–254.

Mahoney, G., Fors, S., & Wood, S. (1990). Maternal directive behavior revisited. *American Journal of Mental Retardation, 94*, 398–407.

Mahoney, G., & Powell, A. (1988). Modifying parent-child interaction: Enhancing the development of handicapped children. *Journal of Special Education, 22*, 82–96.

Marlow, D., & Redding, B. (1988). *Textbook of pediatric nursing* (6th ed.). Philadelphia: W. B. Saunders.

McClannahan, C. (1987). *Feeding and caring for infants and children with special needs*. Rockville, MD: American Occupational Therapy Association.

Meier, P., & Anderson, G. (1987). Responses of small preterm infants to bottle and breast-feeding. *Maternal Child Nursing, 12*, 97–105.

Miller, S. A. (1988). Parents beliefs about children's cognitive development. *Child Development, 59*, 259–285.

Minde, K. K. (1984). The impact of prematurity on the later behavior on children and on their families. *Clinical Perinatology, 11*, 227–244.

Morris, S. (1987). Therapy for the child with cerebral palsy: Interacting frameworks. *Seminars in Speech Language, 8*, 71–86.

Morris, S., & Klein, M. (1987). *Pre-feeding skills: A comprehensive resource for feeding development*. Tucson, AZ: Therapy Skill Builders.

Nelson, C., & Hallgren, R. (1989). Gastrostomies: Indications, management and weaning. *Infants and Young Children, 2*(1), 66–74.

Pilegard, E. (1992, April/May). Tips for parents. *Exceptional Parent*, p. 26.

Phillips, M., & Brostoff, M. (1989). Working collaboratively with parents of disabled children. *Pediatric Nursing, 15*(2), 180–185.

Rehm, R. (1983). Teaching cardiopulmonary resuscitation to parents. *Maternal Child Nursing, 8*, 411–414.

Satter, E. (1992). The feeding relationship. *Zero to Three, 12*(5), 1–9.

Thompson, S. (1983). How to use the heimlich maneuver on choking infants and children. *Pediatric Nursing, 9*(1), 13–16.

Trostle, J. A. (1988). Medical compliance as an ideology. *Social Science and Medicine, 27*, 1299–1308.

Turnbull, A., & Turnbull, H. (1986). *Families, professionals and exceptionality*. Columbus, OH: Merrill.

Wagner, B., & Braun, D. (1992). Infant cardiopulmonary resuscitation for expectant and new parents. *Maternal and Child Nursing, 17*, 27–29.

Weigley, E. (1990). Changing patterns in offering solids to infants. *Pediatric Nursing, 16*(5), 439–441.

Wolf, L., & Glass, R. (1992). *Feeding and swallowing disorders in infancy, assessment and management*. Tucson, AZ: Therapy Skill Builders.

Raising A Child With Developmental Disability: Understanding The Family Perspective

JAN HANDLEMAN, Ed.D.

CONTENTS

The Arnold Family

Judy and Steve Arnold had just celebrated their seventh wedding anniversary when they received the news that Judy was pregnant. Like most couples, the Arnolds had joyfully planned for the exciting addition to their family and made all the necessary preparations. With the maternity leave approved and the nursery painted, Judy and Steve anxiously awaited the birth of their child.

Jodi's first few months brought joy to family and friends. She slept well, was content and seemed to enjoy spending hours playing in her crib. Jodi almost never fussed and rarely demanded attention. Judy and Steve expressed pride with each developmental milestone. While everyone commented on what a perfect child Jodi was at 6 months of age, Judy and Steve grew concerned about their daughter's growth and development. She did not appear to be taking in enough breast milk to to gain weight. Judy had decided to supplement her breast-feeding with solid food and found that Jodi rejected the feedings. Mealtimes soon became increasingly stressful and concern for Jodi's nourishment grew. In addition, Judy and Steve noticed a growing indifference to people by Jodi and increasing unresponsiveness. The Arnolds knew that there was something seriously wrong with their child. As time went on, Jodi rejected foods with texture, failed to learn to chew, and refused the cup. She also spit up frequently and would swallow the regurgitated material.

After of series of multidisciplinary assessments, a diagnosis of developmental disability and dysphagia was made by the staff of a state teaching hospital. A behavioral and dietary regimen was prescribed with regular monitoring by medical and support professionals. Further therapeutic intervention and medical work-up for diagnosis and treatment of the dysphagia were begun.

The Arnolds began to struggle with the devastating news and the challenges presented by the feeding and behavioral program. Judy and Steve found themselves interacting with one another with a frustration they had never experienced in their marriage before. There were many days that Steve could not bring himself to go to work, and Judy spent many hours on the phone crying to her mother. They both felt their dreams for Jodi had been shattered.

In the months that followed, Judy and Steve found it difficult to find friends and family who truly understood what they were going through. Steve found it very hard to accept his father's thoughts that Jodi would grow out of it. Judy became angry with her close friends for canceling play dates for the children. With each week, Jodi's disability became clearer.

Jodi's enrollment in an early intervention program resulted in much needed support for the family. Jodi slowly began to respond to efforts to teach her to tolerate solid foods, and she began to enjoy playful interactions with her parents. She was begun on antacids as well, and her regurgitation slowly decreased. Steve and Judy received support and guidance from professionals to help them cope, made new friendships with parents of other children with disabilities who understood their problems, and began to feel a new sense of control over their lives.

Probably one of the most painful experiences in the life of a parent is learning that his or her child has a disability. The extreme disappointment felt when dreams for a child are destroyed can result in anger and frustration. Although the Arnolds struggled with the challenges that their daughter's diagnosis brought, they were able to combine their strengths and move closer to one another. The support they received from friends, family, and knowledgeable professionals resulted in adapting to their extraordinary situation. The purpose of this chapter is to offer professionals an appreciation of the impact that having a child with a developmental disability can have on the family. It is difficult to fully meet the responsibility of providing professional services for children with developmental disabilities without developing a sensitivity for the complexities families of such children face and a commitment to collaboration with families.

The Nature and Needs of Children with Developmental Disabilities and Their Families

The term developmental disability is multidimensional. The interaction of age of onset, etiology, and type of disability affects a child's level of functioning and results in a spectrum of developmental and behavioral manifestations (Handleman & Harris, 1986). Of recent interest are children whose profiles fall in the severe range of the disability continuum. For example, as a result of confusion of terminology regarding children diagnosed with autism, severe mental retardation, and multiple disabilities, professionals and parents have chosen to refer to these youngsters as displaying severe developmental disabilities (Handleman, 1986; Handleman & Harris, l986; Powers & Handleman, l984). The inclusion of these children under the umbrella of developmental disabilities has resulted in a better understanding of their needs and more effective service provision.

The behaviors of children with developmental disabilities are influenced by a variety of organic and environmental factors, and the population is behaviorally heterogeneous (Handleman & Harris, l986). Diagnosis is a very intricate process com-

plicated by such factors as age of onset, lack of speech, and behavioral challenges. For example, these youngsters may demonstrate multiple difficulties with the acquisition and development of communication skills.

They may have problems with the mechanics of speech or the more complex skill of comprehension, and these deficits in communication may be compounded by social unresponsiveness and serious behavioral challenges such as self-injury. In addition, developmental and cognitive disorders, such as mental retardation or eating difficulties, can further complicate both the diagnostic and habilitation process.

The diagnosis, assessment, and treatment of children with developmental disabilities are among the more challenging issues facing professionals. Service delivery to these children is an intricate task. The diversity of requirements extends beyond traditional concerns and includes their educational, behavioral, medical, home, and community needs. A comprehensive service delivery system is necessary to meet these needs. The expertise and responsiveness of multiple specialists, as well as interdisciplinary assessment and planning, result in the most effective system of services.

Impact of the Child with a Developmental Disability on the Family

Parents

The specialized needs of children with developmental disabilites affect every facet of family life (Fong, 1991; Handleman & Harris, 1986). Although the parents of children with developmental disabilities do not suffer a greater than usual frequency of serious mental disorders (DeMyer, 1979; Gath, 1978), they do respond with measurable distress to the experience of raising a child with a disability. In many cases, they describe greater life discomfort than parents of children without disabilities (Gath & Gumley, 1984) and report that the family environment is less encouraging of stable relationships and personal growth than parents of children without disabilities (Margalit & Raviv, 1983).

Although both parents feel the impact of living with a child with a developmental disability, the stress is often greater for mothers than fathers (Beckman, 1983). Mothers describe more feelings of guilt, suffer more physical complaints, and have more doubts about their parenting abilities than do fathers (Fong, 1991; DeMyer, 1979). In addition, increased symptoms of depression have been identified for mothers of these youngsters (Gath, 1978).

Although less research has been conducted with fathers than mothers, men also experience significant stress in response to the special demands of their son or daughter with a developmental disability. In addition to coping with their own disappointments and loss, fathers may experience distress by witnessing their spouses' pain and feeling unable to help them (DeMyer, 1979). Because fathers typically have less contact with their children than mothers, they may feel that they are limited in their ability to contribute to parenting (Cummings, 1976). As often the primary wage earners, fathers may tend to worry more than mothers about financial burdens (Lamb, 1983).

Recognizing the complexities of maintaining a successful marriage, it is not surprising that the presence of a child with a disability can make this task more challenging (DeMyer & Goldberg, 1983). Although the special needs of the child place extensive demands on the family, there is little evidence that the presence of a child with a developmental disability is directly related to a deterioration of the marriage (Koegel, Schreibman, O'Neill, &

Burke, 1983). Marriages may simply become more complex with the presence of a child with a developmental disability and dysphagia or weakened (Bouma & Schweitzer, 1990; Gath, 1978).

Although little is known about which marriages will be enhanced and which will suffer as the result of the stress of parenting a child with a developmental disability, there appear to be a number of contributing factors. One variable that does seem to be related to marital satisfaction is the sharing of child care responsibilities. Boyle (1985) reported that families that had an equitable distribution of child care reported higher marital satisfaction than those with a greater imbalance of involvement. The sexual relationship also may suffer from the fatiquing demands of physical care of the child or concern about the risk of conceiving another child with a disability.

Siblings

There is some question whether there are either challenges or benefits to growing up with a sibling with a developmental disability (Edmundson, 1985). It has been suggested that it may be more stressful to have a brother or sister with a developmental disability and that sex and birth order may be influencing variables (Ferrari, 1982; Tew & Laurence, 1973). A number of studies have indicated that stress may be especially intense for older sisters and younger brothers (Breslau, 1982; Cleveland & Miller, 1977).

Regardless of birth order or sex, siblings of children with developmental disabilities do seem to have different patterns of interaction with their brother or sister than other children have with siblings without disabilities. There may be differences in general and emotional responsiveness, and these siblings may have few opportunities for the kind of intimate sharing that typically characterizes many healthy sibling relationships. Nonetheless, siblings of children with developmental disabilities, like their parents, do not seem to exhibit more serious adjustment problems than siblings of children without disabilities (Cleveland & Miller, 1977).

Extended Family

Little information is available to help professionals understand the reactions of the extended family to the birth of a child with a developmental disability. Grandparents are central figures in many childhood experiences, but there is limited research on their roles with and perceptions of a grandchild with a disability. Some professionals have suggested that it is important to be sensitive to the disappointments experienced by grandparents who have a grandchild with a developmental disability (Berns, 1980; Handleman & Harris, 1986) and others have written about the potentially useful role these family members can fill in providing support within the family (Rhoades, 1975). Grandparents may not view themselves as being responsible for the shortcomings of their grandchildren (Albrecht, 1954) and may possess a more positive and optimistic view than their children (Harris, Handleman, & Palmer, 1985).

Life Cycle of the Family with a Child with a Developmental Disability

Recently, clinicians have considered the concept of the family life cycle to describe important life transitions that persons experience as members of a family (Carter and McGoldrick, 1980; Figley and McCubbin, 1983). When two people marry they pass from being children in their families of origin to being partners in marriage. Once this relationship has stabilized, couples may choose to take on the transitional task

of having children. Demands and changes continue throughout the life cycle (e.g., children entering adolescence and leaving home). In addition, families must adapt to life cycle events such as the aging of parents and the death of a spouse.

It is useful to be aware of the impact that major transitional events have on all families in order to be sensitive to some of the extraordinary experiences encountered by families of children with developmental disabilities. Parents have dreams about what their children will be like and accomplish. There are few things in life more painful for parents than recognizing that their child has a developmental disability and the limitations that may be placed on the child's future accomplishments.

Dealing with the diagnosis is the first life cycle event that impacts on the family of a child with a developmental disability. Parents of children who have Down's Syndrome will be confronted with their child's disability shortly after birth. For families of a child with autism or mental retardation, the more obvious signs of disability may not appear until months after birth.

Professionals play a major role in the intrinsically difficult process of conveying a diagnosis of developmental disability and dysphagia to families. While physicians often have the first contact with the family, educators and other clinicians may be called upon to convey diagnostic information. Of the few studies that have previously been conducted, results have suggested that many families had disapproved of the way that they were first informed of their children's disability (Abramson, Gravink, Abramson, and Sommers, 1977; Gath, 1978). One critical factor in informing parents, however, seems to be the immediacy of sharing information (Gath, 1978).

For Parents, mourning a child's disability is not an experience that occurs once and is then completed for parents. Rather, there are episodes of sadness stirred by important life events that reawaken a sense of grief (Handleman and Harris, 1986; Olshansky, 1962; Wikler, 1981). This process of episodic mourning is referred to as "chronic sorrow" (Olshansky, 1962). The time of the child's diagnosis is one of the most powerful markers for the family. In addition to this initial event, there are a number of other major life cycle experiences that the family will encounter such as the child entering school and becoming an adult.

Typically a child's entry in kindergarten is one in a series of graded separations in the life cycle of a family. While most parents are pleased to watch their child go off the school, there may also exist feelings of regret that the preschool years are over. For the parents of a child with a developmental disability, this event may be extremely stressful because it serves as a vivid reminder that their child is different from others (Handleman & Harris, 1986).

The need for continuing supervision that the child with a developmental disability requires often has an impact on a parent's development. At a time when options are increasing for other parents such as opportunities for career changes or travel, parents of children with developmental disabilities are faced with balancing personal interests with the special needs of their child.

The special needs of the child with a developmental disability may affect siblings as well as parents. Siblings may feel deep responsibility and love for their brother or sister and yet experience a conflict over the extent to which they should include that sibling in their own adult lives. Brothers and sisters also may miss some childhood experiences because their sibling with a disability is unable to participate in certain activities or family events such as vacations. Siblings may receive less attention from their parents as the result of the special care demands of their brother or sister. Even more difficult for siblings may be learning to deal with the reactions of their friends to the disability of their brother or sister.

A child's adolescence is often a tumultuous time for families (Kidwell, Fischer, Dunhma, and Baranowski, 1983). This life cycle event is frequently viewed as the most demanding transition period and one of the least satisfying times in the life of the family (Ackerman, 1980; Bristol & Schopler, 1983). For the family with a child with a developmental disability, the special demands of child rearing do not end with the closing of childhood. Challenges may grow as social and public support decrease, and stress can intensify when beginning to plan for the adult years (DeMyer and Goldberg, 1983; Marcus, 1984).

A young person's twenty-first birthday is reported to be second only to the time of initial diagnosis as a source of extreme stress for parents (Wikler, Wasow, and Hatfield, 1981). Parents of children with developmental disabilites must deal with their child's continuing need for supervision, potential out-of-home placement, as well as their own physical and emotional fatigue (Handleman and Harris, 1986). In addition, the potential for prolonged dependency on the part of the child may result in concerns by parents of their own death and lack of opportunity to grow beyond their roles as parents.

Creating An Effective Family/Professional Relationship

While the professional cannot eliminate the depression, anger or other responses that parents may experience as they struggle to cope with the special demands of their child with a developmental disability and dysphagia, recognition of how these factors may effect family life is very important. Often, simply hearing some sympathetic words of support may make life considerably easier and lessen some of the burden.

Helping parents understand their child's disability, assisting them in coping with their feelings, and helping them make plans for their child's intervention are the challenges that face the professional. Understanding the complexities of the accommodations that these families must make can enhance the effectiveness of the family/professional relationship. Asking parents what they regard as being helpful can often serve to validate their perspective and promote successful collaboration.

Services can be enhanced by an understanding of the normative experiences involved in the family life cycle and the special needs created by the child with a developmental disability and dysphagia. The professional and the parent can then emerge with an appreciation for the unique, as well as the normative and nonpathological nature of some of the stress experienced as a part of every day living.

Summary

While neither parents, siblings, or extended family members seem to suffer in any sustained way from the complexities of living with a child with a developmental disability, these families typically experience more stress in life than other families. In the case of the Arnolds, Jodi's special needs presented Judy and Steve with many challenges. Responding to their extraordinary demands necessitated personal resolve, emotional strength, family support and professional responsiveness.

The professional who provides services to families with children with developmental disabilities and dysphagia will find it necessary to be sensitive to the range of family experiences. When attention is focused on assisting families to adapt to their situation, family functioning will be enhanced.

References

Abramson, P. R., Gravink, M.J. Abramson, L.M., and Sommers, D. (1977) Early diagnosis and intervention of retardation: A survey of parental reactions concerning the quality of services rendered. *Mental Retardation, 15,* 28–31.

Ackerman, N. J. (1980). The family with adolescents. In E.A. Carter and M. McGoldrick (Eds.), *The family life cycle A framework for family therapy* (pp. 147–169). New York: Gardner Press.

Albrecht, R. (1954). The parental responsibilities of grandparents. *Marriage and Family Living, 16,* 201–204.

Beckman, P. J. (1983). Influence of selected child characteristics on stress in families of handicapped infants. *American Journal of Mental Deficiency, 88,* 150–156.

Berns, J. H. (1980). Grandparents of handicapped children. *Social Work, 25,* 238–239.

Bouma, R., and Schweitzer, R. (1990). The impact of chronic childhood illness on family stress: A comparisom between autism and cystic fibrosis. *Journal of Clinical Psychology, 46,* 722–730.

Boyle, T. D. (1985). *The relationship between marital satisfaction and the distribution of parent involvement with developmentally disabled children.* Unpublished master's thesis, Rutgers University, Piscataway, NJ.

Breslau, N. (1982). Siblings of disabled children: Birth order and age-spacing effects. *Journal of Abnormal Child Psychology, 10,* 85–95.

Bristol, M. M., and Schopler, E. (1983). Stress and coping in families of autistic adolescents. In E. Schopler and G.B. Mesibov (Eds.), *Autism in adolescents and adults* (pp. 251–278). New York: Plenum Press.

Carter, E. A., and McGoldrick, M. (1980). *The family life cycle: A framework for family therapy.* New York: Gardner Press.

Cleveland, D. W., and Miller, N. (1977). Attitudes and life commitments of older siblings of mentally retarded adults. *Mental Retardation, 15,* 38–41.

Cummings, S. T. (1976). The impact of the child's deficiency on the father: A study of fathers of mentally retarded and chronically ill children. *American Journal of Orthopsychiatry, 46,* 246–255.

DeMyer, M. K. (1979). *Parents and children in autism.* New York: Wiley & Sons.

DeMyer, M. K., and Goldberg, P. (1983). Family needs of the autistic adolescent. In E. Schopler and G. B. Mesibov (Eds.), *Autism in adolescents and adults* (pp. 225–250). New York: Plenum Press.

Edmundson, K. (1985). The "discovery" of siblings. *Mental Retardation, 23,* 49–51.

Ferrari, M. (1982). *Chronically ill children and their siblings: Some psycho-social implications.* Unpublished doctoral dissertation, Rutgers University, Piscataway, N.J.

Figley, C.R., and McCubbin, H.I. (1983). *Stress and the family: Vol. 2. Coping with catastrophe.* New York: Brunner/Mazel.

Fong. P. L. (1991). Cognitive appraisals of high and low stress mothers of adolescents with autism. *Journal of Consulting and Clinical Psychology, 59,* 471–74.

Gath, A. (1978). *Down's syndrome and the family: The early years.* New York: Academic Press.

Gath, A., and Gumley, D. (1984). Down's syndrome and the family: Follow-up of children first seen in infancy. *Developmental Medicine and Child Neurology, 26,* 500-508.

Handleman, J. S. (1986). Severe developmental disabilities: Defining the term. *Education and Treatment of Children, 9,* 153–167.

Handleman, J. S., and Harris, S. L. (1986). *Educating the developmentally disabled: Meeting the needs of children and families.* San Diego: College Hill Press.

Harris, S., Handleman, J., and Palmer, C. (1985). Parents and grandparents view the autistic child. *Journal of Autism and Developmental Disorders, 15,* 127–137.

Janicki, M. P., and MacEachron, A. E. (1984). Residential, health, and social service needs of elderly developmentally disabled persons. *Gerontologist, 24,* 128–137.

Kidwell, J., Fischer, J. L., Dunham, R.M., and Baranowski, M. (1983). Parents and adolescents: Push and pull of change. In H.I. McCubbin and C.R. Figley (Eds.), *Stress and the family. Vol. 1: Coping with normative transitions* (pp. 74–89). New York: Brunner/Mazel.

Koegel, R. L., Schreibman, L., O'Neill, R.E., and Burke, J.C. (1983). The personality and family-interaction characteristics of parents of autistic children. *Journal of Consulting and Clinical Psychology, 51,* 683–692.

Kotsopoulos, S., and Matathia, P. (1980). Worries of parents regarding the future of their mentally retarded adolescent children. International *Journal of Social Psychiatry, 26,* 53–57.

Lamb, M. (1983). Fathers of exceptional children. In M. Seligman (Ed.), *The family with a handicapped child: Understanding and treatment* (pp. 125–146). New York: Grune & Stratton.

Marcus, L. (1984). Coping with burnout. In E. Schopler and G.B. Mesibov (Eds.) *The effects of autism on the family* (pp. 311–326). New York: Plenum Press.

Margalit, M., and Raviv, A. (1983). Mothers' perceptions of family climate in families with a retarded child. *Exceptional Child, 30,* 163–169.

Olshansky, S. (1962). Chronic sorrow: A response to having a mentally defective child. *Social Casework, 43,* 190–193.

Powers, M. D., and Handleman, J.S. (1984). *Behavioral assessment of severe developmental disabilities.* Rockville, MD: Aspen.

Rhoades, E. A. (1975). A grandparents' workshop. *The Volta Review, 77,* 557–560.

Tew, B. J., and Laurence, K. M. (1973). Mothers, brothers, and sisters of patients with spina bifida. *Developmental Medicine and Child Neurology, 15*(Suppl. 29), 69–76.

Wikler, L. (1981). Chronic stress of families of mentally retarded children. *Family Relations, 30,* 281-288.

Wikler, L., Wasow, M., and Hatfield, E. (1981). Chronic sorrow revisited: Parent vs. professional depiction of the adjustment of parents of mentally retarded children. *American Journal of Orthopsychiatry, 51,* 63–70.

18

Ethical Issues in Treatment

CYNTHIA J. STOLMAN, Ph.D.

CONTENTS

Families are rarely prepared for or expect to have a child with developmental disabilities and dysphagia. In many ways parents of such a child experience a grieving process similar to the stages of dying that have been elaborated by Elizabeth Kubler-Ross (1979). They may experience feelings of denial and isolation, anger, bargain with God for the child's health, display signs of depression, and finally most parents accept the reality of the situation. Throughout this grieving process, parents usually hope for a good outcome. The unwanted, unexpected news that their child has developmental disabilities and dysphagia slowly becomes part of the everyday reality for the parents. The parents usually have feelings of guilt that they may have caused the child's medical problems and need time to assimilate the medical information about the child's limitations and future prospects.

From the perspective of the health professional, many things must be considered in deciding how to treat and what to recommend in a particular situation. The physician and other health care professionals have the difficult job of first sorting out the medical aspects of the case, considering possible alternative treatments, recommending options that will maximize the child's chances for maintaining health and function, and conveying the appropriate information to the family. The ethical dimension of medical decision making is pervasive in the problem-solving process. At each turn, the values and interests of the decision makers become central in how the medical problem will be solved. The most difficult ethical problems involve children with profound neurologic disabilities. Therefore, this chapter will address ethical decision making in treating children with severe developmental delay and dysphagia and offer guidelines for decision making.

A major part of medical decision making includes the personal value perspectives of the decision makers, related psychosocial issues of assessing the parents' understanding and coping skills, as well as recognizing the ethical dimensions of a particular case (Ackerman, 1989).

Bioethics is concerned mainly with seeking answers to moral questions in the form of what ought to be or what one ought to do in a particular situation. The following ethical principles can be considered basic to ethical decision making: *autonomy*—respecting the competent patient's (or surrogate's) right to make health care decisions; *beneficence*—doing good, the duty to help others, with the primary obligation to serve the child's moral interests; *truth telling*—honesty in informing the competent patient or surrogate decision maker of relevant medical information; *confidentiality*—not divulging information about a child to unauthorized persons; and *justice*—distributing scarce medical resources in an equitable manner. The distribution should be according to need and the ability to benefit from the resource.

Finding the best solution to a bioethical dilemma involves choosing between competing moral principles or interests where the decision makers attempt through open inquiry to reach consensus. One example of a decision model applied to medical ethics discussed by Brody (1981) includes the following elements:

1. Identifying the ethical problem,
2. Defining the issues and the ethical principles that are relevant,
3. Considering alternative solutions and the possible/probable outcomes,
4. Prioritizing the proposed solutions in terms of the principles, and
5. Choosing a solution that is in keeping with the patient's/surrogate's value system.

Frequently, other kinds of moral issues surface that are not strictly bioethical dilemmas, such as social issues, psychological problems, legal issues, and personality or staff problems. Although these problems are not ethical dilemmas, they do require ethically appropriate strategies, such as navigating a bureaucratic social service system to achieve the best treatment for the patient or providing bereavement counseling to a family when the death of a child is inevitable.

Is It Ethical To Start Treatment and Then Stop It?

An important element in medical decision making is consideration of the goals of treatment. A treatment plan should consider the child's present condition, what the health care team hopes to achieve by treatment, and the likelihood of possible and probable outcomes. From an ethical perspective, it is appropriate to start a treatment of uncertain outcome, if it is probable that benefit will occur. Because the likelihood of benefit is unknown, the treatment should be closely monitored and discontinued if and/or when it proves to be nonbeneficial. It is always better to start a treatment and then stop the treatment if it does not do what is expected, than not to start for fear of not being able to stop. This applies to a variety of situations, such as when the medical team is considering gastrostomy, placement of an endotracheal tube, or provision of total parenteral nutrition.

The Symbolic Meaning of Providing Nutrition

Feeding an infant or a child is a basic human act, if not an instinct, that has great cultural as well as psychological and symbolic meaning. The practice of offering visitors and even strangers food and drink is pervasive in most cultures and a familiar social custom. There are classic references to mothers who continually try to feed or offer their grown children food and will not graciously accept "no" for an answer. Hostesses are judged by the amount and variety of food they offer guests. We feed the sick, the infant, the child, and the elderly who can not feed themselves. We also offer food to loved ones as a sign of loving and caring. When a mother or caregiver cannot do this simple act in a natural manner for the child and obtain satisfactory feedback, a variety of negative behaviors are triggered. Extensive training and positive reinforcement methods have to be used to overcome such negative behaviors. On a psychological level, the caregiver may have feelings of guilt and inadequacy related to the inability to successfully satisfy the child's basic nutritional needs. These feelings of inadequacy may interfere with the caregiver's ability to make ethically appropriate treatment decisions that affect the child. For example, the parent may decide against medically indicated tube feedings, because this decision reduces the caregiver's role in providing nutrition.

The emotional attachment we as a society have for providing nutrition to patients is reflected in the case law of a number of states that expressly forbid withholding or withdrawing of artificially provided nutrition and hydration from dying patients. However, in the 1990 Cruzan decision, the Supreme Court of the United States found that there is no substantial difference between artificially provided nutrition and hydration and other forms of medical treatment, and that artificially provided nutrition and hydration can be withheld or withdrawn in the same manner as other treatments, if such treatment is ineffective in improving the patient's condition or is harmful.

On What Basis Should Medical Decisions Be Made?

The general rule in medicine is to treat if possible, even if the outcome is uncertain.

This is usually the appropriate course of action. If the treatment will provide benefit to the patient, it should be provided. But when the patient is seriously neurologically delayed, the automatic response to treat can become a way of avoiding difficult decisions. The problem is how to make decisions that are both patient-centered and avoid imposing painful, uncomfortable procedures on a child or procedures that actually do harm to the child, when there is little or virtually no chance for improvement. When the patient is an adult and competent (has decision making capacity), there is seldom a problem. The health care professional discusses treatment options with the competent patient as part of informed consent. This discussion usually includes the alternatives to treatment, the efficacy of the proposed treatments, possible outcomes, and side effects. Then the patient has the information necessary to make an informed decision.

Decision making for minors who are severely neurologically impaired involves two competing ethical principles—the "sanctity of life" and the "quality of life" principles. According to the sanctity of life principle, human life in whatever form is sacred, of equal value to other human life, and is always good to be preserved no matter what the state or condition or the length of remaining life. Because all life is precious, according to this formulation it may not be shortened regardless of the motives. In keeping with this principle, there is a moral duty to provide treatment to all affected children without exception. In contrast to this, the quality of life principle considers the degree of human suffering, pain, discomfort, and inability to enjoy or experience life to be factors that should be considered when making decisions to limit or forgo life-sustaining treatment. Some would consider it doing harm to a child to engage in acts that cause pain and suffer-

ing in order to keep the child alive with no realistic chance for improvement. According to the principle of nonmaleficence, stated by the maxim of medical ethics, *primum non nocere,* first, one should do no harm (Weir, 1984).

When the patient is a minor he or she is considered incompetent (lacking decision-making capacity) by definition. A surrogate decision maker must be identified or appointed to make decisions on behalf of the child. The surrogate is usually a close family member, usually a parent. There is a large body of common law or case law supporting informal clinical decision making for minors by family members together with the attending physician.

Competence and Surrogacy

In most jurisdictions there is no express law giving parents authority to make decisions on behalf of their minor child, but common law precedent recognizes parents as natural guardians of their children and as such they have authority to make decisions on their behalf. There is the assumption that, unless there is evidence to the contrary, parents have the best interest of their children in mind and at heart and should be recognized as appropriate decision makers. Health care professionals have traditionally recognized parents as surrogate decision makers and usually try to accommodate their wishes. When the patient, who lacks decision-making capacity, reaches legal age, the parents must apply to the court to be named legal guardians of the patient.

The Doctrine of Informed Consent

The doctrine of informed consent is basic to the health care worker's relationships with patients and expresses the principle of autonomy. Competent patients have the right to accept or refuse treatment according to common law precedent, and health care professionals have the responsibility to respect the patient's rights in medical decision making. Patient autonomy, or self-rule, has become a standard in medical care over the last few decades. This trend has been bolstered recently by the Patient Self-Determination Act of 1990 (Omnibus Reconciliation Act 1990.) which mandates all institutions that receive Federal funds provide information to patients at admission concerning the rights of competent patients to make advance directives for health care. Advance directives include living wills (a statement of the patient's wishes to accept or refuse life-sustaining treatments) and durable powers of attorney (the appointment of a medical health care proxy). An advance directive becomes operative at the time the patient is no longer able to make health care decisions. The Patient Self-Determination Act, unfortunately, does not address the case of the minor or the never competent patient. But American jurisprudence and ethical opinion supports the idea that, if the competent patient has the right to accept or reject medical treatment, then the patient who lacks decision-making capacity has that same right. The problem of how to exercise this right is solved by turning to a surrogate decision maker. A surrogate decision maker is someone who is entrusted to make medical decisions on behalf of the patient and to act in the best interests of the patient (American College of Physicians Ethics Manual, 1992). In the case of a child, the surrogate is usually a parent or involved guardian.

The Right to Refuse Treatment

Many state courts have ruled that there is a right to privacy that encompasses the competent patient's right to refuse life-sustaining treatment, including the right to refuse nutrition and hydration. In addition, the Supreme Court of the United States in the Cruzan decision (*Cruzan v. Director, Missouri Department of Health,* 1990) decided that competent patients have the right to refuse unwanted medical treatment and that states have the right to require "clear and convincing evidence" of the patient's wishes. Only New York State and Missouri have laws to date requiring "clear and convincing" evidence of the patient's wishes to refuse medical treatment. Although the Supreme Court did not define what it meant by clear and convincing evidence, other courts have generally accepted as evidence written documents such as living wills or statements by reliable witnesses as to the persons stated wishes.

Emancipated minors (those living outside the home), if they have decision-making capacity, have the right to make decisions about their care and treatment and to refuse medical treatment, even life-sustaining treatment.

Decision making for the previously competent patient most often uses the substituted judgment standard, which many courts have adopted. This standard recognizes the patient's surrogate and requires the surrogate decision maker to choose as the patient would and asks the question, "What would the patient have wanted?"

According to the President's Commission for the Study of Ethical Problems in Biomedical and Behavioral Research (1983) for competent and once competent patients, the right to refuse life-sustaining treatment is regarded as an exercise of personal autonomy. For the never competent patient, the courts have not been decisive. However, it would seem reasonable to consider that only treatment that will "restore or preserve health, minimize or relieve pain, or otherwise promote the patient's well being" should be employed (McKnight & Bellis, 1992).

Making medical decisions for patients who lack decision-making capacity, where there is no evidence of the patient's wishes, should be done according to what is considered to be in the best interests of the patient. The patient's best interests are defined as that which will provide the greatest amount of benefit over harm. This is a subjective judgment, difficult to quantify, that is made by the decision makers concerning the quality of life of the child. The main point is that the decision should be made from the child's perspective. Even if the child has never communicated any thoughts, according to the *Guidelines on the Termination of Life-Sustaining Treatment and the Care of the Dying: A Report by the Hastings Center* (Hastings Center, p. 134, 1987), the decision making should consider "what a reasonable person in the patient's circumstances would want."

For a severely affected dysphagic child, medical decision making often centers on trying to find the most effective, noninvasive, safe method of providing nutrition. The choice of tube feeding (nasogastric or gastrostomy) or hyperalimentation when feeding by mouth has failed to provide adequate nutrition is fraught with emotional, medical, and ethical problems. Health care professionals should be thorough in evaluating the child's alimentary tract to identify any treatable causes for nutritional failure prior to decision making. Providing nutritional support to a child who cannot survive may merely prolong dying, whereas using a gastrostomy tube temporarily until the child is recovered from surgery will improve the child's chances for normal function. It is also well known that dehydration in the dying patient leads to "azotemia, hypernatremia and hypercalcemia, all of which produce sedative, and therefore, an anesthetic effect on the body" (Groher, 1990, p 105). Those who are well hydrated appear to suffer more pain and discomfort in comparison to dehydrated dying patients. The courts have repeatedly held that artificial feeding and hydration are medical interventions to be withheld or withdrawn as medically appropriate.

Who Has the Right to Make Treatment Decisions?

Because the developmentally disabled dysphagic child is incapable of making treatment decisions, we turn to the family as natural guardians to make treatment decisions in cooperation and consultation with the attending physician. The child's parents should be regarded as the primary decision makers. We assume parents care the most for the child's welfare, have the same or similar values and interests as the child, and will act in the child's best interests. However, parents, because of guilt feelings or other psychological and emotional problems of dealing with a developmentally disabled dysphagic child, may want overtreatment from benevolent motives. It is not uncommon to hear of situations where physicians acquiesce to parents who request aggressive treatment for marginal gain.

The physician has great power to influence treatment decisions by recognizing the situation and exposing the reasons motivating the parent's decision making. The most difficult thing for the physician and other health professionals is to separate professional responsibilities toward the patient from personally held value systems which may not be in accord with the patient's best interests. Health professionals should be honest with themselves and the family when discussing treatment options, carefully separating their personally held values and biases from the known medical facts and putting the facts into perspective. If the physician counsels the family that, in her opinion, the proposed treatment is a viable option (the glass is half full, rather than half empty), the family should be made aware that this is an opinion rather than a medical fact. It is not uncommon to hear disappointed parents blame the physician when surgical procedures fail to provide expected results, saying "the doctor did not prepare us for this." "We did not expect this to happen. If he had told us that this might happen we probably would not have agreed."

Should Children Be Included in Experimental Research?

For a severely dysphagic child whose parents and physicians have exhausted conventional modes of therapy, it is natural to turn to experimental research for some hope of a cure or to ameliorate or solve a difficult feeding problem. It is important for physicians to explain to parents that a particular treatment is not "standard treatment" and the purpose of the experimental study. There are two different kinds of research involving human subjects—therapeutic research, which is for the direct benefit of the patient who suffers from a disease, and nontherapeutic research where the study population is normal, and therefore, the participants do not stand to directly benefit from the results. In general, children should not be excluded from therapeutic research because of their status as minors who cannot consent to treatment. The blanket exclusion of children would be discriminatory and deny an entire population from the potential benefits of research. Indeed, the development of many vaccines against childhood diseases and successes in treating childhood leukemia are directly linked to using children as experimental subjects in well designed research. Before entering a child into an experimental study, physicians and parents should consider the scientific merit of the research and any ethical issues. They should weigh the potential risks and benefits to the child of the proposed experimental procedure, including considerations of possible conflicts of interests. The proposed research should be designed so that it maximize the ratio of benefit to risk.

Federal regulation of research involving minors identifies four categories of research. The first category is that of direct benefit and minimal risk to the child, such as that normally encountered in the daily life of the child. Procedures that are considered of minimal risk would be obtaining a blood sample, an x-ray, or minor diet changes. The second category includes research that promises direct benefit to the child and proposes greater than minimal risk. Examples of research procedures that pose greater than minimal risk to the child are spinal taps, biopsies, and drugs whose side effects have not been established in the pediatric population. Research that involves greater than minimal risks to the child requires specific justification, such as a situation where no efficacious alternative treatment exists. The third category of research offers no direct benefit to the subject and involves more than minimal risk. Such research would need to be specifically justified and reviewed by the Internal Review Board (IRB) of the institution. The fourth category offers no direct benefit to the child and involves minimum risk. This research could lead to better understanding of disease processes and improve the health and welfare of children in general. All research conducted on human subjects is subject to review by IRBs of health care institutions that engage in scientific research. IRBs review research protocols for scientific merit, risk to the patient, informed consent, safety and efficacy. Children according to law are unable to consent to treatment due to their status as minors. However, when the parents and the physicians agree it is appropriate, the child should be asked to assent to treatment, especially for nontherapeutic research. This shows respect for the child and recognizes the child as the central figure in the research. Information about the research should be imparted according to the child's ability to comprehend and level of maturity. The child should be given an age-appropriate explanation of the nature of the experimental treatment, its purpose, how long it will last, the expected outcome, and any risks (Grodin & Alpert, 1988).

Futility of Treatment

It is well established legally and morally that physicians do not have to perform useless or futile treatments. A narrow definition of futility, from the physician's perspective, is that the proposed intervention offers no physiologic benefit to the patient. This means that the medical treatment will not be able to reverse the physiologic process it is intended to act on. A second definition of futility that involves a value judgment would consider certain treatments futile if they are "nonbeneficial" to the patient. A physician might argue that a permanently comatose child cannot benefit from a treatment because there is no awareness. Another definition of futility is where the treatment is considered experimental or unlikely to be effective. For example, it might be considered futile to continue to treat a child with chemotherapy who is in constant pain and terminally ill from metastatic disease, when this treatment has failed in the past (Miles, 1992).

The term "medically futile" has been subjected to lengthy analysis without any consensus as to a common definition of the term. This may be because futility arguments tend to be used when health care professionals are seeking to withhold or withdraw treatment from a patient where quality of life is the main issue. Such subjective value judgments made without the express involvement of the family are disrespectful of the patient's autonomy and right to consent to treatment which in the case of a minor is expressed through a surrogate decision maker.

In situations where a social service agency is involved decision making for the child becomes more problematic. Social service agencies appear to be committed to overtreatment. This position is justified by the state's interest in preserving life without consideration of quality of life issues such as amount and duration of pain, suffering, discomfort, or pleasure or of appreciable benefit. If involved family members can be found to act as surrogate decision makers for the child, this is preferable because they are more likely to know the child and his special needs.

Only recently have acute care hospitals acknowledged that ethical issues occur routinely and that there should be a systematic method of dealing with the ethical problems that arise. In response to this need, acute care hospitals are now required by the Joint Commission on Accreditation of Health Care Organizations to have in place hospital ethics committees that consider ethical problems that arise in the health care setting. These committees can be helpful in elucidating the ethical issues, providing an opinion, and supporting the health care team and the family.

Rarely should the courts be involved in medical decision making. Court proceedings for other than select emergency situations tend to be impartial, adversarial, long, involved, expensive, and seldom of benefit to the individual child.

Do Not Resuscitate Orders (DNR) and Forgoing Life-sustaining Treatment

The family of the developmentally delayed dysphagic child is placed in the lifetime role of providing care with little realistic hope for dramatic improvement. For such children the realities of daily life include frequent trips to the physician and the hospital, including occasional admission to the acute care unit as well. For such children medical decision making should include consideration of whether or not it is appropriate to provide cardiopulmonary resuscitation (CPR) or other life-prolonging measures (e.g., dialysis, surgery, transfusions, nutritional support) if the need arises. Without an order to the contrary, it is standard practice in acute care hospitals and some long-term care facilities to provide CPR. The question is when should a do not resuscitate order or forgoing life-sustaining treatment order be considered with severely developmentally delayed children with dysphagia?

A DNR order or forgoing life-sustaining treatment order should be considered in situations where the child is:

1. Imminently dying and the provision of treatment would not be medically beneficial,
2. Terminally ill and is expected to die within a year,
3. In a persistent vegetative state, and/ or
4. Chronically ill with a debilitating disorder where the burdens of treatment clearly outweigh the benefits according to the parents and physicians.

Discussion of the DNR/forgoing life-sustaining treatment order is best done not at a time of crisis, but as part of a general discussion of what should be done if something unforseen occurs. Such discussions should first explore the parent's knowledge and perceptions of the child's medical problems and the parent's expectations for the future. Discussion of what the family considers ordinary care versus aggressive treatment helps the health care professional to be specific when writing a DNR order. It is not unusual for physicians to write "qualified" or "limited" DNR orders where the physician requests "do not intu-

bate only" or "no compressions, use emergency meds." Such orders are confusing and often reflect the ambivilence of the physician or failure to fully discuss the fact that, even in the best of circumstances, CPR has a poor success rate. When a partial resuscitative effort is used, it is most likely to fail. It is more respectful of the family to say that CPR does not work most of the time rather than give false hope.

A decision to forgo (either withhold or withdraw) life-sustaining treatment and allow a child to die is an uncommon event. This kind of decision making should be thoroughly discussed with all involved members of the medical team and the family. The decision should be unanimous by the attending physician, the parents or court appointed guardian, and at least two independent physicians with relevant expertise (or a prognosis committee) who confirm the diagnosis and prognosis. All such determinations should be carefully documented in the medical record.

Decision Making

The physician and the family are the usual decision makers for the child. If the parents and the physician agree that treatment is in the best interests of the child, it should be provided. If the parents and the physician agree that treatment is not in the best interests of the child, then it is not necessary to proceed with treatment. If in the attending physician's best judgment the treatment is not appropriate or not medically beneficial, but the parents disagree, transferring care to another physician or facility that will honor the parents' request is an appropriate option. If the physician feels that the treatment is beneficial, but the parents disagree, the physician should refer the case to the hospital bioethics committee for consideration. Occasionally, the physician may feel uncomfortable in not providing life-sustaining procedures, even in clearly futile cases, where the family feels that the child has suffered enough. In such situations the bioethics committee of the institution should be consulted for an opinion. The bioethics committee consultation serves as an impartial forum for case presentations in which there is an opportunity to present the facts of the case and hear different perspectives and information is raised that might not otherwise have been considered. In addition, the bioethics committee process can be helpful in ensuring that a well reasoned, reflective decision process has occurred, and this process can provide guidance for those rare cases that may require judicial intervention.

Should Children with Developmental Delay and Dysphagia Be Provided with Scarce Medical Resources?

The use of technology in medicine has extended the life span of children with developmental disabilities and dysphagic conditions, so that these children are often living to maturity and beyond. Where dysphagia is accompanied by neurological impairment, the medical problems are more severe, the complications more frequent, and the solutions less apparent. The use of medical, economic, and human resources for the child with physical and neurological disabilities is often great, and the benefits to the individual child have to be questioned.

Allocation of Scarce Medical Resources

Children with developmental delay and dysphagia consume enormous amounts of health care time, energy, and resources, and these children seldom have the ability to live independently. At a time when the health care dollar is shrinking, many would say that resources should be allocated in favor of preventive health care programs rather than to maintain the severely impaired. Can society continue to provide unlimited, expensive maintenance care for children who are severely developmentally delayed and dysphagic when the outcome is that many will die and those who survive are totally dependent and permanently childlike? This is one argument that is made on the "macromolecular level" by health policy makers as a reason to limit health care for certain categories of patients. But health care professionals (e.g., physicians, nurses, therapists, psychologists, social workers) who function on a "micromolecular" level have direct responsibility for the health care needs and welfare of the patient. The physician owes a duty of care toward the child to provide what is in the best interests of the child, without regard to health care policy issues, cost, or other market forces that would compromise his or her responsibilities toward the child.

Case Study

In concluding the discussion in this chapter of the ethical issues of severely affected children with dysphagia, the following case is offered as an example of a difficult ethical dilemma. The patient , GD, was 9 years old when she was brought by her parents to see the physicians at a Dysphagia Clinic associated with a major university teaching hospital. She was diagnosed with microcephaly, hypotonia, cortical blindness, seizure disorder, and profound mental retardation. She had chronic breathing difficulties, vomiting, and recurrent respiratory infections. Additionally, she had failure to thrive, weighed 9 kilograms, and was quite pale in appearance. During team evaluation it was noted that GD had oral preparatory and oral phase dysphagia. Her breathing was noisy. She had excessive thick mucus draining from her nose that interferred with feeding, and she frequently vomited mucus and food. In addition, she had gum bleeding. Because she was unable to tolerate food that was too thick or too thin, she was maintained on a pureed diet. Meals took approximately 1 hour and actual intake was approximately 50–75% of the food offered. She received one can of Ensure per day given by her mother via dropper. Nutrition consultation revealed that her average daily intake was 505 Kcals/day with 28.4 grams of protein. Her needs were estimated at 1100–1500 Kcals/day. The dysphagia team recommended nasogastric tube feeding until her intake was improved. The team agreed that a gastrostomy should be considered only after a trial period with the nasogastric tube. These recommendations were discussed with the parents who requested referral to another center closer to home, as the mother was expecting their third child. A 7-year- old sibling did not have any medical problems.

Mrs. D appeared to be quiet, reserved, and resigned to GD's situation. She deferred to her husband for all medical decisions regarding GD's care and treatment. The staff felt that the reason the parents brought GD to the clinic was because of the impending birth of their third child and Mrs. D's inability to continue to devote approximately 6 hours a day to GD's feeding routine. Mr. D, by all accounts, was an unpleasant person, usually hostile and belligerent toward the medical staff. He accused the staff of not treating his child properly or causing her to suffer more through their ineptitude. He appeared angry most of the time and at best was difficult to deal with.

The gastroenterologist at the referral center noted that GD had the findings described above. She was extremely cachectic

in appearance, had respiratory difficulties and severe halitosis. During discussion with the parents and the gastroenterologist, both parents agreed to a trial period of nutritional rehabilitation to be followed by percutaneous gastrostomy placement. However, Mr D. was at first reluctant to agree and expressed the thought that, if his wife would spend more time attempting to feed his daughter, the gastrostomy would not be needed. After the team suggested that he try to feed GD himself and he was unable to, he agreed to the plan.

The patient was admitted to the hospital and given a thorough work up including cine esophagram and gained weight slowly on nasogastric feeding over a period of 2 weeks. A pH probe was negative for appreciable gastroesophageal reflux. The gastrostomy tube was placed. While in hospital she was seen by an ENT surgeon who felt that tracheostomy placement was advisable. But both parents refused this procedure. GD was transferred to a long-term care facility at the request of the parents who expressed an inability to care for her at home due to the mother's impending delivery. At the chronic care facility, GD could not be maintained on a high caloric diet due to persistent diarrhea that was felt to be the result of chronic malnutrition.

The parents were upset by GD's declining condition and refused further attempts at intervention such as hyperalimentation or evaluation via small bowel biopsy and absorption studies. After GD had been at the long-term care facility for 3 months, Mrs.D. delivered another child with severe neurologic impairment of unknown etiology.

With the birth of another impaired child, prior plans for GD to eventually return home were dropped. After several months at the chronic care facility GD died in her sleep, presumably of upper airway obstruction. Both parents were most distressed at this, and Mr. D in particular blamed the physicians for his daughter's death. Mr. D felt that he should not have agreed to the gastrostomy. He did not accept the physician's explanation that it was GD's upper airway problems that caused her death.

Case Discussion

This case contains ethical as well as psychosocial issues that have direct bearing on the outcome. Several questions can be asked. Did the physicians discuss the treatment goals and possible outcomes with the parents at the time the patient was evaluated for gastrostomy? Was continued treatment in this child's best interests? Should the medical team have insisted on further investigative studies and ventilator support regardless of parental refusal?

To analyze this case the following key factors should be considered (1) relevant medical facts, (2) patient or surrogate wishes, (3) best interests of the patient, and (4) psychosocial considerations.

Relevant Medical Facts

In the case of GD we do not know if the parent's decision not to permit the tracheostomy was made in light of medical information or largely in terms of emotional and psychological factors of personality. We are told that the father was angry, unpleasant, and hostile toward the staff. Could the father's hostile manner have influenced the physician's judgment in recommending treatment approaches for the patient? Most important, did the physician discuss treatment goals with the family and explain the necessity for further diagnostic tests and the tracheostomy? Unfortunately, there was never a specific reason found for this child's constellation of problems. The lack of a definitive diagnosis or underlying cause undoubted created anxiety for the parents who were seeking answers as to why this tragedy occurred .

Patient or Surrogate Wishes

We have no way of knowing how GD felt about her quality of life or if she had any enjoyment of life since she was unable to communicate. Her parents as surrogate decision makers appeared to be devoted to her and wanted her to continue to live. However, after she entered the nursing home and her condition deteriorated, the family may have reached their limit in accepting her compromised situation. Some families, when they are questioned about forgoing life-sustaining treatment give, their reason as simply "she has had enough." No doubt GD's parents felt that her life was becoming exceedingly burdensome to her after transfer to the nursing home.

Best Interests of the Patient

The central ethical issue was whether or not it was in the patient's best interests to have had further diagnostic tests and a gastrostomy. There appears to have been ambivalence on the part of the medical team to pursue permission for the testing and tracheostomy after the parents refused. We do not know if the father's behavior influenced the physician's decision not to pursue tracheostomy, or if it was the physician's feelings about the patient's quality of life that influenced decision making.

Earlier in the chapter, four categories or conditions were offered for consideration of a DNR order or for forgoing life-sustaining treatment. According to the fourth condition, it is considered ethically appropriate to withhold or withdraw life-sustaining treatment if such treatment is not in the best interests of the patient. Best interest judgments are based on both the medical facts of the case and the values of the decision makers, so that if, on balance, providing treatment would be overwhelmingly burdensome to the patient then it does not have to be provided. Although there appears not to have been any indepth discussions of these issues, still we can surmise from the case that this criterion can be applied. Given the child's chronic debilitating situation, the parents' judgment to withhold further diagnostic tests and tracheostomy was reasonable. Moreover, no members of the health care team objected or opposed the parents' decision.

Psychosocial Considerations

There appears not to have been any discussion among the physicians and the parents as to the parents' feelings about their child, their hopes for her future, their disappointment at having a severely neurologically damaged child, and the nature and extent of their guilt feelings. The family developed methods of coping with their daughter's severe problems that may have been stretched to the limit. The third pregnancy no doubt interfered with this precariously balanced system. Although GD's father agreed to the gastrostomy, he may have agreed to the idea intellectually, but emotionally it is evident that he remained opposed to it. We do not know what his expectations were for the gastrostomy placement. But he was obviously unprepared for the complications that followed. Psychologically, anger is regarded as a secondary emotion, probably masking the father's feelings of guilt and impotence at not being able to help his child or improve her health. Addressing the emotional needs of families in crises can be an effective tool for avoiding ethical dilemmas. In this case, more effective psychosocial support for the family and establishing a better relationship with the father might have resulted in his support

for the gastrostomy and permission for diagnostic studies and the recommended tracheostomy. Even though the projected outcome was uncertain and the burdens of continuing treatment increasingly weighty, at the heart of this case was the failure of effective communication between GD's parents and the medical team to deal with the issue of recommended treatment. A more concerted effort to listen and communicate with this family, might have served better their needs.

Summary

In general, for the child with severe developmental disabilities and dysphagia the central ethical principle is respect for the patient's autonomy. This principle encompasses respect for the patient's right to make health care decisions and the right to informed consent. A close family member is usually recognized as the appropriate surrogate to act on behalf of a minor child. The surrogate decision maker is enjoined to further the child's best interests which may lead to decisions to accept or refuse medical treatment. Decision making for the chronically ill dysphagic child is complex, and heath professionals should consider psychological issues of guilt and personal value preferences that may underlie such decisions. For any proposed treatment, there should be an assessment of the potential benefits and risks to the patient. Discussions of difficult end-of-life decisions, including DNR or forgoing life-sustaining treatment orders, need to be planned so that they occur prior to anticipated crises, when family members are more likely to be receptive. Finally, health care professionals have direct obligations to further the welfare of the child by improving health, extending life, and preventing suffering.

References

Ackerman, T. F. (1989). Conceptualizing the role of the ethics consultant: Some theoretical issues. In J. C. Fletcher, N. Quist, & A. R. Jonsen (Eds.), *Ethics consultation in health care* (pp. 37–52). Ann Arbor, MI: Health Administration Press.

American College of Physicians Ethics Manual (3rd ed.). (1992). *Annals of Internal Medicine, 117,* 947–960.

Brody, H. (1981). *Ethical decisions in medicine.* Boston: Little, Brown.

Cruzan v. Director, Missouri Department of Health. (1990). 110 S. Ct. 2841.

Grodin, M. A., & Alpert, J. J. (1988). Children as participants in medical research. *Pediatric Clinics of North America, 35,* 1389–401.

Groher, M. E. (1990). Ethical dilemmas in providing nutrition. *Dysphagia, 5,* 102–109.

Hastings Center. (1987). *Guidelines on the termination of life-sustaining treatment and the care of the dying: A report by the Hastings Center.* New York: Author.

Kubler-Ross, E. (1979). *On death and dying.* New York: Macmillan.

Miles, S. H. (1992). Medical futility. Law, *Medicine, and Health Care, 20,* 310–315.

McKnight, D. K., & Bellis, M. (1992). Foregoing life-sustaining treatment for adult, developmentally disabled, public wards: A proposed statute. *American Journal of Law and Medicine, 18,* 113.

Omnibus Reconciliation Act of 1990. Title IV. & 4206. *Congressional Record,* October 26, 1990, 12638

President's Commission for the Study of Ethical Problems in Biomedical and Behavioral Research. (1983). *Deciding to forgo life-sustaining teatment.* (pp.132–33). Washington, DC: Government Printing Office.

Weir, R. (1984). *Selective nontreatment of handicapped newborns.* New York: Oxford University Press.

CHAPTER

APPENDIX

Pharmacology

CATHY Y. POON, PHARM.D.

MEDICATION DOSING GUIDELINE

Abbreviation Key:

im = intramuscularly
iv = intravenously
po = orally, by mouth
pr = per rectum
sc = subcutaneously

bid = twice a day
qd = daily
qid = four times a day
qod = every other day
tid = three times a day

q4hr = every four hour
q6hr = every six hour
q8hr = every eight hour
q12hr = every twelve hour
prn = as needed

Drug	Indications	Doses	Adverse Effects	Comments
Acetaminophen Acephen®, Panadol®, Tempra®, Tylenol®	Fever Mild to moderate pain	**Children:** 10–15 mg/kg/dose po q4-6hr maximum 2.6 (gm/24hr) 15–20 mg/kg/dose pr q4-6hr **Adults:** 325–650 mg po q4-6hr or 1000 mg 3-4 imes/24hr (maximum 4 gm/24hr)	Rash and hypersensitivity reactions (rare) Hypatotoxicity with chronic use and overdose	Toxic concentration > 200 µg/mL 4hr or 50 µg/mL at 12hr (probable hepatotoxicity)
Acetazolamide Diamox®	Hydrocephalus Edema/water retention Seizures Glaucoma	**Infants:** *Hydrocephalus* Initial: 25 mg/kg/24hr po/iv tid Increment: 25 mg/kg/24hr daily Maximum: 100 mg/kg/24hr or 2 gm/24hr **Children:** *Edema/water retention* 5 mg/kg/dose or 150 mg/m² po/iv qd or qod *Seizure* 8-30 mg/kg/24hr po q6-8hr (maximum 1 gm/24hr) *Glaucoma* 20–40 mg/kg/24hr im/iv q6hr 8-30 mg/kg/24hr po q6-8hr **Adults:** *Edema/water retention* 250–375 mg po q4-6hr or qod *Seizure* 8-30 mg/kg/24hr po q6-12hr (maximum 1 gm/24hr) *Glaucoma* 250-500 mg im/iv, may repeat in 2-4hr prn 250 mg po 1-4 times/24hr	Gastrointestinal irritation Anorexia Dry mouth Paresthesias Muscle weakness Drowsiness Fatigue Transient hypokalemia Renal calculi	Tablet may be crushed and suspended in cherry or chocolate syrup

Drug	Indication	Dosage	Side Effects	Administration
Acetylcysteine Mucomyst®	Excessive abnormal viscid mucous secretions Adjunct therapy for patients with cystic fibrosis (mucolytic) Meconium ileus equivalent Acetaminophen overdose	**Infants:** *Pulmonary mucolytic* 2 mL of 5% solution by nebulization tid-qid *Meconium ileus* Contraindicated **Children:** *Pulmonary mucolytic* 3–5 mL of 5% to 10% solution by nebulization tid-qid *Meconium ileus* 5–30 mL of 5% to 10% solution po/pr 3–6 times/24hr **OR** 100–200 mL of 5% to 10% solution by irrigation bid **Adolescent:** *Pulmonary mucolytic* 5–10 mL of 5% to 10% solution by nebulization tid-qid **Children and Adults:** *Acetaminophen Poisoning* 140 mg/kg po/ng x 1, followed by 70 mg/kg/dose q4hr beginning within 10hr of ingestion x 17 doses or until nontoxic acetaminophen level	Local irritation Bronchospasm Nausea Vomiting Rhinorrhea Stomatitis Hemoptysis with prolonged use	**Pulmonary administration** Give via nebulizer or instill direc tly via endotracheal tube Dilute 10% and 20% solution with water. Patient should receive an aerosolized bronchodilator 10-15 minutes prior to nebulization **Gastrointestinal administration** Give undiluted solution by rectal enema or via an indwelling catheter OR dilute 1:4 with water, saline, cola, or orange juice for oral administration. Use within 1 hour of preparation.
Albuterol Proventil®, Ventolin®	Asthma Bronchospasm	**Oral:** *2-6 yrs old* 0.1–0.2 mg/kg/dose tid (maximum 4 mg tid) *6-12 yrs old* 2 mg/dose tid-qid (maximum 24 mg/24hr (divided qid) *> 12 yrs old* 2–4 mg/dose tid-qid (maximum 32 mg/24hr divided qid) **Nebulization:** (0.5% Solution) 0.01–0.05 mL/Kg q2-6hr (minimum 0.1 mL & maximum 1 mL diluted in 1–2 mL normal saline) **Metered Dose Inhaler (MDI)** (90μg/puff) *< 12 yrs old* 1–2 puffs qid (use with spacer) *> 12 yrs old* 1–2 puffs q4-6hr	Tachycardia Palpitations Dizziness Tremors Nausea Hyperactivity Insomnia	Rinse mouth with water after inhalation

Drug	Indication	Dosage	Side Effects	Comments
Baclofen Lioresal®	Treatment of reversible spasticity	**Children:** *Initial* 10–15 mg/24hr po q8hr *Increment* 5–15 mg/24hr po at 3 day intervals *Maximum* 2–7 yrs old—40 mg/24hr ≥ 8 yrs old—60 mg/24hr **Adults:** 5 mg po tid-qid, increase b 5 mg/dosed at 3 day interval (maximum 80 mg/24hr)	Drowsiness Fatigue Sedation Confusion Headache Hypotension Insomnia Nausea Constipation Urinary frequency	Use with caution in patients with seizure disorder and rental impairment
Beclomethasone Dipropionate Beclovent®, Beconase®, Beconase AQ®, Vancenase®, Vancenase AQ®, Vanceril®	Bronchial asthma Seasonal or perennial rhinitis and nasal polyposis	**Children (6–12 yrs old):** *Oral inhalation* 1–2 inhalations tid-qid (maximum 10 inhalations/24hr) *Aerosol inhalation (nasal)* 1 spray each nostril tid *Aqueous inhalation (nasal)* 1–2 sprays each nostril bid **Adults:** *Oral inhalation* 2 inhalations tid-qid (maximum 20 inhalations/24hr) *Aerosol inhalation (nasal)* 1 spray each nostril bid-qid **OR** 2 sprays each nostril bid- *Aqueous inhalation (nasal)* 1–2 sprays each nostril bid	Oropharyngeal and nasal candidiasis Hoarseness Dry mouth Cough Local irritation Epistaxis	Oral inhalation is used for asthmatics who require chronic corticosteroids. Nasal aerosol spray is used for symptomatic treatment of seasonal rhinitis and nasal polyposis. Gargling and rinsing mouth after administration will reduce the incidenc e of oropharyngeal candidiasis
Benztropine Mesylate Cogentin®	Acute dystonic reactions Drug-induced extrapyramidal effects Parkinsonian symptoms	**Children (> 3 yrs old):** *Drug-induced extrapyramidal reaction* 0.02–0.05 mg/kg/dose im/iv/po qd-bid **Adults:** *Drug-induced extrapyramidal reaction* 1–4 mg/dose im/iv/po qd-bid *Parkinsonian symptoms* Initial—0.5 mg/24hr im/iv/po qd-qid Increment—0.5 mg at 5–6 day intervals to achieve desired effect Maximum—6 mg/24hr	Central nervous system depression or stimulation Confusion Nervousness Hallucinations Weakness Ataxia Dryness of the mouth Blurred vision	

Drug	Indications	Dosage	Side Effects	Comments
Bethanechol Chloride Urecholine®	Gastroesophageal reflux Abdominal distention Urinary retention due to neurogenic bladder	**Children:** *Gastroesophageal reflux* 0.1-0.2 mg/kg/dose po 30-60 minutes before each meal (maximum qid) **OR** 3 mg/m²/dose po q8hr *Neurogenic bladder* 0.15-0.2 mg/kg/day sc tid-qid **Adults:** *Abdominal distention or urinary retention* 10-50 mg po bid-qid 2.5-5 mg sc tid-qid (maximum 10 mg q4hr for neurogenic bladder)	Abdominal cramps Vomiting Diarrhea Flushed skin Sweating Hypotension Bronchial constriction Bradycardia Cardiac arrest	Contraindicated in patients with peptic ulcer or bronchial asthma. Contraindicated for im or iv use.
Brompheniramine Maleate Bromphen®, Dimetane®, Nasahist B®, Oraminic®	Allergic rhinitis	**Children:** *< 6 yrs old* 0.125 mg/kg/dose po q6hr (maximum 6-8 mg/24hr) *6-12 yrs old* 1-4 mg po q6-8hr (maximum 12-16 mg/24hr) **OR** 8-12 mg (sustained released) po q8-12hr **Adults:** 4-8 mg po q6-8hr **OR** 8 mg (sustained released) po q8hr **OR** 12 mg (sustained released) po q12hr	Paradoxical excitability Drowsiness Dizziness Dry mouth Nausea Anorexia	Do not crush or chew sustained released tablets.
Carbamazepine Tegretol®	Seizure disorder Trigeminal neuralgia Diabetic neuropathy	**Children:** *< 6 yrs old* Initial—5 mg/kg/24hr po qd or bid Increment—increase up to 20 mg/kg/24hr po bid-qid at 5-7 day intervals *6-12 yrs old* Initial—100 mg po bid **OR** 10 mg/kg/24hr po bid Increment—increase by 100 mg/24hr at weekly intervals until therapeutic concentration is achieved Usual maintenance dose—15-30 mg/kg/24hr po bid-qid **Adolescents and Adults:** Initial—200 mg po bid Increment—increase by 200 mg/24hr at weekly intervals until therapeutic concentration is achieved Usual maintenance dose—800-1200 mg/24hr po tid-qid	Sedation Drowsiness Rash Stevens-Johnson syndrome Nystagmus Ataxia Aplastic anemia Agranulocytosis Anorexia	Monitoring Trough level drawn prior to the next dose Therapeutic range Monotherapy: 8-12 μg/mL Polytherapy: 4-8 μg/mL

Drug	Indication	Dosage	Side Effects	Comments
Chloral Hydrate Noctec®	Sedation Anxiety Hypnotic	**Neonates:** *Sedation* 25 mg/kg/dose po/pr prior to procedure **Children:** *Sedation and anxiety* 25–50 mg/kg/dose po/pr q6-9hr (maximum 500 mg/dose) *Hypnotic* 20–40 mg/kg/dose po/pr (maximum 50 mg/24hr **OR** 1 gm/dose **OR** 2 gm/24hr) **Adults:** *Sedation and anxiety* 250 mg po/pr tid *Hypnotic* 500–1000 mg po/pr at bedtime **OR** 30 minutes prior to procedure (maximum 2 gm/24hr)	Gastric irritation Nausea Vomiting Sedation Disorientation Ataxia Paradoxical excitement Headache	Not recommended for long-term use.
Chlorpheniramine Maleate Chlor-Trimeton®	Rhinitis	**Children:** 0.35 mg/kg/24hr po q4-6hr (maximum 12 mg/24hr) **OR** 2-6 yrs old—1 mg po q4-6hr 6-12 yrs old—2 mg po q4-6hr **Adults:** 4 mg po q4-6hr (maximum 24 mg/24hr) 8-12 mg (sustained released) po q8-12hr	Excitability Drowsiness Dry mouth Nausea Polyuria Diplopia	Do not crush or chew sustained released tablets
Chlorzoxazone Parafon Forte™ DSC	Muscle spasm	**Children:** 20 mg/kg/24hr po tid-qid **OR** 600 mg/m²/24hr po tid-qid **Adults:** 250-500 mg po tid-qid (maximum 750 mg tid-qid)	Drowsiness Dizziness Paresthesia Nausea Vomiting Gastrointestinal bleeding Granulocytopenia Anemia	Contraindicated in patients with impaired liver function

Drug	Indications	Dosage	Adverse Effects	Comments
Cimetidine Tagamet®	Gastroesophageal reflux Duodenal ulcer Gastric ulcer Gastric hypersecretory states	**Neonates:** 5–10 mg/kg/24hr po/iv q8–12hr **Infants:** 10–20 mg/kg/24hr po/iv q6–12hr **Children:** 20–40 mg/kg/24hr po/iv q6hr **Adults:** *Active ulcer* 300 mg po qid **OR** 800 mg po at bedtime **OR** 400 mg po bid **OR** 300 mg iv q6hr for 8 weeks *Duodenal ulcer prophylaxis* 400–800 mg po at bedtime *Gastric hypersecretory condition* 300–600 mg po/iv q6hr (maximum 2.4 gm/24hr)	Diarrhea Dizziness Myalgia Gynecomastia Mental confusion	Adjust dosing interval in renal impairment
Cisapride Propulsid®	Gastroesophageal reflux Chronic intestinal pseudoobstruction Chronic idiopathic constipation Gastrointestinal motility disorders	**Infants and Children:** 0.15–0.33 mg/kg/dose po tid–qid **Adults:** 5–10 mg po tid–qid	Abdominal cramping Borborygmi Diarrhea Somnolence Fatigue	Administer 15 minutes prior to a meal.
Clonazepam Klonopin™	Seizure disorder	**Infants and Children (≤ 10 yrs old or ≤ 30 kg):** Initial—0.01–0.05 mg/kg/24hr po bid–tid Increment—0.25–0.5 mg/24hr at 3 day intervalsx Usual maintenance—0.1–0.2 mg/24hr po tid Maximum 0.2 mg/kg/24hr **Adults:** Initial—1.5 mg/24hr po tid Increment—0.5–1 mg/24hr at 3 day intervals Usual maintenance—1.5–20mg/24hr o tid Maximum—20 mg/24hr	Drowsiness Ataxia Slurred speech Behavioral changes Hypersalivation	Relationship between serum concentration and seizure control is not well established

Drug	Indications	Dosage	Side Effects	Comments
Clorazepate Dipotassium Tranxene®	Seizure disorder General anxiety and panic disorder	**Children:** *< 9 yrs old* Not recommended *9-12 yrs old* Initial—3.75-7.5 mg po bid: Increment—3.75 mg /24hr at weekly intervals Maximum—60 mg/24hr bid-tid *< 12 yrs old* Initial—7.5 mg po bid-tid Increment—7.5 mg / 24hr at weekly intervals Maximum—90 mg/24hr tid **Adults:** Initial—7.5 mg po bid-tid Increment—7.5 mg / 24hr at weekly intervals Maximum—90 mg/24hr tid	Drowsiness Dizziness Confusion Depression Ataxia Blurred vision Diplopia Dry mouth	Long-term use may be associated with hepatic and renal injury. Abrupt discontinuation may cause withdrawal symptoms and seizures. Reference range: 0.12–1μg/mL
Corticotropin ACTH®, Acthar®	Infantile spasms	**Infants:** *Aqueous preparation* 20-40 units im/sc qd *Gel preparation* 80 units im qod	Allergic reaction Cushing syndrome	
Cromolyn Sodium Intal®, Nasalcrom®, Opticrom®	Allergic disorders, rhinitis Asthma Exercised-induced bronchospasm Food allergy Inflammatory bowel disease (IBD)	**Children:** *Inhalation* > 2 yrs old—20 mg via nebulization qid > 5 yrs old—2 inhalations via metered spray qid **OR** 20 mg via Spinhaler® qid For exercise-induced bronchospasm—2 inhalations (aerosol) prior to exercise *Nasal* > 6 yrs old—21 spray in each nostril tid-qid *Ophthalmic* > 4 yrs old—1-2 drops 4-6 times/24hr *Oral (food allergy and IBD)* 100 mg po qid '15-20 minutes before meals (maximum 40 mg/kg/24hr) **Adults:** *Inhalation* 2 inhalations by metered spray qid *Nasal* 1 spray in each nostril tid-qid *Ophthalmic* 1-2 drops 4-6 times/24hr *Oral (food allergy & IBD)* 200 mg po qid '15-20 minutes before meals (maximum 400 mg qid)	Cough Wheezing Throat irritation Dizziness Hoarseness Nasal burning	

Cyclobenzaprine Hydrochloride Flexeril®	Muscle spasm	**Children:** Dose not established **Adults:** 20–40 mg/24hr po bid-qid (maximum 60 mg/24hr)	Drowsiness Dry mouth Fatigue Asthenia Unpleasant taste Headache Blurred vision Tachycardia Hypotension	
Dantrolene Sodium Dantrium℠	Spasticity Malignant hyperthermia	**Children:** *Chronic Spasticity* Initial—0.5 mg/kg/dose po bid Increment—increase frequency to tid-qid at 4–7 day intervals, then increase dose by 0.5 mg/kg to maximum dose Maximum—3 mg/kg/dose bid-qid **OR** 400 mg/24hr *Malignant hyperthermia* Prevention—4–8 mg/kg/24hr po qid Treatment—1 mg/kg/dose iv; may repeat dose up to cumulative dose of 10 mg/kg, then switch to po **Adults:** *Chronic Spasticity* Initial—25 mg po qd Increment—increase frequency to tid-qid, then increase dose by 25 mg every 4–7 days to maximum dose Maximum—100 mg bid-qid **OR** 400 mg/24hr *Malignant hyperthermia* Same as for children	Hepatitis Seizures Muscle weakness Dizziness Diarrhea Confusion	Contraindicated in active liver disease. Monitor liver function tests.

| Dexamethasone Decadron® | Inflammation Airway edema Cerebral edema Bacterial meningitis Nausea | **Children:** *Airway edema* 0.5–1 mg/kg/24hr po/im/iv q6hr beginning 24hr prior to extubation and continuing for 4–6 doses post-extubation *Cerebral edema* Loading dose—1–2 mg/kg/dose iv x 1 Maintenance dose—1 mg/kg/24hr iv q4–6hr (maximum 16 mg/24hr) *Bacterial meningitis (> 2 months old)* 0.6 mg/kg/24hr iv q6hr for 4 days (concurrent with antibiotic therapy) *Emesis* First dose—10mg/m²/dose Maintenance dose—5 mg/m²/dose q6hr prn **Adults:** *Inflammation* 0.75–9 mg/24hr po/iv/im q6–12hr *Cerebral edema* First dose—10 mg iv stat x1 until Maintenance dose—4 mg im/iv q6hr response is maximized, then switch to po, then taper | Muscle weakness Growth suppression Glucose intolerance Edema Gastrointestinal upset/bleed Nausea Vomiting Seizures Vertigo Pituitary-adrenal axis suppression | With long-term use, must taper appropriately. |

Drug	Indications	Dosing	Side Effects	Comments
Diazepam Valium®	Status epilepticus Sedation Anxiety Muscle spasms	**Neonates::** *Status epilepticus* 0.5–1 mg/kg/dose iv q15–30 minutes for 2–3 doses **Children:** *Status epilepticus* Infants 30 days to 5 yrs old—0.05–0.5 mg/kg/dose iv over 2–3 minutes q15–30 minutes for 2–3 doses (maximum total dose = 5 mg) > 5 yrs old—0.05–0.5 mg/kg/dose iv over 2–3 minutes q15–30 minutes or 2–3 doses ff maximum total dose = 10 mg) Rectal—05 mg/kg then 0.25 mg/kg in 10 minutes if needed *Sedation/anxiety/muscle spasms* 0.12–0.8 mg/kg/24hr po q6–8hr 0.04–0.3 mg/kg/dose iv/im q2–4hr maximum (0.6 mg/kg over 8hr period) **Adults:** *Status epilepticus* 5–10 mg iv q10–20 minutes (maximum 30 mg in an 8hr period), may repeat in 2–4hr *Anxiety* 2–10 mg po bid-qid 2–10 mg im/iv, q3–4hr pm *Muscle spasms* 2–10 mg po bid-qid 5–10 mg im/iv q2–4h pm	Drowsiness Ataxia Respiratory depression Apnea Impaired coordination Laryngospasm Paradoxical excitement or rage	In children, do not exceed 1–2 mg /minute IVP; in adults, 5 mg/minute. Rapid iv administration may cause respiratory depression and hypotension.
Diphenhydramine Hydrochloride Benadry®, Benylin®, Cough Syrup, Diphen® Cough	Allergic symptoms Sedation Cough	**Children:** 5 mg/kg/day po/im/iv q6-8hr 150 mg/m²/day po/im/iv q6-8hr Maximum 300 mg/day **Adults:** 25–50 mg po q4–6hr 10–50 mg iv/im q2–4hr (maximum 400 mg/24hr)	Paradoxical excitement Sedation Dizziness Hypotension Dry mucous membrane Fatigue Palpitations Tremor	Should not be used in acute attacks of asthma

Epinephrine Hydrochloride Adrenalin® Primatene® Mist	Bronchospasm Hypersensitivity reactions Cardiac arrest	**Neonates:** *Cardiac arrest* 0.01–0.03 mg/kg or 0.1–0.3 mL/kg (1:10,000) (iv/et q3–5 minutes as needed **Children:** *Bronchospasm* 0.01 mg/kg (0.01 mL/kg 1:1000) sc q15–30 minutes for 3–4 doses or q4hr prn (maximum 0.4 mg/dose) 1–2 inhalations during attack; repeat q4hr prn *Hypersensitivity reactions* 0.01 mg/kg (1:1000) sc q15min x 2 doses, then q4hr prn (maximum 1 mg/dose) *Cardiac arrest* 0.01 mg/kg or 0.1 mL/kg (1:10,000) iv/et q3– 5 minutes prn (maximum 10 mL/dose) Continuous infusion—0.1–4 µg/kg/min **Adults:** *Bronchospasm* 0.1–0.5 mg im/sc q10–15min 0.1–0.25 mg iv q10–15min Single maximum dose = 1 mg *Hypersensitivity reactions* 0.2–0.5 mg im/sc q20min to 4hr (maximum 1 mg/dose) *Cardiac arrest* 0.1–1 mg iv/intracardiac q5min prn 1 mg et q5min prn	Tremor Anxiety Nausea Weakness Tachycardia Pallor	For endotracheal administration, dilute with 1–2 mL of normal saline.
Ethosuximide Zarontin®	Seizure disorder	**Children:** *< 6 yrs old* Initial—15 mg/kg/24hr po qd-bid (maximum 250 mg/dose) Increment—increase by 250 mg/24hr every 4–7 days Usual maintenance dose—15–40 mg/kg/24hr po qd-bid Maximum—1500 mg/24hr *> 6 yrs old* Initial—250 mg po qd-bid Increment—increase by 250 mg every 4–7 days Usual maintenance dose—20–40 mg/kg/24hr po qd-bid Maximum—1500mg/24hr **Adults:** Initial—750 mg/24hr po qd-bid Increment—250 mg/24hr at 4–7 day intervals Usual maintenance dose—750–2000 mg/24hr mg/24hr po qd-bid	Nausea Vomiting Anorexia Abdominal pain Blood dyscrasias Irritability Hyperactivity Lethargy Fatigue Stevens-Johnson syndrome Gum hypertrophy Hirsutism	Therapeutic level: 40–100 µg/mL. Monitor trough levels.

Drug	Indication	Dosage	Adverse Effects	Comments
Glycopyrrolate Robinul®	Excessive salivation Peptic ulcer disease (adjunct therapy) Excessive upper airway secretion	**Children:** *Antisialogogue or control of secretions* 40–100 µg/kg/dose po tid-qid 4–10 µg/kg/dose im/iv q3–4hr *Preoperative* < 2 yrs old—4.4–8.8 µg/kg im 30–60 minutes prior to procedure > 2 yrs old—4.4 µg/kg im 30–60 minutes prior to procedure **Adults:** *Peptic ulcer disease* 1–2 mg po bid-tid 0.1–0.2 mg im/iv tid-qid *Preoperative* 4.4 µg/kg im 30–60 minutes prior to proc edure	Drowsiness Dry mouth Blurred vision Tachycardia Nervousness Insomnia	
Guaifenesin Anti-Tuss®, Humibid® LA, Robitussin®	Cough Viscous and mucoid secretion	**Children:** *< 2 yrs old* 12 mg/kg/24hr po q4hr *2–5 yrs old* 50–100 mg po q4hr (smaximum 600 mg/24hr) *6–11 yrs old* 100–200 mg po q4hr (maximum 1200 mg/24hr) *> 12 yrs old* 200–400 mg po q4hr (maximum 2400 mg/24hr) **Adults:** 200–400 mg po q4hr (maximum 2400 mg/24hr)	Drowsiness Nausea Vomiting	
Haloperidol Haldol®	Severe pediatric behavioral problems (agitation or hyperkinesia) Mental retardation Infantile autism Acute psychosis	**Children:** *3–12 yrs old* Initial—0.25–0.5 mg /24hr po bid-tid Increment—increase by 0.25–0.5 mg every 5–7 days Usual maintenance dose Agitation/hyperkinesia—0.01–0.03 mg/kg/24hr qd Mental retardation—0.05–0.075 mg/kg/24hr bid-tid Psychotic disorder—0.05–0.15 mg/kg/24hr bid-tid *6–12 yrs old (im as lactate)* 1–3 mg/dose im q4–8hr (maximum 0.1 mg/kg/24hr) **Adults:** 0.5–5 mg po bid-tid (maximum 30 mg/24hr) 2–5 mg im (as lactate) q4–8hg pm	Drowsiness Dry mouth Urinary retention Constipation Blurred vision Gynecomastia Tachycardia Hypotension Extrapyramidal reactions Neuroleptic malignant syndrome Tardive dyskinesxia	Safety and efficacy have not been established in children < 3 yrs old.

Drug	Indication	Dosage	Side Effects	Comments
Hydroxyzine Atarax®, Vistaril®	Anxiety Preoperative sedation Itching Emesis	**Children:** 0.6 mg/kg/dose po q6-8hr 0.5-1 mg/kg/dose im q4-6hr prn **Adults:** 25-100 mg/dose po q4-6hr (maximum 600 mg/24hr) 25-100 mg/dose im q4-6hr prn	Dry mouth Drowsiness Dizziness Ataxia Hypotension Weakness	
Ibuprofen Advil®, Motrin®, Nuprin®, Pamprin®, IB, PediaProfen®, Rufen®	Fever Mild to moderate pain Juvenile rheumatoid arthritis Inflammatory conditions	**Children:** *Fever* 5-10 mg/kg/dose po q6-8hr (maximum 40 mg/kg/24hr) *Pain* 4-10 mg/kg/dose po q6-8hr *Juvenile rheumatoid arthritis* 30-50 mg/kg/24hr po qid (maximum 2400 mg/24hr) **Adults:** *Fever/pain/dysmenorrhea* 200-400 mg/dose po q4-6hr (maximum 1200 mg/24hr) *Inflammatory disease* 400-800 mg/dose po tid-qid (maximum 3200 mg/24hr)	Dyspepsia Gastrointestinal bleeding Nausea Vomiting Dizziness Drowsiness Tinnitus Vision changes	
Ipratropium Bromide Atrovent®	Bronchospasm	**Children < 2 yrs:** Nebulization: 250 µg tid **Children 3-14 yrs:** 1-2 inhalations tid (maximum 6 inhalations/24hr) **Children >14 yrs old and Adults:** 2 inhalations q4-6hr prn (maximum 12 inhalations /24hr)	Dry mouth Cough Palpitations Nervousness Dizziness	
Isoetharine Bronkometer®, Bronkosol®	Bronchospasm	**Children:** 0.1-0.2 mg/kg/dose by inhalation q2-6hr (maximum dose = 5 mg) **Adults:** 1-2 inhalations q3-4hr prn	Tachycardia Hypertension Palpitations Nausea Restlessness Excitement	For inhalation, dilute solution with 2-3 mL of normal saline.
Isoproterenol Hydrochloride Isuprel®	Bronchospasm	**Children:** *Nebulization* 0.05-1.25 mg/kg/dose q4hr *Inhalation* 1-2 metered doses up to 5 times/24hr *Intravenous, continuous* 0.1-2 ug/kg/min **Adults:** *Inhalation* 1-2 inhalations 4-6 times/24hr	Tachycardia Nervousness Restlessness Anxiety Tremors Ventricular arrhythmias	For continuous infusion, do not discontinue abruptly; infusion must be tapered over 24 to 48 hrs.

Drug	Indications	Dosage	Side Effects	Comments
Loperamide Hydrochloride Imodium®	Diarrhea Excessive ileostomy secretion	**Children:** *Acute diarrhea* 0.4–0.8 mg/kg/24hr po q6–12hr (maximum 2 mg/dose) *chronic diarrhea* Initial—0.5–1.5 mg/kg/24hr po bid-qid Maintenance—0.25–1 mg/kg/24hr po bid-tid (maximum 2 mg/dose) **Adults:** Initial—4 mg po x 1 Maintenance—2 mg po after each loose stool Maximum—16 mg/24hr	Constipation Nausea Vomiting Abdominal cramping Fatigue Dry mouth Dizziness	Use with caution in patients with pulmonary, hepatic, or renal disorders.
Meperidine Hydrochloride Demerol®	Moderate to severe pain Anesthesia (adjunct therapy Preoperative sedation	**Children:** 1–1.5 mg/kg/dose po/im/iv/sc q3–4hr prn (maximum 100 mg/dose) **Adults:** 50–150 mg/dose po/im/iv/sc q3–4hr prn	Central nervous system and respiratory depression Nausea Vomiting Constipation Sedation Tachycardia Tremors Seizures	
Metaproterenol Sulfate Alupent®, Metaprel®	Bronchospasm	**Infants:** *Oral* 0.4 mg/kg/dose q8–12hrs *Nebulization* 0.01–0.02 mL/kg (5% solution) diluted in normal saline q4–6 hr (minimum dose = 0.1 mL; maximum dose = 1 mL) **Children:** *Oral* < 2 yrs old—0.4 mg/kg/dose tid-quid 2–6 yrs old—1–2.6 mg/kg/24hr q6–8hr 6–9 yrs old—10 mg/dose tid-qid > 9 yrs old—20 mg/dose tid-qid *Nebulization* 0.01–0.02 mL/kg (5% solution) diluted in normal saline q4–6hr (minimum dose= 0.1 mL; mazimum dose = 1 mL) **Adolescents and Adults (> 12 yrs old):** *Oral* 20 mg/dose tid-qid *Nebulization* 0.2–0.3 mL (5% solution) in 2.5-3 mL normal saline q4–6hr OR 5–20 breaths of 5% solution *Inhalation* 2–3 inhalations q3–4hr (maximum 12 inhalations/24hr)	Tachycardia Palpitations Hypertension Nervousness Tremor Nausea	

Drug	Indications	Dosage	Adverse Reactions	Comments
Methylphenidate Hydrochloride Ritalin®	Attention deficit disorder with hyperactivity Narcolepsy	**Children: (≥ 6 yrs old)** *Initial* 0.3 mg/kg/dose or 2.5–5 mg/dose po given before breakfast and lunch *Increment* Increase by 0.1 mg/kg/dose or by 5–10 mg/24hr at weekly intervals *Usual maintenance dose* 0.5–1 mg/kg/24hr po *Maximum dose* 2 mg/kg/24hr or 60 mg/24hr **Adults:** 10 mg po bid-tid (maximum 60 mg/24hr)	Insomnia Nervousness Anorexia Nausea Abdominal pain Weight loss Growth retardation Tachycardia Drowsiness Lowered seizure threshold	Treatment with methylphenidate should include "drug holidays" in order to assess the patient's requirement and to decrease tolerance
Methylprednisolone A-methaPred®, Medrol®, Solu-Medrol®	Status asthmaticus Inflammation Immunosuppression Lupus nephritis	**Children:** *Status asthmaticus* Loading dose—2 mg/kg/dose iv x 1 dose Maintenance dose—0.5–1 mg/kg/dose iv q6hr *Inflammation or immunosuppression* 0.16–0.8 mg/kg/24hr po/im/iv q6–12hr OR 5–25 mg/m2/24hr po/im/iv q6–12hr *Lupus nephritis* 30 mg/kg/dose iv qod x 6 doses **Adults** *Inflammation or immunosuppression* 2–60 mg po qd-qid 10–80 mg/24hr im qd *Lupus nephritis* 1 gm/24hr iv x 3 days	Muscle weakness Growth suppression Glucose intolerance Edema Gastrointestinal upset or bleeding Nausea Vomiting Seizures Vertigo Pituitary-adrenal axis bleeding Acne Fractures	
Metoclopramide Hydrochloride Reglan®	Gastroesophageal reflux Gastrointestinal hypomotility Facilitate intubation of small intestine Nausea associated with chemotherapy Diabetic gastric stasis	**Children:** *Gastroesophageal reflux or hypomotility* 0.4–0.8 mg/kg/24hr po/iv qid *Intubation of small intestine* < 6 yrs old—0.1 mg/kg/dose iv 6–14 yrs old—2.5–5 mg/kg/dose iv *Chemotherapy induced emesis* 1–2 mg/kg/dose iv given 30 minutes prior to chemotherapy and 2hr post chemotherapy and then q2–4hr prn **Adults:** *Gastroesophageal reflux or stasis* 10–15 mg *Chemotherapy induced emesis* 1–2 mg/kg/dose iv given 30 minutes prior to chemotherapy and 2hr post chemotherapy and then q2–4hr prn	Extrapyramidal reactions Drowsiness Fatigue Anxiety Agitation Constipation Diarrhea Gynecomastia	Extrapyramidal reactions occur most often in children and young adults following iv administration of high doses; usually occurs within 24–48 hours after initiation of therapy.

| Mineral Oil
Agoral®, Fleet®
Mineral Oil Enema,
Kondremul® | Constipation
Fecal impaction | **Children:**
5–11 yrs old
5–20 mL po qd or in divided doses
2–11 urs old
30–60 mL pr as a single dose
>12 yrs old
15–45 mL/24hr po qd or in divided doses
Retention enema, 60–150 mL/24hr pr as a
single dose
Adults:
5–45 mL/24hr po qd or in divided doses
Retention enema, 60–150 mL/24hr pr as a
single dose | Nausea
Vomiting
Abdominal cramps
Pruritis ani
Lipid pneumonitis with
aspiration | Do not take with food or
meals. |

Morphine Sulfate Duramorph®, MS Contin®, Roxanol™	Moderate to severe pain Preanesthesia	**Infants and Children:** *Oral* Prompt release—0.2–0.5 mg/kg/dose q4–6hr prn Controlled release—0.3–0.6 mg/kg/dose q12h prn *Intermittent IM or IV or SC* 0.05–0.2 mg/kg/dose q2–4hr prn (usual maximum = 15 mg/dose) Sedation/analgesia for procedure—0.05–0.1 mg/kg/dose iv 5 minutes prior to procedure *Continuous infusion (IV or SC)* 0.01–2 mg/kg/hr (average dose = 0.06 mg/kg/hr) **Adolescents: (> 12 yrs old)** Sedation/analgesia for surgery—3–4 mg/dose iv 5 minutes prior to procedure and repeat in 5 minutes if necessary **Adults:** *Oral* Prompt release—10–30 mg/dose q4hr prn Controlled release—15–30 mg/dose q8–12hr *Intermittent IM or IV or SC* 2.5–20 mg/dose q2–6hr prn (usual dose = 10 mg/dose q4hr prn) *Continuous infusion (IV or SC)* 0.8–10 mg/hr, increase as necessary for adequate pain control or evidence of adverse effects (usual range up to 80 mg/hr) *Epidural* Initial—5 mg/dose in lumber region Increment—if inadequate pain control within 1hr, give 1–2 mg Maximum dose = 10 mg/24hr *Intrathecal (1/10 of epidural dose)* 0.2–1 mg/dose (repeat doses not recommended)	Central nervous system and respiratory depression Sedation Nausea Vomiting Constipation Hypotension Bradycardia Drowsiness Dizziness Dependency Peripheral vasodilation	Start with lowest dose and increase progressively as required to achieve adequate pain control (especially with continuous infusions). Do not crush controlled release tablets.

| Phenobarbital Sodium Luminal | Status epilepticus Seizure disorder Sedation Hypnotic Neonatal hyperbilirubinemia Hyperbilirubinemia due to chronic cholestasis | **Neonates:**
Status epilepticus
15–20 mg/kg/dose iv x 1 dose
Seizure disorder
3–4 mg/kg/24hr po/iv q12–24hr (increase to 5 mg/kg/24hr if needed base on therapeutic concentration and clinical state)
Infants:
Status epilepticus
15–18 mg/kg/dose iv x 1 dose usual maximum 20 mg/kg/dose; may need to give 5 mg/kg/dose every 15–30 minutes until seizure is controlled; total maximum 30 mg/kg)
Seizure disorder
5–6 mg/kg/24hr po/iv q12–24hr
Children:
Status epilepticus
Same as for infants
Seizure disorder
1–5 yrs old—6–8 mg/kg/24hr po/iv q 12–24hr
5–12 yrs old—4–6 mg/kg/24hr po/iv q 12–24hr
> 12 yrs old—1–3 mg/kg/24hr po/iv q 12–24hr
Sedation
2 mg/kg/dose po tid
Hypnotic
3–5 mg/kg/dose im/iv/sc at bedtime
Preoperative sedation
1–3 mg/kg/dose po/im/iv 1–1.5hr prior to procedure
Hyperbilirubinemia
< 12 yrs old—3–8 mg/kg/24hr po bid-tid (doses up to 12 mg/kg/24hr have been used)
Adults:
Status epilepticus
Same as for infants
Sedation
30–120 mg/24hr po/im bid-tid
Hypnotic
100–320 mg/dose po/im/iv/sc at bedtime
Preoperative sedation
100–200 mg/dose im 1–1.5hr prior to procedure
Hyperbilirubinemia
90–180 mg/24hr po bid-tid | Respiratory depression Paradoxical excitation Drowsiness Hypotension Cognitive impairment defects in general comprehension Decreased attention span Ataxia Short-term memory deficits Circulatory collapse |

| Phenytoin Sodium
Dilantin® | Status epilepticus
Seizure disorder
Ventricular arrhythmias
Epidermolysis bullosa | **Neonates:**
Status epilepticus
15–20 mg/kg/dose iv in a single or divided dose
Seizure disorder
Initial—5 mg/kg/24hr iv q12hr
Usual dose—5–8 mg/kg/24hr iv q12hr
Infants and Children:
Status epilepticus
15–18 mg/kg iv in a single divided dose
15–20 mg/kg po in 3 divided doses given every 2–4 hr
Seizure disorder
Initial—5 mg/kg/24 hr iv/po q12hr
Usual maintenance (iv/po q8–12hr)
0.5–3 yrs old—8–10 mg/kg/24hr
4–6 yrs old—7.5–9 mg/kg/24hr
7–9 yrs old—7–8 mg/kg/24hr
10–16 yrs old—6–7 mg/kg/24hr
Arrhythmias
Loading dose
1.25 mg/kg/dose iv q5min (maximum total loading dose=15 mg/kg)
Maintenance dose
5–10 mg/kg/24hr po/iv q12hr
Adults:
Status epilepticus
15–18 mg/kg iv in a single or divided dose
15–20 mg/kg po in 3 divided doses given every 2–4hr
Seizure disorder
300 mg/24hr or 5–6 mg/kg/24hr po q8hr or q12–24hr using extended release preparations
Arrhythmias
Loading dose
1.25 mg/kg/dose iv q5min (maximum total loading dose=15 mg/kg)
Maintenance dose—250 mg po q6hrx1 day, 250 mg po q12hr, then 300–400 mg/24hr po qd–qid | *Dose-related*
Nystagmus
Diplopia
Blurred vision
Ataxia
Lethargy
Coma
Intravenous administration
Hypotension
Bradycardia
Cardiac arrhythmias (especially rapid iv administration)
General effects
Gingival hyperplasia
Rash
Nausea
Mood changes
Osteomalacia
Hyperglycemia
Systemic Lupus Erythematosus-like syndrome
Steven-Johnson Syndrome
Blood dyscrasias | Avoid intramuscular route of administration; irregular and incomplete absorption.
For intravenous administration, do not exceed infusion rate of 0.5 mg/kg/min in children, 1–3 mg/kg/min or 50 mg/min. in adults
Intravenous injections should be followed by normal saline flushes through the same needle or IV catheter to avoid irritation to the vein.
Monitor therapeutic trough levels: 10–20 µg/mL
Toxicity is monitored clinically in addition to drug concentration; toxic level=30–50 µg/mL |

Prednisone Deltasone® Liquid Pred®	Inflammation Immunosuppression Nephrotic syndrome Adrenocortical insufficiency	**Children** *Inflammation or immunosuppression* 0.05–2 mg/kg/24hr po qd-qid OR 6–30 mg/m²/24hr po q6–12 hr *Acute asthma* 1–2 mg/kg/24hr po qd-bid *Nephrotic syndrome* Initial—2 mg/kg/24hr (maximum 80 mg/24hr) po tid-qid until urine is protein free x 5 days (maximum 28 days) Increment—4 mg/kg/dose po qod for an additional 28 days if proteinuria persists Maintenance—2 mg/kg/dose qod for 28 days, then taper over 4–6 weeks *Physiological replacement* 4–5 mg/m²/24hr **Adults:** 5–60 mg/24hr po qd-qid	Muscle weakness Growth suppression Glucose intolerance Edema Gastrointestinal upset/bleed Nausea Vomiting Seizures Vertigo Pituary-adrenal axis suppression Acne Fractures	Dose depends on condition, severity of disease, and response of the patient rather than on strict adherence to dosage indicated by age, weight, or body surface area. Discontinuation of long-term therapy should be gradual.
Ranitidine Zantac®	Duodenal ulcer Gastric ulcer Gastric hypersecretory states	**Children:** *Oral* 1–3 mg/kg/dose q12hr *Intermittent IM or IV* 0.5–1.5 mg/kg/dose q6–8hr (maximum 400) mg/24hr *Continuous infusion* 0.1–0.25 mg/kg/hr **Adults:** *Short-term treatment of ulceration* 150 mg/dose po bid OR 300 mg po at bedtime *Prophylaxis of recurrent duodenal ulcer* 150 mg po at bedtime *Gastric hypersecretory conditions* 150 mg po bid (maximum 6 gm/24hr)	Headache Dizziness Sedation Insomnia Confusion Constipation Diarrhea Gynecomastia Hepatotoxicity	Continuous infusion is preferred for stress ulcer prophylaxis and may be given concurrently with maintenance IVF or TPN.
Simethicone Gas-X, Mylicon®, Phazyme®	Flatulence Gastric bloating Postoperative gas pain	**Infants:** 20 mg po qid **Children:** <12 Yrs Old 40 mg po qid >12 yrs old 40–120 mg po after meals and at bedtime prn (maximum 500 mg/24 hr) **Adults:** Same as for children >12 yrs old		Chew tablets thoroughly before swallowing. Suspension may be mix with water or infant formula.

Sucralfate Carafate®	Duodenal ulcer Stomatitis (topical suspension)	**Children:** 40–80 mg/kg/24 hr po q6hr **Adults:** 1 gm po qid, 1hr before meals and at bedtime **Stomatitis:** 2.5–5 mL swish and spit or swish and swallow qid	Constipation Diarrhea Nausea Gastric discomfort Dry mouth Dizziness Sleepiness Vertigo	
Terbutaline Sulfate Brethaire®, Brethine®	Bronchoconstriction Asthma	**Children < 12 yrs old:** *Oral* 0.05 mg/kg/dose q8hr, increase gradually to maximum of 0.15 mg/kg/dose or 5 mg/24hr *Subcutaneous* 0.005–0.01 mg/kg/dose q15–20min x 3 doses (maximum 0.4 mg/dose) **Children > 12 yrs old and Adults:** *Oral* 2.5–5 mg/dose q8hr *Subcutaneous* 0.25 mg/dose repeated q15–30min x 1 doses (maximum total dose 0.5 mg within 4 hr period) **Inhalation** 2 inhalations q4–6hr **Nebulization** <2 yrs old 0.5 mg in 2.5 mL normal saline 2–9 yrs old 1 mg in 2.5 mL normal saline > 9 yrs old 1.5 mg in 2.5 mL normal saline	Tremor Nervousness Tachycardia Headache Nausea Arrhythmias Palpitations	Injectable product may be used for nebulization.

Theophylline Ethylenediamine Elixophyllin®, Slo-bid™, Somophyllin®-T, Theo-Dur® Theolair™, Uniphyl®	Bronchoconstriction Bronchospasm Asthma Neonatal apnea/bradycardia	**Neonates:** *Apnea/bradycardia* Loading—4–6 mg/kg/dose Maintenance <36 weeks—1–2 mg/kg/24hr po q8–12hr >36 weeks to 1 month old—2–4 mg/kg/24hr po q8–12hr *Asthma* Loading—0.8 mg/kg/dose for each 2µg/mL desired increase in theophylline level Maintenance (0–2 mo)—3–6 mg/kg/24hr q8hr **Children:** *Loading* 1 mg/kg/dose for each 2 µg/mL desired increase in theophylline level *Maintenance (dosing interval is dependent on the oral formulation selected)* 2–6 mo: 6–15 mg/kg/24hr 6–12 mo: 15–22 mg/kg/24hr 1–9 yr: 22 mg/kg/24hr 9–12 yr: 20 mg/kg/24hr 12–16 yr: 18 mg/kg/24hr **Adults:** Loading—Same as for children Maintenance—13 mg/kg/24hr (maximum 900 mg/24hr)	Nausea Vomiting Anorexia Gastroesophageal reflux Nervousness Tachycardia Hallucinations Seizures Arrhythmias	Therapeutic levels Apnea/bradycardia: 5–12 µg/mL Bronchospasm: 10–20 µg/mL Monitor steady state levels Half-life is age-dependent Newborns: 20–30hrs Children: 1.5–9.5hrs adults: 3–9.5hrs Dosing intervals Immediate release products: q6hr Sustained release products: q8–24hr
Thioridazine Hydrochloride Mellaril®	Severe behavior problems in children Psychotic disorders Depressive neurosis	**Children (> 2yrs old):** *Range* 0.5–3 mg/kg/24hr po bid–tid (usual dose 1 mg/kg/24hr; maximum dose 3 mg/kg/24hr) *Behavior problems* 10 mg po bid–tid, increase gradually *Severe psychoses* 25 mg po bid–tid, increase gradually **Adults:** *Psychoses* Initial—50–100 mg po tid Increment—gradual increases Maximum—800 mg/24hr po bid–qid *Depressive disorders* Initial—25 mg po tid Maintenance—20–200 mg/24hr	Central nervous system Sedation Extrapyramidal effects Drowsiness Anxiety Restlessness Seizures Anticholinergic effects Dry mouth Urinary retention Constipation Blurred vision Cardiovascular Hypertension EKG changes Gastrointestinal upset	Dilute oral concentrate with water or juice before administration.

Thiothixene Navane®	Psychotic disorders	**Children (< 12 yrs old):** Dose not well established 0.25 mg/kg/24hr po bid-qid has been used **Children (> 12 yrs old) and Adults:** *Oral* Initial—2 mg tid Increment—up to 20-30 mg/24hr Maximum—60 mg/24hr *Intramuscular* Initial—4 mg bid-qid Increment—increase gradually Usual dose—16-20 mg/24hr Maximum—30 mg/24hr	Central nervous system Sedation Exqtrapyramidal effects Drowsiness Anxiety Restlessness Seizures Anticholinergic effects Dry mouth Urinary retention Constipation Blurred vision Cardiovascular Hypotension EKG changes Gastrointestinal upset	
Valproic Acid and Derivatives Depakene®, Depakote®	Seizure disorders	**Children:** *Oral* Initial—10-15 mg/kg/24hr qd-tid Increment—5-10 mg/kg/24hr at weekly intervals until therapeutic concentrations are achieved Maintenance—30-60 mg/kg/24hr qd-tid *Rectal* Loading—17-20 mg/kg x 1 dose Maintenance—10-15 mg/kg/dose q8hr beginning 8hr after loading dose **Adults:** *Oral* 1-3 gm/24hr qd-tid	Nausea Diarrhea Vomiting Gastrointestinal upset Hepatotoxicity Sedation Temporary alopecia Weight gain or loss Impaired platelet function Headache	Children requiring polytherapy (>1 anticonvulsant) may need doses up to 100 mg/kg/24hr po tid-qid. Rectal preparation Dilute syrup 1:1 with water for use as a retention enema. Severe hepatotoxicity is frequently fatal and occurs most often within first 6 months of therapy and in children <2 years old. Therapeutic levels 50-100µg/mL Monitor trough levels

Sources:

1. Alexander, K. S., Haribhakti, R. P., & Parker, G.A. (1991). Stability of acetazolamide in suspension compound from tablets. American Journal of Hospital Pharmacy, 48(6), 1241-1244.

2. Benitz, W. E., & Tatro, D. S. (1988). The pediatric drug handbook. Chicago: Year Book.

3. Bond, W. S. (1987). Recognition and treatment of attention deficit disorder. Clinical Pharmacy, 6(8), 617-624.

4. Carroccio, A., Iacono, G., Li Voti, G., Montalto, G., Cavataio, F., Tulone, V., Lorello, D., Kazmierska, I., Aciemo, C., & Notarbartolo, A. (1992). Gastric emptying in infants with gastroesophageal reflux: Ultrasound evaluation before and after cisapride administration. Scandanavian Journal of Gastroenterology, 27, 799-804.

5. Farrinton, E. (1990). Drugs used in the pediatric intensive care unit. In D. L. Levin (Ed.). Essentials of pediatric intensive care: A pocket companion (pp. 101-199). St. Louis: Quality Medical Publishing.

6. Gilman, J. T. (1991). Carbamazepine dosing for pediatric seizure disorders: The highs and lows. Drug Intelligence and Clinical Pharmacy, 25(10), 1109-1112.

7. Hrachoby, R. A., & Frost, J. D. Jr. (1989). Infantile spasms. Pediatric Clinics of North America, 36(2), 311-329.

8. Lambert, J., Mobassaleh, M., & Grand, R. J., (1992). Efficacy of cimetidine for gastric acid suppression in pediatric patients. Journal of Pediatrics, 120(3), 474-478.

9. Lee, C. K. K. (1991). Drug doses. In M. G. Greene (Ed.). The Harriet Lane handbook (pp. 141-244). St. Louis: Mosby Year Book.

10. Mann, N. P., & Hiller, R. G., (1982). Ipratropium bromide in children with asthma. Thorax, 37(1), 72-74.

11. Rachelefsky, G. S., & Siegel, S. C., (1985). Asthma in infants and children - Treatment of childhood asthma: Part II. Journal of Clinical Immunology, 76(3), 409-425.

12. Rhode, H., Stunden, R. J., Millar, A. J. W., Cywes, S. (1987). Esophageal pH assessment of gastroesophageal reflux in 18 patients and the effect of two pro-kinetic agents: Cisapride and metoclopramide. Journal of Pediatric Surgery, 22(10), 931-934.

13. Rhode, H., Stunden, R. J., Millar, A. J. W., Cywes, S. (1987). Pharmacologic control of gastro-esophageal reflux in infants with cisapride. Pediatric Surgery International, 2, 22-26.

14. Serrano, A. C., (1981). Haloperidol - Its use in children. Journal of Clinical Psychiatry, 42(4), 154-156.

15. Taketomo, C. K., Hodding, J. H., & Kraus, D. M. (1992). Pediatric dosage handbook. Hudson: Lexi-Comp Inc.

16. Yaffe, S. J., & Aranda, J. V. (Eds.). (1992). Pediatric pharmacology. Philadelphia: W. B. Saunders.

Index

DATE DUE

5/02/00			
11-11-10			

UNIVERSITY PRODUCTS, INC. #859-5503